# PRAISE FOR *PEAK*

"*Peak* is one of the most impressive and detailed books on applied sports science ever published — a must-have for any practitioner in performance."

— **Dr. Fergus Connolly**, PhD, performance expert;
author of *Game Changer* and *59 Lessons*

"*Peak* is an essential read for anyone looking to reach their full potential! Dr. Bubbs has synthesized the research and practices that you can use to amplify your health and performance as an athlete."

— **Dr. Greg Wells**, PhD, human performance expert;
exercise medicine researcher; best-selling author of *The Focus Effect*

"You have two options: You can either not read this book and miss invaluable tips on how to become a more efficient and effective athlete and human being (or coach others to do the same), or you can read *Peak* as soon as possible and be that much closer to your quest for total world domination. To anyone who wants to enhance their performance, read this book and thank me later!"

— **Jimmy Conrad**, World Cup veteran and
former captain of the US Men's National Soccer Team

"A must-read for athletes and everyone alike. *Peak* is an immeasurable tool for becoming the best you can be!"

— **Kelly Olynyk**, forward, Miami Heat, NBA

"*Peak* pushes the envelope. If you want to better understand the numerous ways you can positively impact your athletes, this is a must-read!"

— **Mike Robertson**, MS, CSCS, co-owner, IFAST,
named one of America's 10 Best Gyms by *Men's Health Magazine*

"Dr. Bubbs's advice on nutrition, health, and recovery for peak performance has been a game changer!"

— **Kevin Pangos**, point guard, Barcelona FC Basketball

"Dr. Bubbs is an amazingly knowledgeable health professional who is able to translate highbrow science into practical, applicable gems that athletes and sports nutrition practitioners can use to fuel body and mind for peak performance. I'm very excited about *Peak*, and you should be, too!"

— **Miguel Mateas**, PhD(c), clinical neuroscientist;
doctoral researcher in gut-brain communication

"In *Peak*, Dr. Marc Bubbs has produced one of the most comprehensive and practical resources on human performance, nutrition, and recovery available in print form. Whether you are the performance director of a professional sports team, a coach of a youth sports club, or an individual looking to improve your overall health and wellness, *Peak* will provide you a road map for enhancing your overall probability of success. This well-researched and clearly presented book should be in the libraries of anyone who is guiding the development of athletes and fitness enthusiasts."

— **Derek Hansen**, international performance consultant,
NFL, NBA, MLS, NCAA

"*Peak* is a masterpiece of nutritional science from one of the world's leading authorities on athletic health and performance. It's a fantastic resource that provides a road map to reaching true wellness."

— **Dr. Rocco Monto**, orthopedic surgeon; physician,
Team USA; author of *The Fountain*

"*Peak* is a highly informative, interesting, useful, and all-encompassing performance enhancement book I wish I had when I started coaching."

— **Jorge Carvajal**, strength and conditioning coach
for NFL players, elite military personnel, and big wave surfers

"In today's world of human performance, it is becoming harder and harder to blaze new trails. However one of those trails is the model of common language and consistent service from a multitude of specialists, as highlighted by Dr. Bubbs in his new book *Peak*. With this model of teamwork, we can expect the whole is greater than the sum of its parts. *Peak* should yield excitement to achieve greater success with your own systems and methods."

— **Dr. Charlie Weingroff**, DPT, Strength and Conditioning Coach,
Canadian men's national basketball team; member,
Nike Executive Council; consultant to professional athletes

"An accomplished contributor to the field of sport performance in his own right, Dr. Bubbs possesses a unique ability to ask relevant questions and identify practitioners and researchers generating the most current and effective solutions pertaining to athlete readiness. Dr. Bubbs is a connector, and *Peak* is an incredibly comprehensive resource that addresses many of the variables that influence performance — conveniently in one place."

— **Dr. Doug Kechijian**, DPT, performance coach;
US Air Force Outstanding Airmen of the Year

# PEAK

The New
Science
of Athletic
Performance
That Is
Revolutionizing
Sports

## Dr. Marc Bubbs

### ND, CISSN, CSCS

Chelsea Green Publishing
White River Junction, Vermont
London, UK

Editor: Makenna Goodman
Project Manager: Alexander Bullett
Copy Editor: Diane Durrett
Proofreader: Caitlin O'Brien
Indexer: Linda Hallinger
Designer: Melissa Jacobson

Printed in the United States of America.
First printing May 2019.
10 9 8 7 6 5 4 3      22 23 24 25 26

**Library of Congress Cataloging-in-Publication Data**
Names: Bubbs, Marc, author.
Title: Peak : the new science of athletic performance that is revolutionizing sports / Marc Bubbs.
Description: White River Junction, Vermont : Chelsea Green Publishing, 2019. | Includes
    bibliographical references and index.
Identifiers: LCCN 2019000511| ISBN 9781603588096 (hardback) | ISBN 9781603588102 (ebook)
Subjects: LCSH: Physical fitness — Health aspects. | Exercise — Physiological aspects. | Nutrition.
    | BISAC: HEALTH & FITNESS / Exercise. | SPORTS & RECREATION / Training. | MEDICAL
    / Physical Medicine & Rehabilitation. | HEALTH & FITNESS / Nutrition. | MEDICAL / Sports
    Medicine. | SPORTS & RECREATION / Triathlon. | MEDICAL / Holistic Medicine.
Classification: LCC RA781 .B823 2019 | DDC 613.7--dc23
LC record available at https://lccn.loc.gov/2019000511

Chelsea Green Publishing
85 North Main Street, Suite 120
White River Junction, Vermont USA

Somerset House
London, UK

www.chelseagreen.com

# CONTENTS

**PART ONE**

# Foundation

### PART FOUR

# Supercharge

# The Revolution in Performance

T here is a revolution happening in sports. The financial boom in professional sports over the last decade has led to phenomenal investment in research on athlete health, nutrition, training, recovery, and mindset in an attempt to beat the competition. Multimillion-dollar team complexes, partnerships with universities, the latest advances in technology like sleep pods, GPS, wearable tech; nothing is spared, it seems, in the pursuit of high performance. Unfortunately, the evidence-based fundamentals, the expert treatment from PhDs, the support of academic institutions, and the professional performance protocols used by staffs can be in stark contrast to what many athletes follow in practice. The noise of social media, old-school traditions, and broscience makes it difficult to separate fact from fiction.

*Peak* takes you behind the scenes and unveils the experts who influence the games' top performers. What will you uncover? A heavy emphasis on the fundamentals (not the fads), the importance of consistency (not extreme effort), and the value of patience (not rapid transformation). It might not seem sexy at first, but the mind-blowing feats of athleticism and record-breaking performances you see on TV highlight reels are rooted in this approach. I'll connect you with the "best of the best" experts in sport and show you how they achieve world-class success. Regardless if you're trying to improve your physique, propel endurance performance, or improve team sport athlete success, *Peak* will lay out the blueprint for how elite sport scientists, performance nutritionists, and coaches unlock athlete potential.

This book also attempts to clarify common confusion among popular topics. For example, ketogenic diets are incredibly popular at the moment, but is becoming fat-adapted really the best strategy for fueling endurance performance? Well, legendary cyclist Chris Froome won multiple Tour de France titles, and many on social media believe he was following a low-carb approach to diet. Is this really true, or was Froome's approach much more strategic, planned, and purposeful? I'll connect you with the experts who fueled him to victory. And what about the constant drive for optimization? Do your nutrition, recovery, and supplementation strategies match-up with (or detract from) your optimization goal? And at what cost? Optimization comes with consequences (sometimes significant), something world-leading experts are quick to point out. This dovetails into a conversation about inflammation — is it really the enemy? The world's number one tennis star, Novak Djokovic, removed gluten from his diet a few years back and went on a historic and remarkable run of winning. Did a gluten-free diet play a role in his ability to compete and recover? Did it simply create an environment for better food choices? Or perhaps was the only effect on his mindset? We'll explore this complex connection between inflammation, nutrition, and emotions. Inflammation is certainly a powerful signal for adaptation; without it, you cannot adapt. But what happens when the noise of poor health or your nutrition, supplementation, or training strategy drowns out this essential signal? Know your context; understand the nuance. Quarterback Tom Brady recently released his book *The TB12 Method* with trainer Alex Guerrero, who cited "muscle plasticity" as a key to his success. Is this an evidence-based statement? How about Brady's claims that his success comes in part from avoiding acidic foods, such as beef and salmon, that raise acid levels in the blood? Do the experts on the front lines agree with these theories? Can some people succeed despite what they do (rather than because of them)? You'll find out from the best evidence-based experts in the world.

There are many fantastic books written about nutrition, mindset, or athletic performance and recovery. However, many of these current books are either too steeped in theory or not sufficiently evidence-based to meet the needs of today's athlete. What is lacking is a cohesive book that links deep nutrition with peak performance — for they need to be considered together — and synthesizes the salient points from expert specialists into actionable guidance. *Peak* covers the four pillars — Foundation, Fuel, Recovery, and Supercharge — to make the fittest, healthiest, and most resilient modern athlete. It is about beating odds, extending careers, and maximizing time-tested and experimental technologies. It's about being an expert in the fundamentals. It is about knowing the difference between fads and real science, assessing the research, and differentiating between the data. It assumes that while top athletes are born, they're also *made*.

If you're a recreational athlete who wants to improve how you look, feel, or perform, this book is for you. If you're a more competitive athlete looking for that performance advantage to get you over the hump, this book is for you. If you're a personal trainer or strength coach looking for an evidence-based summary of health, nutrition, recovery, and mindset strategies to help your clients achieve their goals, this book is for you. If you're a practitioner or doctor looking for a deeper understanding of these core areas and how they directly impact your patients every day, this book is for you.

## What You'll Find in This Book

In Part One: Foundation, you'll learn how athlete health is essential for success and how frequent illness is incompatible with elite performance. Struggle with poor sleep and you're more likely to get sick. Struggle with digestive issues and your health will suffer. Struggle with blood sugar peaks and valleys and your health will be compromised. This concept of "Human First" has emerged recently in performance circles, highlighting how athletes must first be healthy to achieve their performance potential. Until quite recently, athletic performance and an athlete's health were almost considered mutually exclusive. As long as they were fit enough to play or compete, that was sufficient. Today, research shows athletes who fail to complete 80 percent of their training sessions do not hit their performance goals. In other words, if you're too sick, too tired, or too rundown to train, you'll never achieve elite performance. Athlete health is also crucial to supporting longevity, meaning sustaining elite performance over multiple seasons and throughout a career.

In Part Two: Fuel, you'll learn the fundamental principles of successful nutrition strategies common across all athletes. These fundamentals make up the bulk of every elite athlete's protocol. You'll also see how the experts *individualize* nutrition for elite athletes, and you'll get an exploration into the evolution of sports nutrition and health over the past few decades. That said, many practitioners still fall victim to putting the icing on the cake with exotic supplements and deep testing before firming up the foundation with sound nutrition principles. You'll learn how this is a recipe for failure. Building more lean muscle, making weight for competition, winning a triathlon, or playing pro basketball are distinct goals that require different nutritional strategies. I'll connect you with the experts in each domain.

You cannot simply blindly apply strategies to athletes; you must constantly reassess and be nimble enough to change course when needed.

In Part Three: Recovery, you'll learn the new science of recovery and how "over-recovery" can be as problematic as a lack of adequate rest. You'll learn the latest blood tests, biomarkers, and baseline assessments that performance staffs use with athletes, and how elite coaches prioritize nutrition, sleep, and stress management above all else. You'll learn the fundamental importance of athlete immunity, the emerging field of immunonutrition, and why simple activities like handwashing can make all the difference in the world. You'll also see how monitoring athletes can be very helpful (or sometimes harmful), the value of subjective data, and the evidence-based periodized recovery strategies to extract the marginal gains athletes need to reach the podium.

In Part Four: Supercharge, you'll learn how the brain and mood are deeply impacted by nutrition, the consequences of concussions, and strategies to support cognitive function. You'll learn how expert psychologists build emotional intelligence, the pitfalls of *too much* confidence, and how to build a resilient mind. You'll also get a look at the mindset of elite leaders, the value of simple heuristics, if intelligence trumps wisdom, what team culture really means, and the value of consistency in achieving elite outcomes.

## A Little about Me

I've played sports for as long as I can remember. I was an athlete growing up; I played basketball, baseball, volleyball, golf, and more. I loved everything about sports: the challenge, the camaraderie, the coaching, and the competition. I dreamed of playing in the NBA. (Like many of you reading this book, going "pro" was the ultimate goal.) I had pictures of Canadian All-Star Steve Nash lining my walls, as well as local legends like Rowan Barrett and Greg Francis. Of course, as the years went by I realized I wasn't going to make it to the NBA. So what was next? An unexpected health challenge in high school steered me in a new direction.

In my senior year of high school, my efforts to bulk up and add more muscle resulted in struggles with persistent digestive and immune problems. I was constantly sick and it hampered my ability to perform. In the end, it wasn't a medication or invasive technique that got me back on track, it was nutrition. It made me realize how interconnected diet and health were to performance. This led me to take an interest in nutrition, health, and medicine. Unfortunately, the institutions of nutrition and medicine didn't seem to go hand in hand (as crazy as that sounds, since they're so inextricably linked). While getting my undergraduate degree at university, I discovered that the role of nutrition in chronic medical conditions seemed to be completely ignored. Unsure what to do next, I did what my peers were doing at the time — I went backpacking! My travels around the globe exposed me to new environments, new people, new languages, and new ways of looking at the world. I worked as a personal trainer along the way, and it further cemented my beliefs that nutrition, movement, and lifestyle factors (such as lack of sleep and stress management) were absolutely crucial factors for health and weight loss. With more than two-thirds of the population overweight and obese, and the trickle-down effects leading into all types of chronic degenerative conditions, it seemed that diet, exercise, and lifestyle were the keys to improved health. (Today, the research shows 9 out of 10 chronic conditions are lifestyle-related.)

When I returned to Canada to do my naturopathic medicine studies, I realized health problems impact high-level athletes as well. I worked at renowned strength coach Charles Poliquin's high performance center in Toronto and saw firsthand how poor health could lead to poor performance. It also opened my eyes to how intensely elite athletes train, day after day, in preparation for their competitive season. Because of my background in naturopathic medicine, I would get referred athletes who were struggling with immunity issues, digestive complaints, or unexplained fatigue. Getting back to basics — ensuring adequate energy availability, resolving dysbiotic digestive systems, ensuring adequate macro- and micronutrient intakes, and the like — was often enough to resolve their problem. Adding a little bit of objective data from blood tests, combined with the subjective experience from the athlete, also helped get things back on track. It was an important realization: Despite that these guys and gals are superheroes in the gym and on the playing field, they could succumb to health-related problems just like everybody else. In fact, it could even be *the* major roadblock standing between them and success. This is a fundamental concept behind *Peak*: In order to unlock your athletic potential, you need to be a healthy person first.

Of course, just being healthy doesn't make you an elite athlete. You need talent, a disciplined work ethic, and a vision. You also need support. The same goes for trainers, practitioners, and coaches. This is one of the lessons I've learned working at Canada Basketball with the men's national teams, alongside the integrated support team leader (aka performance director) and head athletic therapist, Sam Gibbs. Sam's vision of high performance was refreshing: a hierarchy of athlete health first and foremost, followed by physical outputs, and topped off with elite skill development — all while bringing together knowledge of how the body and brain are constantly communicating via the myriad systems in the body. A similar mindset was shared by Canada Basketball's strength and conditioning coach and renowned physical therapist Charlie Weingroff, another deep thinker in the athlete space. Charlie is always trying to connect the dots from various fields to uncover the true roadblocks to athlete success. The idea of experts in a specific field capable of wearing multiple hats, of understanding performance problems through the lens of another practitioner with a different expertise, illuminated for me how complex problems can be effectively solved, and how they *should* be solved. This environment supported creative thinking, independence, and ultimately very positive outcomes. It's an environment shared by high performance staffs around the world in elite sport. The revolution is happening.

## What Is Peak Performance?

It takes a long time to be elite. It's planned, periodized, and purposeful. You need to show up every day and put in the work. Inspiration and motivation are great to get started on your journey, but they will fizzle out long before you make it to the finish line. I've seen it time and time again in the athletes I work with, as well as when observing the best of the best practitioners, PhDs, and coaches up close from the sidelines. Observation and environment are powerful learning tools. This book is about connecting you with world-leading experts and the research, the insights, and the methods they use (and perhaps more important, don't use) to help athletes achieve world-class success.

Unfortunately, you can't be an expert in everything. There is too much information out there about nutrition, training, recovery, health, and cognitive function. You'll never be able to read it all. As the old saying goes: "Jack of all trades; master of none." But does this really have to be true, particularly as it relates to complex problems like upgrading athletic performance or reversing chronic disease? Complexity comes from interactions. Professor Sidney Dekker, PhD, an expert in complexity and systems thinking, says, "You cannot reduce a complex system to one of its parts, because if you do, you will tragically and dramatically oversimplify things." By taking a certain perspective, you obscure some things and make others highly visible. The outcome of a system is never produced by one single part; rather, the outcome is produced via the interactions of all the parts. In this book you'll find it is the interrelation of disciplines that unlocks our true potential. No longer can we look at sports and nutrition apart. No longer can we think that stress and mindset are separate from performance. Sleep matters. The food you eat during halftime matters. It all matters.

### The Rise of the Expert-Generalist

The general assumption is if you study in multiple areas or participate in multiple different domains, you're only learning at a surface level and never delving deeply enough to truly gain mastery. The term *expert* is typically applied to individuals with very specific knowledge, in contrast to a generalist whose knowledge is broad and more fundamental. It takes a high degree of intelligence to be a specialist, and specialists have revolutionized modern-day living.

All of the major advancements in the last century — the automobile, the airplane, rocketry, nuclear power, antibiotics, radio and television, the personal computer, the internet, and so on — have been the result of brilliant specialists. In the 1940s, Alexander Fleming discovered penicillin — the world's first true antibiotic — whose introduction into general medical practice was one of the century's greatest advances in medicine. It kicked off the dawn of the antibiotic age and dovetailed with development of vaccines to treat infectious diseases and rapid technological advancements in surgery that have saved millions of lives. Specialists are essential for innovation and advancement, both in medicine and athlete performance. There will always be a role for the specialist. But there's a problem with overspecialization, too.

The amount of scientific research is doubling every nine years and the number of disciplines is growing exponentially as well. These are two crucial findings from the field of scientometrics (the science of science), which studies the evolution of scientific knowledge. This growth has created an enormous challenge. Each discipline has their own culture and language, and as the realm of science grows seemingly similar domains divide to such a degree that specialists in one subfield know very little to nothing about what is going on in another subfield. For example, many geneticists have limited understanding of the application of epigenetics. Similarly, medical doctors receive very little training in nutrition, movement, and lifestyle modification even though modern chronic diseases are rooted in nutrition, movement, and lifestyle modification. What's wrong with this picture? For the first time in human history, chronic conditions such as obesity, type 2 diabetes, cardiovascular disease, and dementia kill more people than infectious diseases. What's the response to this current state of affairs? Sadly, the answer has been more and more subspecialization in the hopes it will yield groundbreaking results. While it might in certain areas, there are still too many opportunities being missed *between* areas of expertise. Whoever can bridge these gaps will trigger the next wave of innovation and solutions. This is what *Peak* aims to do — break down the barriers between once-thought-as-separate disciplines and look for the links.

In the wake of overspecialization, let's consider the *expert-generalist*, a term coined by Orit Gadiesh, chairman of Bain & Company, to describe "someone who has the ability and curiosity to master and collect expertise in many different disciplines, industries, skills, capabilities, and topics." Why is collecting expertise in different fields important? Gadiesh highlights that the expert-generalist can draw on a palette of diverse knowledge to recognize patterns and connect the dots across multiple areas. Rather than delving deeply into one subject, the expert-generalist casts a wide net across multiple disciplines, expanding the *breadth* of their knowledge rather than simply plumbing the depths (see figure 0.1).

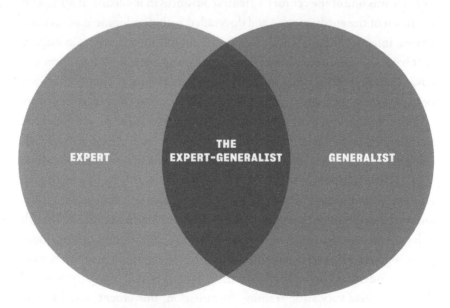

**FIGURE 0.1.** The Expert-Generalist.

Studying across many different fields, identifying the deeper principles, and then applying them back into their own core area is a major advantage of an expert-generalist. They can often see problems more accurately because they aren't as susceptible to the established biases or assumptions within a specific field. Expert-generalists also develop relationships with people from a variety of backgrounds. Knowing people from a wide cross section of disciplines enables them to acquire a better understanding of problems via various perspectives, which means they're more likely to see problems from another person's point of view. Expert-generalists also tend to connect more effectively with people, and most important, connect with people from *different* groups. This style is referred to as having an "open network" and has been cited as the number one predictor of career success.[1] For an athlete or a coach implementing this open network model, embracing the identity of an expert-generalist is crucial.

Learning across multiple fields gives you an information advantage, because most people focus solely on their own field. This multiple-field learning style is referred to as *learning transfer*, which is when you learn something in one context and then apply it to another. For example, if you're a doctor who rarely reads exercise literature, you might be completely unaware that grip strength, leg strength, and lean muscle mass are three evidence-based predictors strongly associated with longevity. Doctors with a wider knowledge base are able to make those connections and achieve better patient outcomes. Not convinced? The *Journal of the Association of American Medical Colleges* recently published a paper called "The Expert-Generalist: A Contradiction Whose Time Has Come" and concluded, "The expert-generalist would benefit both the quality of the patient experience and the bottom line."[2] The prestigious *British Medical Journal* (BMJ) is also in agreement. The BMJ's recent review titled "Celebrating the Expert Generalist" sums things up as follows: "Generalists are no less expert simply because their skills and value aren't defined by an organ system or procedure."[3] Looks like the expert-generalist might be the magic bullet the medical system has been looking for to solve the chronic disease epidemic. This is critical because the rates of obesity, type 2 diabetes, and heart disease have reached epidemic levels, and 9 out of 10 chronic diseases are due to diet, exercise, and lifestyle factors.

For specialists, enhancing their expert-generalist skillset yields major benefits. A recent study at the University of Pennsylvania investigated how the best opera music composers of the twentieth century mastered their discipline. Contrary to the popular belief, they didn't spend 10,000 hours of deliberate practice to hyper-specialize in their field. They expanded their knowledge to other styles and genres. Researchers found the master composers "were able to avoid the inflexibility of too much expertise by cross-training."[4] Expanding the breadth of their musical knowledge, rather than simply the depth, separated them from the competition.

You might be asking yourself at this point, how does this relate to sports? Let's take the example of a collegiate strength coach or personal trainer. As one of these coaches, you spend all your time focusing on and learning the fundamentals and intimate details of strength and conditioning, and as a result, little time is devoted to learning the fundamentals of nutrition, sleep, health, or behavior change. Also, because your skillset is rooted in training alone, you're far more likely to think exercise is the solution to a problem you're confronted with. You might think your client is struggling to perform due to inadequate strength or poor aerobic capacity, because that's where your mind is focused (consciously or unconsciously), even if the reason might be a result of inadequate sleep, or poor nutrition, or a chronic health condition. A general understanding of the fundamentals of nutrition, sleep, or mental performance can provide the strength coach with the tools to help the athlete get back on track, thereby maintaining progress and performance. Even a decade ago this concept was largely ignored: trainers trained athletes, nutritionists talked only nutrition, doctors prescribed medications, and so forth. That said, we're still not all the way there. Just because you have a dietitian, doctor, strength coach, athletic therapist, and psychologist, working under the same roof doesn't guarantee they're still not working as if they are siloed in their own domains.

## The Revolution in Peak Performance

A revolution is defined as "a dramatic and wide-reaching change in conditions, attitudes, or operation." In high performance, the revolution is a reemphasis on the evidence-based *fundamentals* as a foundation. The revolution is an attitude toward *individualized* athlete health, nutrition, training, recovery, and psychology. The revolution is not only technology driving innovation and operation in sport, but the people *analyzing* and *interpreting* the data. Kevin Hartman of Google highlights this importance best, stating: "Invest 10 percent of your budget in technology and 90 percent in analysis." It's not just Big Data, but the value of the coach's eye and knowing when to trust your instincts when faced with complex problems.

This book is just the tip of the iceberg. Entire textbooks are written about each individual chapter in this book, so it would be impossible to give you all the information out there. You can pursue deeper learning in any of the areas through the work of the subject matter experts noted in this book, and via the 600-plus references listed. My goal is to connect you to the leading experts, sport scientists, and coaches out there, so you can learn the key fundamentals of their success and apply them in your practice. You get the insights directly from the performance professionals who spend lifetimes in the trenches working with high-performers. They rarely have 100,000 followers on Instagram, but they are truly blazing the trails and making a difference.

*Peak* is about these fundamentals. But you won't find recipes or lengthy discussions about food quality, sourcing, and so forth in these pages. I will say, however, that I have a Food First approach to performance nutrition. An athlete's diet should be made up primarily of whole, unprocessed foods such as quality meats (beef, fish, seafood, chicken, and the like), plentiful vegetables (cruciferous, leafy, and everything in between), fresh fruit (all colors of the rainbow), complex carbohydrates, and healthy fats from grass-fed meats and natural oils. Diet can become very nuanced and complex, or it can be very simple. Build your diet around "real" food and limit your intake of processed foods. A healthy diet rooted in whole foods is achievable. The Mediterranean dietary strategy is a great example — people in Mediterranean countries such as Spain, France, and Italy spend a paltry 20.3, 14.2, and 13.4 percent of household income respectively on processed foods. Comparably, individuals in the United States, United Kingdom, and Canada spend more than 50 percent of household income on processed foods. Not surprisingly, the former have some of the lowest incidences of chronic disease, while the latter struggle mightily. That said, *performance* nutrition is different than nutrition for health, even though optimal health is crucial for performance. The difference is that performance nutrition is about *winning*. An athlete might need to include more processed foods to achieve their required energy intake during training, two-a-days, or when trying to make weight. An athlete might need supplementation, nutrient timing, and specific fueling strategies (that might appear at first glance extreme or even unhealthy) to get them over the hump. This is not to say they should be ignoring a Food First nutritional strategy, but simply that in high performance sports, certain strategies need to be implemented in order to compete at an elite level. In these pages you'll learn the big rocks: the total caloric intake for athletes to target; the amounts or "grams per day" of proteins, fats, and carbs; and the therapeutic dose of a supplement. It's up to you as the athlete or sports professional to round out the diet and select a quality supplement. (Check out my website DrBubbs.com if you'd like more support, or stay tuned for my next book).

## The Next Greatest Gains

The success of expert-generalists throughout history is impressive. Albert Einstein was trained in physics, but to formulate his law of general relativity he taught himself an area of mathematics far removed from his expertise. Rosalind Franklin, James Watson, and Francis Crick combined discoveries in X-ray diffraction technology, chemistry, evolutionary theory, and computation to solve the puzzle of the DNA double helix. Steve Jobs drew on insights from his study of calligraphy and a rich understanding of design to create a new breed of computing devices. Expert systems theorist, inventor, architect, and legendary expert-generalist Buckminster Fuller (born in 1895) perhaps best highlighted the importance of general expertise long ago when he said: "We are in an age that assumes the narrowing trends of specialization to be logical, natural, and desirable. . . . In the meantime, humanity has been deprived of comprehensive understanding. . . . It has also resulted in the individual's leaving responsibility for thinking and social action to others."

In the world of high performance, most experts are in agreement that the next revolution is unlikely to come from traditional channels and that you must be open-minded to new opportunities and a changing landscape. "The intersection of where modalities meet is where the next greatest gains will be made," says renowned performance expert Fergus Connolly, PhD. Empowering people to take ownership of their health, nutrition, training, recovery, and mindset is the ultimate goal. This is why I do what I do — to help the patient, to help the athlete, to help the team — to be part of something bigger than myself. It's a feeling all practitioners, personal trainers, and coaches have felt at some point when they work with clients who overcome challenges to achieve their goal. But make no mistake — it's the clients who do all the work. The Chinese philosopher Lao Tzu sums it up best: "A leader is best when people barely know he exists. When his work is done, his aim fulfilled, they will say: we did it ourselves."

# PART ONE

# Foundation

*Health is the greatest of human blessings.*

— HIPPOCRATES

# CHAPTER 1

# Sleep and Circadian Rhythms

Roger Federer was bent over in pain. It was 2013, and Federer was struggling with chronic back injuries, failing to reach a major tournament final for the first time in 15 years. It was the start of a decline for the greatest tennis player of all time. In 2016, he saw another setback. As Federer began to rediscover his game and gain some momentum, he was sidelined by a knee injury that required surgery. The questions started reverberating around the tennis world. Will Federer even win another major? Is Federer finished? After more than a decade of total domination in tennis and winning major championships at an unprecedented rate, it looked as though time had caught up to Federer. It looked like the competition had also caught up to him; tennis isn't kind to athletes over 30. Then something surprising happened: In 2017, at the age of 35, Federer turned back the clock. It seemed as if he had found the fountain of youth. He won the Australian Open major championship, his first major since five years earlier. Did he catch lightning in a bottle? Then Federer had another major win in 2017 at Wimbledon, in totally dominating fashion. He defended his title to win the Australian Open again in 2018, which reaffirmed him at the top of tennis. How was this possible at the age of 36, when contemporaries of his vintage were in the booth calling the action and not on the court? Rumors emerged that Roger Federer had discovered a secret weapon to preserve his stamina, accelerate his recovery, sharpen his quickness, and keep his mind agile. Rumors were, this secret weapon was so impactful in the years building up to his reemergence that Federer refused to talk about it. But what was it? In the end, we found out: The secret was Federer's relentless focus on *sleep*. And now, when the focus on sleep is ubiquitous in high-level sport, is it actually translating to athletes taking action and getting more sleep? Does training intensely impact your sleep quality? And what about the time of day you train – how does that affect performance? In this chapter, we will take a deeper dive into the science of sleep, circadian rhythm, and performance.

First of all, it is important to note that sleep is universal. All living organisms on the planet sleep. It's fundamental to life. There are very few things shared across all species, but sleep is one of them. Ironically, in today's modern culture we wear lack of sleep like a badge of honor. If you can work all hours of the day and tolerate little sleep, you're celebrated as the strongest. A culture of sleeplessness seems common across almost all domains. Doctors doing their residency in hospitals are notoriously sleep-deprived, a practice seen as a rite of passage in the field despite the research highlighting the potential harms to patient care. Coaches log incredibly long days, often sleeping less than 5 hours a night to watch game film and stay ahead of the competition, despite the harmful effects on their health. Athletes who balance training with school or work trade sleep for more time studying or punching the clock. The average adult today gets approximately 6.5 hours of sleep per night, which falls short of the National Sleep Foundation's recommendation of 7–9 hours per night.[1] Approximately 30 percent of the population survive on less than 6 hours of sleep, and incredibly, about 10 percent on less than 5 hours.[2]

The fascination with and addiction to social media is no doubt fueling this fire. For it's not just uncontrollable factors like training, school, or work schedules leading to lack of sleep, it's that being "busy" is a new form of social status. The typical young person aged 18–24 checks their phone 74 times per day, adults 25–34 check their devices 50 times per day, and those between 35–44 check about 35 times per day. We can't go more than 12 minutes without checking our phones (on average). Both American and British people will check their phones 10,000 times in one year.

This addiction to social media is not just a social phenomenon; it has significant consequences to our health and sleep. In fact, lack of sleep has now become a global problem, the World Health Organization (WHO) declaring it a new epidemic throughout industrialized nations. Insufficient sleep is strongly associated with an increased risk of diabetes (type 2), cardiovascular disease, cancer, dementias, depression and anxiety, and mortality.[3] On a day-to-day basis lack of sleep wreaks havoc on your health. It pummels your immune system, increasing your risk of catching a nasty cold or flu. It worsens your blood sugar control, causing a constant rollercoaster of highs and lows in response to your meals (even healthy options). If you don't get enough shut-eye, appetite-stimulating hormones such as ghrelin ramp up, causing strong cravings for sugar, sweets, and processed foods while satiety hormones, such as leptin, are blunted. Insufficient sleep impacts your cognition, impairs decision-making, and negatively influences your ability to problem solve and consolidate memories. In short, there is virtually no area of health unscathed by lack of sleep. The need for sleep has not changed in more than two million years of evolution; that is how essential it is to human health.

If sleep is fundamental to health and how well we think, move, and perform, then what are the consequences for the athlete? Because, as I discuss in this book, to perform your best as an athlete and truly reach and sustain your performance potential, you need to be a healthy person first. This idea is referred to in sports as the Human First paradigm. Insufficient sleep is perhaps the greatest limiting factor to human health, and therefore, it follows that it might also be one of the greatest limiting factors in athletic performance. In this chapter, you'll learn from the world-leading experts how enhancing an athlete's sleep quality, duration, and timing can upgrade health, performance, recovery, and cognition.

## Sleep, Performance, and the Twenty-First-Century Athlete

Research on sleep and athletic performance has exploded over the past decade. Sleep scientists have found that total sleep time and sleep quality are both highly associated with virtually every athletic quality: speed, endurance, strength, power, injury risk, immunity, attention, decision-making, learning, and so on.[4] This can be the difference between winning and losing. If you're spending long hours in the gym, on the playing field, and in the film room trying to be the best you can be, do you really want to ignore the low-hanging fruit of sleep and all the potential benefits? Sleep expert Cheri Mah, MD, of the University of California San Francisco (UCSF) Human Performance Center and sleep consultant in all four major American sports (NBA, NFL, NHL, and MLB) was one of the first researchers to quantify the effects of lack of sleep on athletic performance almost a decade ago. Her work at Stanford with collegiate basketball players exposed the tremendous impact sleep extension could have on athletic performance. Mah's research revealed how extending sleep from 6.6 hours to 8.5 hours nightly produced significant performance gains — a 5 percent increase in speed, a 9 percent increase in free throw percentage and a 9.2 percent increase in three-point shooting percentage — in only two months.[5] It wasn't just basketball players; athletes across all sports were performing better. Football players had better reaction times, tennis players had greater first serve percentage, swimmers had faster sprint times, baseball players had better reaction times, and on it went. It seemed that every athlete who extended sleep time performed better.

Mah's initial research was not aimed at athletic performance but rather at assessing the cognitive effects of sleep extension in athletes. Interestingly, the athletes returning to her lab were reporting significantly improved performances in practice or hitting new personal best times in competition. As a result, Mah shifted her research focus to performance. Based on her work, it became apparent athletes should be aiming for 8–10 hours of total sleep per night. The impact of sleep on recovery and performance is so profound, Dr. Mah says, that "sleep should be a nonnegotiable." Since then a huge focus has shifted to sleep in the context of performance. Yet while athletes and coaches are aware of the tremendous importance of sleep on performance, the question remains: How much sleep are athletes *actually* getting?

Adult and youth recreational athletes consistently report less than 8 hours of sleep per night, with no differences between men and women.[6] Elite athletes must be better, right? Unfortunately not. In fact, they fare even worse. A recent study of more than 800 elite athletes in South Africa found 75 percent were not getting at least 8 hours of sleep per night.[7] Alarmingly, they also found 11 percent were not even getting 6 hours of sleep nightly! Less than 6 hours of sleep per night is when health and performance really start to nosedive, and incredibly 1 out of 10 athletes is performing at the highest level *despite* this performance shackle. Olympic athletes are the same story; they are human too and also struggle to get enough shut-eye. Olympic athletes consistently show poorer sleep quality and more fragmented sleep as compared to age- and sex-matched controls.[8] Plus, if you're a female athlete or perform in an aesthetic sport like gymnastics, you're even *more likely* to struggle. We all assume Olympic-level athletes (the most elite in the world) have all aspects of training and recovery dialed in. Unfortunately, the reality is they're people, too, and sometimes life gets in the way. If you don't identify it as a problem, and prioritize it, it can easily go unnoticed. For Olympic athletes, many are at the mercy of their training schedules while balancing work (often multiple jobs to support training costs), family, and social commitments. It's a lot to take on. It's also a testament to their resiliency that they can still perform at a world-class level. At the same time, it's incredible to think they could potentially unlock an extra 2–5 percent of performance gains by simply getting more rest.

There are four key domains to maximize athletic performance: physical abilities (speed, strength, and the like); technical skills (such as dribbling and lifting technique); tactical skills (during the game or competition), and psychological mettle (mindset, drive, and so on). The lack of sleep can sabotage all four (probably faster than any other factor). Sleep is perhaps the ultimate performance enhancer, yet despite the research and increased public awareness, it is not a fully tapped resource. But before we discuss a variety of sleep solutions from world-leading experts, let's take a closer look at why sleep is so crucial.

## The Evolution of Sleep

How old is sleep? Really, really old. The earth is approximately 3.8 billion years old, and the oldest living things on the planet, single-celled bacteria called prokaryotes, undergo a form of sleep. They have distinct "on" and "off" phases of their cell cycles that mimic sleep. Five hundred million years ago, before the first vertebrates appeared on the scene, worms existed — and they sleep, too. In fact, if you deprive a worm of sleep for a night, it will sleep longer the following night. In his terrific book *Why We Sleep*, Matthew Walker, PhD, sleep expert and professor of neuroscience at the University of California, Berkeley, explains how the same phenomenon occurs in humans, and how this natural effect of sleep extension (after deprivation) is evolutionarily hardwired.[9] Dr. Walker also highlights that we share 99 percent of our DNA with our primate ancestors like chimpanzees, and yet our sleep requirements are almost half. How could this be? Despite existing for five million years before humans, Walker notes chimpanzees didn't acquire the ability to reason, problem solve, or create societies to the level of humans; nor did they achieve the equivalent brain size. In fact, chimpanzees are still functioning under the same set of rules they have for millions of years. Dr. Walker argues that sleep is one of the strongest factors that *made us human,* and believes REM sleep played a fundamental role in shaping the human brain.

REM sleep is the dream state, when our bodies become paralyzed and our brains are hurled into a frenzy of sporadic activity. REM sleep promotes more rational control, dials in emotional connections, and facilitates recognition and intelligent decision-making. REM sleep also supports creativity, connecting all of your brain networks to help you form new ideas and curiosities. In short, REM sleep enhances our *emotional intelligence*, a key piece of the puzzle in the evolution of humans. Incredibly, humans dedicate 20–25 percent of sleep time to REM sleep, compared to only 9 percent in other primates.[10] How did humans evolve this ability to amplify REM sleep? Dr. Walker believes it was our early ancestors' ability to use fire. *Homo erectus* was the first of our hominid ancestors (the great apes family of orangutans, gorillas, chimpanzees, and humans) to come down from the trees and sleep on the ground. Sleeping in trees doesn't afford you the luxury of a lot of REM sleep; during REM sleep, your body is in a state of paralysis, so falling out of a tree at night was not good for survival. Once on the ground, the sleep of our early ancestors got shorter and much more intense. (Sleeping on the ground by a campfire also likely served as a deterrent to keep predators at bay.) Walker believes sleeping on the ground ramped up REM sleep, triggering an explosion of neural circuitry and complexity that has become our human brains. In short, REM sleep is fundamental to both our health and athletic performance.

## Pushing the Limits: The Impacts of Sleep Quality and Duration

To be the best, you need to train frequently and train hard. This is the reality of high-level sport. Athletes are constantly pushing the limits to trigger the training adaptations that allow them to get bigger, faster, stronger, and so forth. But how does intense training impact sleep? Football and soccer players, for example, both show significant drops in sleep duration when acutely ramping up training load.[11] There appears to be a "sleep cost" to pushing yourself hard. And if you don't balance this cost with adequate recovery, you're destined to struggle. In fact, the evidence is clear: Athletes who push themselves hard during heavy training blocks tend to experience a reduction in total sleep time.[12] This reduction can compromise recovery and capacity to adapt if not taken into account. Plus, your sport might also be contributing to your sleep debt. Sports such as swimming and rowing are traditionally practiced in the early morning hours, and research shows swimmers and rowers sleep less and feel more fatigued before early morning training sessions.[13] Early mornings also negatively affect your training (or competition) in the evening.[14] This is important to consider if you work with teenage or collegiate athletes, or high-level athletes with early morning practices before evening games. It seems you can't escape the performance pitfalls of lack of sleep.

Endurance athletes might need more sleep than team or strength sport athletes. Sleep expert Amy Bender, PhD, from the Canadian Sport Institute in Calgary highlights how the typical longer duration of endurance sessions, the trend toward earlier morning workouts, and the heavier toll of high training volume on the nervous systems of endurance athletes all likely play a role in the need for more sleep. The mechanism of how insufficient sleep impairs endurance performance isn't clear, but some research suggests it might inhibit exercise capacity through an increase in perceived exertion.[15]

Sleep loss has been found to have a negative effect on a number of measures of subjective well-being, including fatigue, mood, soreness, depression, and confusion. Lack of sleep adds up: If you don't get enough sleep through the week, it can affect your performance on the weekend, because accumulated weekday sleep debt is associated with poorer reaction times by the end of the week.[16] Sleep debt also gets exposed before major competitions. Seventy percent of athletes report having poor sleep the night *before* competition (typically due to competition-related anxiety). So if you're already in a sleep debt before the big game, another night of poor sleep can negatively impact game day performance, too. Sleep time is also lower *after* competition, says sleep expert and researcher Ian Dunican, PhD, who points out that athletes are always trying to dig themselves out of the sleep debt accrued from two consecutive nights of poor sleep and that it typically takes 2–3 days to recover from this lost sleep.

## SLEEP QUALITY MATTERS

It's not just your total sleep time that's crucial to your health and performance; sleep *quality* matters, too. In general, athletes seem to have better quality of sleep compared to age-matched sedentary folks, but once again, pushing the limits of training volume and intensity starts to impair sleep quality, too.[17] In Brazil, approximately 600 elite male and female athletes were asked to rate their sleep quality and mood immediately before a national or international competition. Researchers found the majority assessed their sleep quality as normal or good, but after the matches they found athletes with poorer sleep quality actually performed worse at the competition.[18] In fact, poor sleep quality was an independent predictor of lost competition (even after accounting for the effects of anger, vigor, and tension). That's a high price to pay for poor sleep quality!

An athlete's age and sport might potentially predict their likelihood of poor sleep as well. Sleep experts found that for players of individual sports — runners, cyclists, weight lifters, tennis players, and others — the chances of experiencing sleep problems increases with age, compared to team sports where it decreases with age. In younger athletes, academic pressures have also been found to be a major threat to sleep quality (and duration).[19] Athletes face a unique set of roadblocks when it comes to optimal sleep. They're at the mercy of training schedules, traveling frequently to training and competitions, balancing training with work, academic, and family commitments, as well as experiencing the natural precompetition anxiety — all can impair sleep. In the general population, physical activity is usually helpful for improving sleep. If you don't get enough movement in your day, or you spend most of your time sitting at a desk, then being more active is a great way to support better sleep.

### TRICKLE-DOWN EFFECTS: PAIN, INJURY, AND INFECTION

Alarmingly, athletes are remarkably poor at assessing their own sleep duration and quality! But it is important to know what trickle-down effects sleep has on performance. For starters, in elite sport, you need to be able to push through pain. A lot of pain. Anything that impairs your ability to fight through discomfort could limit your training intensity (or frequency), thus limiting your ability to adapt. Lack of sleep clobbers your capacity to push through pain, reducing your pain tolerance by almost 10 percent.[20] If your sport requires grueling efforts (such as Ironman training, long CrossFit WODs, or hard physical contact), this should definitely be on your radar. If you don't get 8 hours of sleep per night, you're at 1.7 times greater risk of injury compared to those who get at least 8 hours per night.[21] Experts aren't clear on the mechanisms, but they believe reduced reaction time and cognitive function are likely to blame. Young athletes (and young adults in general) are at the greatest risk of sleepiness-related accidents.[22] A recent study of 496 adolescent athletes from 16 different individual and team sports found that increased training load and decreased self-reported sleep duration were independently associated with an increased risk of injury. The greatest overall risk for injury resulted when both occurred; training load increased and sleep duration decreased simultaneously.[23] This risk for injury is often seen during competition travel and training camp-type settings. Therefore, added sleep and recovery support should be emphasized during these periods.

If you're an athlete and you don't get a sufficient amount of sleep, you can be more susceptible to colds and flu as well. Lack of total sleep time suppresses your immune system and increases your risk of upper respiratory tract infections (URTI).[24] If you're always struggling with niggling colds throughout your training block and missing sessions, it will be a lot harder for you to keep up with the competition. The importance of sleep for maintaining a robust immune system was best highlighted by Professor Sheldon Cohen, director of the Laboratory for the Study of Stress, Immunity, and Disease at Carnegie Mellon University, and his team who took a group of athletes and deliberately inoculated them all with a cold virus. To assess the impact of inadequate sleep on immunity, Cohen then divided the groups into varying sleep times to see who got sick the most. The group getting less than 7 hours a night were three times more likely to get sick (compared to at least 7 hours nightly); the group getting less than 6 hours of sleep really got hammered, showing a 4.5-fold increased risk of infection.[25] Keep this in mind if you are a coach or practitioner working with younger adolescent athletes, as the data clearly supports longer sleep times translating to far fewer illnesses. Lastly, team doctors must remember that lack of sleep can compromise the effectiveness of vaccines, which is important to note before athletes require vaccinations for travel or infection.[26] Before I discuss common roadblocks to sleep and the experts' sleep solutions, let's review the physiology of sleep and how circadian rhythms fit into this protol.

## Understanding Sleep Architecture

Sleep occurs in two distinct phases: non-rapid eye movement (NREM) and rapid eye movement (REM) sleep. The NREM phase occurs first and is divided into four stages, progressively getting deeper from one to four. Upon completion of the NREM stages, your brain then shifts into dreamy REM sleep, the second phase of sleep. This is considered one complete sleep cycle. Throughout the night, your brain repeats these cycles — alternating between NREM and REM sleep stages — over and over again until you wake in the morning. This is known as your sleep architecture. NREM sleep dominates the first half of the night, then as you transition into the second half of the night the REM stages get progressively longer (at the expense of NREM sleep). Your last sleep cycle before waking is dominated by REM sleep, so if you get to bed too late at night or wake up too early, you'll cut into this REM-rich last sleep cycle. This, in turn, compromises your ability to consolidate all the information you took in the day before.

Sleep scientists believe the primary role of NREM sleep early in the night is to trim unnecessary or less useful neural connections. There isn't enough memory space in the brain to keep all the information, thus sleep is a time to consolidate and organize all the meaningful data. Just like a sculptor working on a piece of art, your brain cuts away the useless material and adds finer details over and over again. When you're awake, things change, and your brain wave activity is fast and chaotic. Then during sleep, it slows down dramatically and becomes more synchronized, like your neurons are all marching quietly in rhythm to the same beat. At this point, you're in deep sleep.

To achieve this state of deep sleep, a small structure within your brain called the thalamus acts as a sensory blocker. The thalamus is located deep in the middle of your brain (just above the brainstem) and prevents all perceptions of sound, sight, touch, and so on from reaching the outer cortex of your brain. The cortex is the "thinking" part of your brain, and when the thalamus shuts it down, you relax and lose consciousness. As your brain waves slow during deep sleep, you're better able to communicate information from distant areas of the brain, converting short-term memory to long-term memory. After a cycle of NREM sleep stages, you move into a period of dreaming REM sleep. During REM sleep, your body is actually completely paralyzed as your thalamus opens the gate back to the outer cortex of your brain, where your emotions, memories, and internal drives are unleashed. The primary role of REM sleep is to strengthen and consolidate your existing neuronal connections. If you're learning new information, skills, or techniques, a lack of REM sleep will undoubtedly stall progress. REM sleep is also crucial for developing emotional intelligence, which, as you'll see in Part Four: Supercharge, plays a massive role in your athletic (and life) success, too.

## One Bad Night's Sleep

Can just a single night of poor sleep impact your sleep architecture and your ability to compete and perform? The simple answer: yes. In competitive cyclists, one sleepless night after a heavy training session reduced time trial performance the following morning, suggesting insufficient sleep might hamper recovery between strenuous exercise bouts.[27] In volleyball players, similar effects were observed as they were unable to maintain their work capacity during progressive testing after partial sleep loss.[28] What about pulling an all-nighter? Not surprisingly, it's been shown to impair your ability to cover the same distance in an endurance time trial test, but it doesn't seem to impact strength sports the same way.[29] Collegiate weight lifters didn't see any dip in performance after a total night of sleep loss, despite feeling fatigued and sleepy (oh, the benefits of being in your early 20s!).[30] Sport scientists believe lack of sleep impacts your physiology via increasing your heart rate and oxygen consumption, as well as ramping up lactate levels. All of these metrics suggest your body must work harder under sleep loss conditions compared to normal conditions.[31] Your muscle glycogen status also takes a hit with sleep loss, promoting a shift in your fuel availability during training that could lead to poor endurance efforts.[32]

But one bad night's sleep doesn't just impact you peripherally, it also impacts you centrally. That is, your mental game suffers, too. Numerous studies have shown insufficient sleep blunts neurocognitive function, specifically attention, learning, and executive function (the higher-level thinking you need to apply strategy, make decisions, and maintain attention — all important factors for athletes).[33] All of these areas are central to elite athletic performance. If you've been up all night or are sleep deprived from one night's bad sleep, your inhibitory control is reduced, which means you're more likely to engage in risk-taking behavior.[34] (I guess it's no accident casinos are open 24 hours a day in Las Vegas!) Sleep deprivation also undermines your decision-making skills and your ability to make split-second decisions during competition. A night of poor sleep is also a big problem for skill execution. For example, tennis players competing on less than 5 hours of sleep see dramatic reduction in first serve accuracy.[35] Likewise, professional dart players (they're athletes, too, right?) competing on 5 hours of sleep also suffered from significant accuracy deficits compared to those who had a full night's rest.[36] The bad news is, even after you catch up on your sleep, there seems to be a major lag time before your full cognitive performance is restored.[37] This is important to consider before a major competition, because most athletes think they can simply catch up on a missed night a few days out. The research says they can't.[38] Dr. Dunican says it takes his athletes about 2–3 days to reverse the effects of a few nights of reduced sleep time and quality.

## Sleeping Pills, Alcohol, and Health

If you've struggled with sleep in the past, chances are you've used a prescription medication. While acute use is not a problem, chronic use can heavily compromise health and performance. Incredibly, the use of prescription sleeping pills like Ambien are common go-to strategies for many athletes (and coaches) to get some sleep when they're too buzzed from a busy day of work or training. This is a dangerous strategy. "No drugs we currently have will help the patient sleep," says Matthew Walker, professor of neuroscience at the University of California, Berkeley, summing up the current state of evidence-based research. Another common misconception is that alcohol is a great sleep aid. While alcohol makes you feel tired in the short-term, and acts as a nervine that relaxes your nervous system after a stressful day, it also *directly* impairs sleep quality. After you consume alcohol, your liver must process it, which raises your body temperature, hindering your sleep quality and often leading to more frequent waking through the night. As you get older, lack of quality sleep due to regular alcohol consumption in the evening is strongly associated with increased risk of neurological degenerative disorders, cardiovascular disease, and cancer. In fact, the use of sleep drugs and alcohol often go hand in hand, with disastrous results. This is something legendary college football coach Urban Meyer found out the hard way. Despite winning two national championships with the University of Florida, from 2005 to 2010, he was miserable and his health was a mess. Meyer admits getting less than 4 hours of sleep a night and relying heavily on sleep medications to get any shut-eye at all. He often forgot to eat, lost 40 pounds, and stopped working out altogether. He was on a road to disaster before getting help from his wife and doctors, and he now openly speaks about the importance of taking care of yourself. This is the key to peak performance: health matters.

## Sleep Pressure and Circadian Rhythms

Now that you have a better understanding of how decreased sleep time, poorer sleep quality, and even a single night of bad sleep can hamper performance, let's circle back to sleep physiology and discuss the two driving factors that trigger sleep onset: circadian rhythm and sleep pressure. Sleep pressure is a simple phenomenon — the longer you've been awake, the sleepier you feel and the greater your drive to seek sleep. Sleep pressure helps to promote sleepiness in preparation for sleep and recovery via the buildup of a compound called adenosine in your brain. The longer you've been awake, the more buildup of adenosine and the sleepier you feel. Have you ever wondered exactly why coffee keeps you awake? It produces its stimulant effect via caffeine, which inhibits the binding of adenosine to receptors in the brain, delaying how sleepy you feel. This is important to consider because caffeine can clearly support superior athletic performance, but it might also come at a cost (depending on timing, dose, and your individual genetic response to caffeine). If you don't use caffeine judiciously and personalize the frequency and dose, it can quickly compromise your sleep quality, health, recovery, and ultimately performance.

It's not just sleep pressure that influences wakefulness; circadian rhythms — your internal body clock that runs on an approximate 24-hour cycle — also play a fundamental role. After billions of years of evolution, the only predictable cue for our brains has been the rising and setting sun, which happens every day without fail. The light and dark cycles are hardwired into the deepest parts of our brain. The suprachiasmatic nucleus (SCN), located at the intersection of your optic nerves behind your eyes, samples the incoming light from each eye as it travels to the back of your brain for interpretation. The SCN in your brain is like the offensive coordinator on a football team, relaying information from one input to another. The SCN relays the incoming information from the light and dark cycles of the day to your brain using melatonin as its key messenger. Not long after the sun goes down, the SCN programs the release of melatonin from the pineal gland deep in your brain, signaling that it's time to wind down and prepare for sleep. Melatonin helps to regulate the timing of your sleep, telling your brain that darkness is coming. Throughout the night, your melatonin levels gradually decline. As the first morning light hits your eyelids, production of melatonin is blunted, and your pineal gland effectively turns off the melatonin tap. This gives the signals to your brain that it's time to start the day.

Daylight is a primary cue to keep your body clock running on time, but it isn't the only external circadian cue. Your brain's SCN is a major multitasker, also coordinating your daily body temperature, which fluctuates throughout the day as well. Your body temperature drops in the evening, reaches a low point a few hours after you fall asleep, rises again in the morning, and peaks during the day. This occurs in sync, which changes in light and darkness and would still happen even if you pulled an all-nighter and didn't sleep a wink. In fact, in a recent interview with sleep expert Dr. Dan Pardi, PhD, he explained that researchers believe temperature changes in our fingertips might be the first external trigger to the brain to set waking patterns. Other external cues include your first meal of the day, caffeine intake, movement, and even socializing with friends. These are called *zeit-gebers*, from the German word for "synchronizing." While daylight is the most powerful of these external cues, these other variables can be manipulated and timed to support healthy circadian rhythms or when adjusting to a new time zone.

Finally, each person also has a degree of variability in their individual chronotype, which is the time of day they naturally prefer to wake and sleep. I have many clients who love to get up as early as 4:30 a.m. to exercise or get started on work, long before most people even get out of bed. These uberachievers, oftentimes CEOs and high-level executives, aren't staying up until last call at the bar, but rather tuck into bed early around 9 or 10 p.m. In the research, morning people are referred to as morning lark chronotypes, and they make up about 40 percent of the population. But not everyone runs on this pattern. Teens and adolescents are more genetically hardwired to stay up later and sleep in longer; this chronotype is called a night owl, making up approximately 30 percent of the population (the remaining 30 percent are intermediates, somewhere in between). In fact, the night owls can often suffer from social jetlag, which occurs when their late night–preferred pattern doesn't fit in with society's typical 9 to 5 workday. This can be a major problem for cognition. The prefrontal cortex area of your brain sits directly above your eyes and acts a little bit like the quarterback of the brain, coordinating high-level thought, reasoning, and emotional control. If you regularly go to bed late and wake up early, your prefrontal cortex is slow to get up to the line of scrimmage and call the plays, and it can take some time before it hits its stride. This makes sleep debt a bigger problem for late sleepers than early risers, with research showing higher rates of anxiety, depression, diabetes, heart attack, and stroke.[39] Thankfully, while your chronotype appears to be strongly genetically linked, the zeitgeber strategies previously discussed can help to shift your patterns.

## Circadian Timing and Athletic Performance

Circadian rhythms are interesting from a science perspective, but as an athlete you might be wondering how it impacts your ability to perform. Actually, circadian rhythms can play a major role in athletic performance, as the time of day seems to have a big influence on your ability to achieve success. Research on Olympic athletes has uncovered that the chance of breaking an Olympic record is highest in the early afternoon, the natural peak of the human circadian rhythm.[40] Not convinced? In the NFL over the last 40 years, researchers have analyzed the impact of circadian rhythm on performance for the West Coast teams traveling to the East Coast to play night games. The sport scientists included 106 games played at 8 p.m. Eastern Time (by West Coast teams traveling east) in order to assess the impact of an earlier circadian "home body clock" on performance. The results were staggering. During the evening games, the West Coast teams beat the point spread in 66 percent of those games![41] The experts believe it's because West Coast teams are operating on a 3-hour time difference, and their body clock is tuned in to a late afternoon West Coast time, which tends to be correlated to superior performance. So what about day games? Interestingly, visiting West Coast teams experienced no such advantage in daytime games played on the East Coast. These results highlight the dramatic effects late afternoon and early evening circadian rhythms have on physical performance.

Sleep expert Michele Lastella, PhD, provides more evidence of a circadian performance effect. He highlights some of the earliest research in athlete chronotypes, noting that morning larks have significantly higher batting averages in day versus night games.[42] The time of day professional dart players compete also has a significant impact on their performance, as throwing accuracy is strongly associated with time of competition. Researchers believe there is an opportunity in circadian timing, and that playing close to the circadian peak in performance might demonstrate a palpable athletic advantage over those who are playing at other times. In fact, if you compare aerobic and anaerobic fitness on a cycle ergometer between morning and afternoon training sessions, both men and women perform better in the afternoon, improving by 5.1 percent and 5.6 percent respectively.[43] Dr. Lastella also highlights how chronotypes can impact coaching decisions like training times or which athletes share rooms together. Pairing a night owl and morning lark as roommates will have disastrous effects on sleep quality, and if your roster is made up of younger athletes who are typically night owls, scheduling early morning practices will likely hinder adaptation and recovery. In baseball spring training, morning start times have recently been pushed back in an effort to support better sleep and circadian timing.

## Roadblocks to Maximizing Sleep

It is now quite clear in evidence-based research that athletes who get enough total sleep time, quality of sleep, and maintain a healthy circadian rhythm experience improvements in health and performance. Of course, it's the application that's still difficult. Even after reading the data, athletes still don't get enough sleep and are very poor at rating their own sleep. Let's review some of the top sleep and circadian rhythm roadblocks.

### CAFFEINE

Too much caffeine in the evening can delay sleep onset and reduce your total sleep time and quality. Caffeine delays sleep pressure by acting as an adenosine inhibitor, preventing the binding of adenosine receptors in the brain. Athletes who consume too much caffeine in the late afternoon or evening, or who rely on highly caffeinated preworkout formulas (exceeding 6 mg/kg for the day), or those who are genetically slow to metabolize caffeine might be doing themselves more harm than good (more on this in Part Two: Fuel). If you struggle with sleep, keep your caffeine consumption to before noon.

### ALCOHOL

Contrary to popular belief, athletes drink *more* alcohol than the general population. When you drink alcohol late in the evening or too close to bedtime, it leads to an increased body temperature as your liver begins to metabolize the alcohol. This temperature alteration can impair your sleep architecture and quality of rest. Alcohol is also particularly harmful to your precious REM sleep, a crucial time when your brain is synthesizing and consolidating new information. In fact, scientists have identified alcohol as one of the most powerful suppressors of REM sleep.

## BLUE LIGHT

Using tablets or phones before bed is another way to pummel your REM sleep. The light receptors in your eyes are highly sensitive to the short wavelength light in the blue light spectrum, and blue light blocks melatonin output twice as much as incandescent lightbulbs. If you use your laptop or tablet for 2 hours before bed, it can blunt melatonin output by a whopping 23 percent.[44] Not only does the use of these devices suppress REM sleep and melatonin output, it also will reduce your feeling of being rested the following day. Teens and young adults in particular are at higher risk. Sleep expert Amy Bender, PhD, says to power down at least 1–2 hours before bed. If you do have to work late using such devices, she suggests using blue-light-blocking glasses to reduce the harmful effects of blue light.

## JET LAG

Long-haul plane travel and jet lag are strongly associated with fatigue, disorientation, impaired sleep, and general discomfort.[45] If you travel frequently for sport or work, all of these are threats to your performance potential. Interestingly, traveling east to west is generally easier for your circadian system to acclimatize to compared to traveling west to east. This is because your daily internal circadian clock is approximately (but not exactly) 24 hours, which makes it easier for you to stretch out your day and stay up a little longer when travelling westward. When you go east, you need to fall asleep before your body clock is ready to rest. Making things worse, when a West Coast–based person wakes up in the East the next morning, it's far earlier in your new time zone compared to your natural home time. Your brain is capable of recalibrating approximately 1 hour for every day in your new environment. For example, if you fly 4 hours from New York to LA it would take you around 4 full days to completely adjust, whereas a 7-hour flight from New York to London (U.K.) would take a full week to reboot your circadian rhythm. All things considered, jet lag takes a tremendous toll on your body. Studies in pilots and cabin crew doing regular long-haul flights found changes in areas of the brain related to learning and memory had shrunk, suggesting a mild form of brain damage, as well as short-term memory loss.[46] Even more troubling, their rates of type 2 diabetes and cancer were also much higher than the average population. To minimize the negative effects of jetlag, Dr. Dunican suggests preflight, in-flight and postflight strategies (see table 1.1).

## Supporting Circadian Rhythms in Winter: Light Box Therapy

Light exposure is key to a healthy circadian clock. During winter months, the shorter and darker days are tougher to handle as you get up in the dark and come home after the sun's gone down. Most people will also spend their day inside, further compounding the strain on their internal clocks. A pro tip to support your circadian clock during the short, cold, and dark days of winter is to use Light Box Therapy (LBT). The Society for Light Treatment and Biological Rhythms (SLTBR), a collection of the world's leading experts, support the use of LBT for maintaining healthy circadian rhythms during winter. Light exposure in the morning hours is a big win for increasing alertness and maintaining your sleep and wake cycles. Countless athletes have reported that 15 minutes of LBT in the morning over breakfast or coffee does wonders for energy levels and mood for the day.[47]

### ADDERALL AND NICOTINE

Adderall is a prescription medication for attention-deficit hyperactivity disorder (ADHD), which affects 4.4 percent of the adult population. Alarmingly, nearly 1 out of 10 players in Major League Baseball has been granted a therapeutic exemption to use Adderall or other ADHD medication, more than double the rate of the general population.[48] Dr. Doug Richards, a physician and professor of sports medicine at the University of Toronto says "it's highly suspicious that they're over-diagnosing it or [the players] are faking it so they can use these drugs." Regardless, stimulants like Adderall or nicotine should be avoided in the afternoon due to the sleep-impairing nature of these products (this is, of course, one of many reasons to avoid smoking and chewing tobacco). Other medications that can disturb REM sleep include nasal decongestants, aspirin and headache medications, pain relievers that contain caffeine, cold and allergy medications containing antihistamines, as well as antidepressants and diet pills. If you notice an athlete regularly consuming these products in the evening, it should be a red flag.

### SLEEP APNEA AND RESTLESS LEGS SYNDROME

It's important to screen athletes for medical conditions. Although sleep apnea affects only 4 percent of the general population, this form of sleep-disordered breathing impacts 14 percent of professional American football players (rugby players likely fall into a similar category). The research shows that the larger a persons' BMI or neck circumference, the higher their risk of sleep apnea.[49] Restless legs syndrome, which affects 13 percent of marathon runners, is another example of a medical condition that can impair sleep.[50] Of course, remember your scope of practice. If you suspect an athlete might have a medical condition impairing quality sleep, refer them to a medical professional.

### FOREIGN ENVIRONMENT

We've all had a bad night's sleep during travel. It's not just you; the research supports that half of your brain experiences lighter REM sleep when you're in a foreign environment. Interestingly, after a few nights in the new environment, this phenomenon dissipates and both sides of the brain register REM uniformly. Sleep experts believe this is evolutionary evidence that our brains are still "on guard" for predators or threats in a new and foreign environment. For athletes, this highlights the importance of getting to competition venues or hotels a few days early. If the first night of sleep in a new bed is destined to be poorer, it's best to hedge your bets and get a few more nights at the new accommodation if possible. When you add the psychological loads of mood, stress, and the anxiety of long distance travel, this can make a huge difference.[51]

## Sleep Solutions: Straight from the Experts

Sleep is fundamental to human health, and as you've learned in this chapter, it's essential for recovery and elite performance. When you consider sleep experts suggest that 50 percent of athletes still do not get enough sleep, it hammers home the important point that sleep should be a nonnegotiable. Let's review the fundamentals for sleep — they're not as obvious as you might think.

### THE FUNDAMENTALS OF SLEEP

Sleep expert Cheri Mah, MD, emphasizes three fundamental areas, or "buckets," of sleep to focus on when improving sleep in athletes: sleep duration, sleep quality, and sleep timing (see figure 1.1). If you're getting less than 7 hours of sleep per night, Dr. Mah says you should aim to extend sleep by 30 minutes a night each week until you achieve the desired 8–10 hours per day for athletes. When it comes to sleep timing, first anchor the waking time and keep it consistent throughout the week. A consistent waking and bedtime is proven in the research to help set healthy circadian rhythms and keep your internal clock running on time.[52] Ideally, you should address something in each bucket simultaneously, and Dr. Mah points out it's important to drip-feed in changes gradually.

Next, the ideal sleep environment should feel like you're sleeping in a cave: cool, dark, quiet, and comfortable. If the environment is too bright, too warm, or too noisy, it can throw off your circadian clock and impair sleep quality.[53] Unfortunately, the reality for a lot of people is that a comfortable cave isn't a possibility. If you can't control your environment, Dr. Mah suggests you invest in a quality eye mask to block light, some quality ear buds, and a white noise app to dampen background noises.

Finally, once you've dialed in your sleep time and sleep environment, the last piece of the puzzle is to adopt a sleep routine. Just like a professional

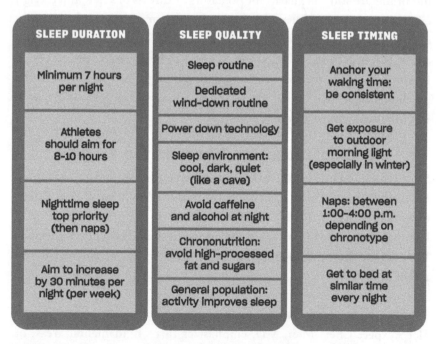

| SLEEP DURATION | SLEEP QUALITY | SLEEP TIMING |
|---|---|---|
| Minimum 7 hours per night | Sleep routine | Anchor your waking time: be consistent |
| | Dedicated wind-down routine | |
| Athletes should aim for 8-10 hours | Power down technology | Get exposure to outdoor morning light (especially in winter) |
| | Sleep environment: cool, dark, quiet (like a cave) | |
| Nighttime sleep top priority (then naps) | Avoid caffeine and alcohol at night | Naps: between 1:00-4:00 p.m. depending on chronotype |
| | Chrononutrition: avoid high-processed fat and sugars | |
| Aim to increase by 30 minutes per night (per week) | General population: activity improves sleep | Get to bed at similar time every night |

**FIGURE 1.1.** Sleep Time, Quality, and Timing Strategies.

## Assess Yourself with the
## Athlete Sleep Screening Questionnaire

You've learned athletes are poor at assessing both their sleep duration and quality, so flagging athletes for potential sleep concerns would be highly beneficial. The problem is athletes don't want to volunteer to go into a sleep lab for assessment, and unfortunately sleep questionnaires have only been geared to the general population — until now. The incredible work of Amy Bender, PhD, and her team over the past five years has recently culminated in the validation of the Athlete Sleep Screening Questionnaire (ASSQ) specific to athletes.[54] This tool is an absolute home run for athletes and coaches because it gives a scientifically validated glimpse into athletes' sleep without too much hassle for them.

golfer adopts a preshot routine to control and relax their nervous system under pressure — using the same number of steps, waggles, and looks at the hole — you can use a similar routine to prep your brain and body to decompress and prepare for deep, restful sleep. Set an alarm for 60 minutes before bed and engage in relaxing activities. Do some light stretching, read a book, take a warm bath, practice meditation or prayer, and so forth. Eating too late at night, in particular too much sugar or foods that are too high in saturated fat (typically processed food), can also negatively impact sleep.

### POWER NAPS AND JET LAG STRATEGIES

Sleep experts are quick to point out that consolidated sleep at night should be everybody's primary goal. However, if you need an energy boost or need to add to your total daily or weekly sleep time, then power naps can be a great strategy. Start by adding a short 20–30 minute nap midday between 1–4 pm, depending on when you wake up. If your chronotype is a morning lark, earlier naps closer to 1 or 2 p.m. would be best, whereas the night owls will do better with later naps at 2:30 or 3:30 p.m. Dr. Bender says short naps are ideal on game and practice days due to the restorative effects on your brain and nervous system. As well, they minimize the risk of waking up groggy due to sleep inertia. Research shows a short nap following partial sleep loss improves sprint time.[55] On rest days, Bender suggests a 2-hour sleep opportunity for athletes to support recovery, especially endurance athletes with greater training volumes. You'll go through a full sleep cycle during a nap of this length, so if possible, sleep in your usual sleep environment. Of course, Bender warns extra naps won't offset lack of total sleep. If you're consistently getting less than 6 hours of sleep per night, you're going to be impairing your ability to produce maximal speed, speed endurance, and skills like accuracy. If you wake up feeling sluggish or groggy from your nap, you've slept too long and are suffering from sleep inertia.[56] Dr. Bender warns not to sleep past 4 p.m., regardless of your chronotype, to avoid sleep inertia as it can hamper performance. Some athletes have started using the "nap-pucino" strategy — having a pre-nap coffee to improve wakefulness when they get up from their rest. However, you must be *highly* sleep-deprived (meaning you fall asleep within 5 minutes) for this to be effective. Bender warns against the negative effects of this practice on sleep architecture and in delaying sleep pressure at night. In short, just nap — don't add coffee.

### Jet Lag Strategies

Sleep expert Ian Dunican, PhD, knows a thing or two about jet lag. He worked with Western Force, an Australian professional rugby union team from Perth, which had the distinction of flying the most miles of any professional sports team in the world. If anybody knows about jet lag strategies, it's Dr. Dunican. Targeted circadian strategies such as specifically time light exposure, meal-timing, altering training schedules, and melatonin supplementation can help support phase shifts during travel.[57] The following list includes Dr. Dunican's tips for preflight, in-flight, and postflight strategies to fight off jet lag so you can perform on the field or in the boardroom (see table 1.1).

### Sleep and Circadian Technology

New sleep and circadian rhythm technologies are emerging in an attempt to make it easier for clients to assess their sleep or support circadian rhythms. The tech company Oura makes a ring that claims to accurately assess your sleep and sleep stages, something no other commercial wearable

**TABLE 1.1.** Strategies to Prevent Jet Lag

| PREFLIGHT | IN-FLIGHT | POSTFLIGHT |
|---|---|---|
| Ensure you get *adequate sleep* before you travel (don't be sleep deprived) | Control light and dark cycles: *Wear sunglasses* during periods of rest or add a blue light stimulus during periods of wakefulness to help prepare you for the new time zone. | *Coffee:* Caffeine is a natural zeitgeber; having a cup upon rising in your new time zone is helpful. |
| Start to *shift your body clock* a few days before you fly. Go to bed 30 minutes earlier and wake up 30 minutes earlier in the days leading up to travel. | *No napping:* If flying west to east (e.g., LA to NY), do not nap in-flight in order to keep your sleep drive high for when you land on the East Coast. | *Meal timing:* Eat breakfast at the natural time in your new time zone. If arriving late on a flight and it's bedtime in your new time zone, abstain from eating until the following morning. |
| If getting up earlier to prep for jetlag, use a *light box* to simulate the sun, and at night, use *blue-light-blocking glasses* to trick your body into thinking it's evening. | *Hydration:* Ensure adequate water intake, as planes are very dry and dehydrating. *Avoid Alcohol:* It will impair REM sleep upon landing and is also dehydrating. | *Physical activity:* Upon rising in your new time zone, exercise is a great zeitgeber to get adjusted. Get outside to add the natural light stimulus. |
| | *Medication:* Temazepam, a class of sedative-hypnotic drug with a short half-life (4 hours), is sometimes used by sports teams to help trigger sleep onset during travel. (Consult doctor before use.) | |

*Source:* Robert L. Sack, "Jet Lag," *The New England Journal of Medicine* 362, no. 5 (2010), https://doi.org/10.1056/NEJMcp0909838.

tech has been able to accomplish to date. Oura's new sleep ring has been validated by independent Harvard researchers and can accurately measure sleep and sleep stages, as well as body temperature, heart rate, and heart rate variability. Most sleep researchers would still argue over the validity of the data, as the gold-standard scientific verification of sleep requires polysomnography, the measurement of brain waves, eye movement, and muscle activity. While you should always be cautious with how you interpret the data of wearable technology, it can provide insights into how your nutrition, training, stress, and the like might be compromising your sleep. Using sleep tech like the ring from Oura to modify behaviors could yield good results for you. But if you think you might get stressed out from poor sleep scores, it's probably not for you. It's best to work with your trainer, coach, and practitioner to analyze the data in order to avoid overreacting or misinterpreting the information. (If you think you have a medical sleep concern, consult your doctor.)

Circadian rhythm technology is also emerging. What would happen if you could control your light exposure on your next flight from San Francisco to London? A new device on the market called the HumanCharger is a light therapy device that might be beneficial for circadian rhythm restoration during long-haul travel or in countries with limited light exposure in winter months. Researchers at the University of Oulu in Finland found that pulsing transcranial bright light (TBL) to specific photoreceptor proteins in the brain sensitive to light — reached via the ear canal — can stimulate the brain and mimic the light and dark cycles of the day. More research needs to be done to validate these technologies, but they might provide a small margin of benefit for athletes who already have their sleep fundamentals firmly in place.

––––––––––

Understanding the fundamentals of sleep and circadian rhythms and their effects on athlete health and performance is crucial. After reading this chapter you will hopefully appreciate the value of extending sleep time, improving sleep quality, and maximizing circadian health to improve your performance and athletic longevity. Like the legendary Roger Federer, there is much evidence that shows good sleep positively impacts athlete recovery and performance at any age. Let's now shift our focus on another crucial area of this approach: the athlete microbiome.

# CHAPTER 2

# The Athlete Microbiome

About 3.8 billion years ago Earth was formed, developing an atmosphere and an ocean. Soon thereafter the first appearance of life arose in the form of blue-green algae bacteria, which were incredibly resilient and could survive in a highly toxic environment. Make no mistake, bacteria are the reason you are here today — they are responsible for oxygen-forming photosynthesis and ultimately the emergence of the genus *Homo*. Humans have always been intimately connected with bacteria. Your gut, for example, contains more than 100 trillion microorganisms, collectively called microbiota, which includes bacteria, viruses, and fungi consisting of over 160 different species and 9 million genes.[1] The human genome, by contrast, only has approximately 24,000 genes. Interestingly, you share about 99.5 percent of the same DNA as the person sitting next to you, but only about 10 percent of the same gut microbiota species.

Your gut microbiome — the collection of your gut microbiota community and their genes — plays a critical role in your health. Scientist Rob Knight, PhD, of the University of California, San Diego, and founder of the American Gut Project, a scientific initiative to map the human gut, refers to the microbiome as a "microbe organ" due to the profound impact it has on virtually all systems of the body. Throughout evolution, we outsourced key roles to our gut microbiota because they could respond more quickly to change than our human genome (which takes generations to adapt). Like the operating system on your laptop, your microbiome plays a fundamental role in your body's own operating system. Without it, your health and performance will crash when faced with the challenges of new environments and stressors.

Our gut microbiota perform an incredible array of essential functions to keep us healthy. This includes setting our metabolism, breaking down and assimilating food, neutralizing drugs and carcinogens, and synthesizing vitamins (like choline, folate, and vitamin $K_2$), as well as short-chain fatty acids (SCFAs) and secondary bile acids, which are key signaling compounds crucial to your health and performance. Our gut bacteria send powerful signals across our entire body, supporting immunity, protecting us from foreign invaders, and regulating oxidative stress.[2] Different areas of the body — skin, mouth, gut, vagina, colon — are home to different species of bacteria. The large intestine is host to the greatest concentration — with about 3 pounds of bacterial biomass living in our guts — as well as the greatest bacterial diversity. A high degree of bacterial diversity is considered one of the best markers of a healthy gut. New research is highlighting this as a potential biomarker for overall health, making it a key player in this approach.[3]

In the mid-2000s, the field of microbiome research — referred to as microbiomics — boomed with researchers' groundbreaking discovery of at Stanford University. While studying the gut microbiota of lean versus obese mice, researchers observed that the microbiota were markedly different from one another. They posed a pivotal question: Is the gut microbiome a cause or effect of weight gain? To test this hypothesis, they decided to transfer the gut microbiota of obese mice into normal, healthy mice to see if the bacteria would trigger weight gain in the host. The results were eye-opening: The gut microbiota of obese mice were making the lean mice fatter.[4] This was the first time it was shown that gut microbiota could affect complex physiologic function outside of the gut. Today, experts can incredibly predict with 90 percent accuracy whether you'll be lean or obese based on your gut microbiota signature, making it far more predictive than even your DNA. Research into microbiomics and the complex interplay of your genome, microbiome, and environment has exploded, linking an array of chronic diseases: celiac and inflammatory bowel disease (IBD), rheumatoid arthritis, type 2 diabetes, and anxiety and depression. Researchers are currently racing to identify specific "microbiome signatures" for each condition.

The microbiome varies dramatically from one individual to the next and can change dramatically over time in a single individual. If you think of your genome (DNA) as a guitar, your microbiome would be the music playing from that guitar. You could have 50 different musicians (representing factors in the environment) play the same guitar and you would get a different melody from each. That's the power and influence of the microbiome. The problem today is the significant loss of gut bacteria diversity, which experts believe is due to our highly processed diets, lack of physical movement, heightened stress levels, and modern environments. Our gut microbiota plays a massive role in how we (and our genes) respond to the food we eat, which is referred to as epigenetic programming.[5] Epigenetics is the study of changes in an organism caused by modifications in gene expression, rather than alterations of the genetic codes itself. The metaphor used by scientists is, "Your genes load the gun, the environment pulls the trigger."

Humans are incredibly complex. In fact, a key concept of modern biology is that genes participate in complex, interconnected networks rather than simple, linear pathways.[6] For example, both flying a plane and performing surgery are highly complicated, but not complex. They can be solved with mathematics and a series of algorithms; in short, computers can do it. However, you can't solve complex problems in the same way. The ability of the microbiome to change and adapt quickly has allowed us as humans to evolve quickly by solving complex problems through outsourcing the things we can't do well (digesting fiber, for example) to our gut bacteria allies.

This modern mismatch is highlighted by a recent groundbreaking study using a new technology — continuous glucose monitoring systems (CGMs) — to assess participants' glucose response to meals. Traditional nutrition dogma states that certain foods have a low, moderate, or high glycemic index (GI), representing the speed at which they enter the bloodstream. Typically, low-GI foods are preferred because it's believed they provide a slower, more sustained release of glucose into the bloodstream. In theory, participants given the same GI meal (be it a low-GI meal or high-GI meal), should all have had similar blood glucose responses. For example, if you eat an apple and I eat an apple, we both should get the predicted low-glycemic response. Or if you eat a cookie and I eat a cookie, we both should get the predicted high-glycemic response. During the weeklong study, 800 participants had CGMs inserted under the skin to analyze blood glucose response to over 46,000 meals. The findings sent a shockwave through the research community.[7] Researchers found massively different glucose responses to *exactly the same meals* between individuals.[8] When some individuals ate an apple, their blood glucose spiked with an unpredictably high response, as if they had eaten a cookie. Alternatively, others eating a high-glycemic cookie revealed slow and steady blood glucose responses. But how is it possible to have markedly different blood glucose response to the same meals? The authors concluded the individual gut microbiota signature of each person was heavily influencing their glucose response to the food and was acting as an interface, amplifying or buffering the glycemic effects of their nutrition choices.

If our gut microbiome plays a pivotal role in our blood glucose response to food, and experts can predict weight gain via a specific microbiome signature in obese individuals, a new question has been emerging in the research: Do elite athletes have a characteristic "microbiome signature" that differentiates them from the general population? Before we review the evidence, let's first try to define a "healthy" gut microbiome.

## The Evolutionary versus Modern Gut

What is a healthy gut? Experts believe understanding the early-human microbiome will help establish a better baseline to assess gut health today. Our ancestors from the genus *Homo* have been walking upright on earth for some two million years. Our closest relatives — *homo sapiens sapiens* — appeared on the scene about 200,000 years ago in East Africa. They were omnivores who hunted, scavenged, and gathered food until the advent of agriculture around 10,000 BC. This period accounts for 99.5 percent of our time on this planet, thus our genome and microbiome (and how our brains are hardwired) have been massively influenced by our natural environment and food choices. Today, remnants of this evolutionary legacy still exist in our gut microbiota. Incredibly, experts have figured out a way to go back in time to study the microbiome of our early ancestors. Researchers did this by investigating coprolite samples — the fancy scientific term for fossilized poop — from early man at various archeological sites around the world. The oldest is called Ötzi, the Iceman, discovered in the Italian-Austrian Alps in the early 1990s. His 5,000-year-old remains were impeccably mummified from the cold winters at high altitude. Analysis of his coprolite samples revealed that approximately 66 percent of his gut microbiota very closely resembled a "primate gut," highlighting the tight connection to our primate past.[9] Fast forward from 5,000 to 1,400 years ago, and another sample collected from the Rio Zape in Mexico revealed the following: a 33 percent similarity to a primate gut, a 33 percent similarity to modern-day hunter-gatherer gut, and 33 percent unknown species.[10] You can see how the gut microbiota signature is changing over time and adapting to the new environment. Finally, the research team examined samples from a World War I soldier found frozen in a glacier. He also had a mixed primate and hunter-gatherer gut microbiota signature. But perhaps the most interesting finding is what he *didn't* have. The World War I soldier showed no signs of a modern twenty-first century gut. The authors concluded our modern gut microbiota, in just the last 100 years, have dramatically changed.

Of course, this doesn't answer the question, "What is a healthy gut?" Scientists believe modern-day hunter-gatherer tribes who more closely resemble our early ancestors might provide some clues. Today, the Hadza hunter-gatherer tribe in Tanzania are thought to most closely resemble our early ancestors. The Hadza people practice no cultivation or domestication of plants and animal; they hunt and gather their food on a daily basis, and their diet consists mainly of meat, honey, baobab fruit, berries, and fiber-rich tubers. Researchers analyzing their microbiome have found largely two dominant phyllum (categories) of bacteria: *Firmicutes* (72 percent) and *Bacteroidetes* (17 percent).[11] The Hadza's very high-fiber, plant-based diet is reflected by the presence of several well-known fiber-degrading *Firmicutes* species in their gut: *Roseburia, Blautia, F. prausnitzii,* and a *Bacteroidetes* species called *Prevotella. Prevotella* in particular is characterized for its ability to break down tough fiber-rich starches and is characteristic of a healthy gut. Experts believe this more closely resembles what our gut microbiome would have looked like throughout evolution (with obvious differences depending on a tribe's geographic location, environment, and food staples).

In the last 100 years, the story has changed dramatically. Like the mass extinctions seen on planet Earth, our intestinal ecosystems have seen a mass extinction of its microbial diversity over the last century, with potentially significant consequences to our health. Experts believe the major factors reshaping our intestinal ecosystem are a lack of exposure to soil and dirt (both via our food and our own exposure to nature); lack of fermented foods (since the advent of refrigeration); the explosion of sugar and processed food consumption; and our chronic overuse of antibiotics for medical conditions and in our livestock.[12] Research at Stanford University highlights this modern mismatch. The recently aggregated data on the gut microbiome signature from traditional hunter-gatherer communities across the globe — in Burkina Faso, Malawi, Mongolia, Cameroon, Tanzania, Venezuela, Central African Republic, Peru, and Papua New Guinea — reveal the communities all cluster into a similar pattern. Most important, they have a much higher *diversity* of gut bacteria. Comparably, Western populations living in suburban and urban areas experience a dramatic reduction in overall microbial diversity and stability.[13] A common metaphor used by experts to highlight how this impacts your health is a rainforest. The massive diversity of flora and fauna is essential for its health and sustainability, but the modern practice of clear-cutting leaves little diversity and compromises the ecosystem. It looks like our modern industrial lifestyle has significantly impacted the mutually beneficial relationship between us and our "old friends" in the gut.

## Can You "Re-Wild" Your Gut?

Emerging evidence suggests the more diverse the community of bacteria in your gut, the better your health and the more resilient you might be to chronic disease. This has potentially big implications for athletes. Experts also believe diet plays the biggest role in influencing the health and diversity of our gut microbiota. A recent poll on consumer spending found that in America and Great Britain over 50 percent of the household grocery bill is spent on ultra-processed food.[14] This makes you wonder, what are the trickle-down effects on the gut? Tim Spector, MD, professor of genetic epidemiology at King's College London, asked himself a similar question when he was an undergraduate student. Tim decided to test out the hypothesis that processed food consumption hammers gut bacteria diversity. His method involved eating nothing but McDonald's fast food for 10 days. Spector tested his gut microbiota signature before and after to assess the impact. What happened? The results were pretty staggering. The diversity of his gut microbiota species plummeted after only 10 days of the fast food diet.[15] Think about the implications for young high school and collegiate athletes (who often eat highly processed diets) or the typical weight-loss client who always eats on the go and struggles to lose weight.

If eating fast food could totally change your microbiome in just over a week, could living and eating with a modern-day hunter-gatherer tribe provide a healthy reboot? Can you "re-wild" your gut? Spector also put this hypothesis to the test. Internationally recognized microbiome researcher Jeff Leach, PhD, and his research team at King's College took Spector into Tanzania, home of the Hadza hunter-gatherer tribe, to investigate how 3 days of living, eating, and trekking around with the tribe would impact his microbiome. During his stay with the Hadza, Spector ate baobab fruit pods for breakfast (full of fiber, fructose-based carbs, and vitamins), snacked on wild Kongorobi berries (containing 20 times the polyphenols of Western berries), ate fiber-rich tubers, and cooked and ate local animals such as porcupine for dinner. He even got a treat for dessert: luscious golden honey from a honeycomb that was loaded with fat and natural sugar.

The Hadza have one of the most diverse gut microbiota signatures on the planet, a widely recognized marker of good health; so how did Spector's 3-day sojourn with the Hadza in the rural African savanna impact his gut diversity? Remarkably, after only 3 days Tim's gut diversity increased by 20 percent, a tremendous shift considering Tim was already healthy at the outset.[16] This experiment highlights how adaptable gut bacteria are to our food and our environment (and perhaps the lack of certain stressors of modern living). Of course, one of the big questions Dr. Leach and his team wanted to answer was if his new upgrade in gut microbiota diversity would hold up once he returned home to the U.K. Unfortunately, after only a week back in London, Dr. Leach's gut testing revealed Tim's intestinal microbiota had almost completely shifted back to baseline. While experts still agree diet is the biggest influencer we can control to build a diverse gut microbiota, it looks like environment still trumps all. The real question for athletes and coaches is if this can directly impact athletic performance or recovery.

## Microbiome-Mitochondria "Cross Talk"

There is an intimate connection between your microbiome and mitochondria, the earliest prokaryotic cells having evolved from alphaproteobacteria over 3.5 billion years ago.[17] Although the vast majority of these ancestral alphaproteobacteria genes have disappeared from the mitochondria's genome, the lineage can still be seen in the molecular machinery they use in the aerobic energy system.[18] This deep connection between bacteria and our energy-producing mitochondria has sparked a lot of interest, as it might unlock potential benefits for the athlete.

You might recall that your DNA differs by less than 1 percent compared to the person next to you, yet the diversity in your gut bacteria species differs by up to 30 percent.[19] Researchers have described humans as "super-organisms" made up of the trillions of microorganisms that outnumber our human cells. But here's where it gets truly interesting: Our microbiome and mitochondria converse via cellular signaling. This special language is an inter-kingdom communication system that allows bacteria, fungi, yeasts, and other cells to all talk to one another.[20] Your microbiome uses this language to positively impact your health via multiple mechanisms. Three key areas to consider in this "cross talk" follow.

### Supports Energy Production

A healthy gut produces significant amounts of the short-chain fatty acids (SCFAs) called butyrate, which is then burned in the mitochondria of intestinal cells to produce adenosine triphosphate (ATP) energy.[21] Butyrate is also a key regulator of mitochondrial function via PGC-1alpha gene expression in muscle and brown fat (mitochondria-packed fat cells that burn energy and produce heat), supporting fatty acid oxidation via the AMPK (an enzyme inside your cells that triggers energy utilization) pathway.[22] In short, it helps to improve your fuel efficiency, which is crucial for all types of athletes. The specific types and amount of SCFAs produced by your gut microbiota depends on the existing composition and diversity of your gut microbiota, as well as the metabolic interactions between your gut bugs and your diet.[23] Athletes eating too many simple sugars, processed foods, or pro-inflammatory omega-6 fats might be compromising this system.

### Cools Excessive Inflammation

Intense training lights up your sympathetic nervous system, raising adrenaline and blood cortisol levels that promote an acute inflammatory response and an influx of neutrophils from your immune system in defense. In dramatic contrast to light exercise, strenuous training causes a significant increase in the number of pro-inflammatory cytokines — TNF-alpha, IL-1, IL-6, and the like — that occurs in a dose-dependent manner.[24] The harder you train, the bigger impact on your gut microbiota and immune system. In particular, elevated levels of IL-6 cytokines are associated with exercise-induced muscle injury and intestinal permeability.[25] This can be a major problem for endurance athletes, where IL-6 can increase up to 100-fold in marathon runners.[26]

### Strengthens Your Gut Barrier

Healthy gut microbiota produce the SCFA propionate, which is highly beneficial for the integrity of your gut wall because it increases the number of tight junction proteins and down-regulates pro-inflammatory TNF-alpha in colon cells. A diverse gut microbiota is crucial for athletes because it helps to keep their gut barrier strong, which in turn prevents harmful lipopolysaccharides (LPS) (endotoxins) from penetrating into the bloodstream and triggering an exaggerated inflammatory immune response. A leaky gut leads to an inflamed microenvironment in the digestive system, creating an open vacuum for blooms of pathogenic renegade bacteria like *E. coli*, *Klebsiella*, and *Proteus*, which are commonly overgrown in the inflamed Western gut.[27] Chronic gut inflammation also increases oxygen in the intestinal lumen, increasing blood flow and hemoglobin levels and promoting the growth of more gut pathogens and creating more mitochondrial dysfunction. Building healthy gut diversity contributes to a strong gut barrier by triggering SIRT1 activity, which stimulates the gut gatekeeper zonulin (as well as gut stem cells) to seal your gut and keep it impenetrable to renegades.[28]

It's not just the "talk" from the gut microbiota to the mitochondria that influences gut health. Mitochondria also talk to the gut and immune system. This is exactly why it's so important for the general population to exercise, as the improvements in mitochondria help to maintain a strong gut barrier and diverse community. Both are essential for a diverse and resilient gut. Your mitochondria play a key detective role in immunity, spying for infectious foreign invaders that might be penetrating the gut and looking for any signs of cellular damage, as well as consequently relaying the message to your innate "first line of defense" immune system to get the soldiers ready to defend the body.[29] (This is a good reason for strength-based athletes to maintain a minimum level of aerobic fitness.) Our mitochondria also support a highly diverse gut microbiota via maintaining the protective mucous layer of the intestines.[30] This is important for athletes because intense training leads to significant stress on their gut walls. Other factors that can compromise gut integrity are high-sugar diets, processed foods, regular "fat bomb" coffees or snacks, chronically taken painkillers, and the like. Gut barrier function is critical to both our health and athletic performance.

## The Athlete Microbiome Signature

What does all this mean for the athlete? Is there an "athlete microbiome signature" that could support improved health, performance, or recovery? It's an incredibly complex question that researchers are racing to try to answer. Nic West, PhD, renowned exercise immunologist at Griffith University in Australia, has been researching the gut microbiota in recreational and elite Olympic athletes for many years. West and his team recently compared the gut microbiome signatures of recreational and elite athletes (as well as healthy controls) to attempt to tease out any significant differences.[31] Here is what they found: *Bifidobacterium longum* (*B. longum*) levels were very high in elite athletes, almost *double* that of recreational and healthy controls. Bifidobacterium dominates the GI tracts of healthy breast-fed infants, compared to adults where levels are lower but relatively stable. The presence of different species of bifidobacteria changes with age, from childhood to senior years, and *B. longum* is most prevalent in adults. If you don't consume dairy products, evidence is emerging of the potential beneficial effects of supplementation for health and performance (if you avoid dairy, your *B. longum* levels are more likely to be low). The *Bifidobacterium animalis* species was also much higher in elite athletes, a strain highly prevalent in fermented milk products.

*Bacteroides* species were also found in very high concentrations in both recreational and elite athletes. The bacteroides bacteria are anaerobic, bile-resistant, and have a complex and typically beneficial relationship with your gut microbiota. Bacteroides levels can increase on higher fat, higher protein diets, which are often followed by athletes. They're passed from mom to baby during vaginal birth and become part of your microbiota at the earliest stages of life.

*Akkermansia* levels were high across the board, in elite and recreational athletes as well as the healthy control. Foods rich in the fiber oligofructose (found in garlic, onions, and bananas) help to feed *Akkernmansia* in the gut. Low-carb diets, periods of fasting, and diets high in polyphenols (such as berries, cherries, and coffee) have also been shown to increase levels. *F. prausnitzii* levels were also in abundance in the athlete gut, which is very interesting considering it plays a special role in the intestinal ecosystem; it's located right up against the gut lining, allowing it to interface very closely with the body and other gut microbiota. *F. prausnitzii* specializes in fermenting dietary fiber, stimulating healthy mucus production, and exerting potent anti-inflammatory effects. Finally, some other notable species higher in elite athletes compared to recreational and healthy controls include *L. fermentum*, a species that demonstrates antimicrobial activity against gut pathogens as well as high antioxidant effects, and *Prevotella*, a species highly proficient at breaking down carbohydrates that is considered to be a keystone bacteria in a healthy gut microbiome.

Another leader in the field of microbiomics currently trying to map the athlete microbiome signature in endurance athletes is Lauren Petersen, PhD, formerly of the prestigious Jackson Laboratory. Dr. Petersen notes that a dominant driver of the gut microbiome in the general population is the jack-of-all-trades *Bacteroides* group that is capable of breaking down everything in the diet. This is in contrast to her high-level and elite cyclists who have a *Prevotella*-dominant community.[32] Interestingly, Dr. Petersen also notes the microbiomes of athletes tend to cluster around how they race. Her research revealed that regardless if they were meat eaters, vegetarians, consumers of alcohol, or avoided gluten, athletes tended to have more similar gut microbiome signatures if they performed similar type of races (aerobic versus anaerobic). She also found a dose-response relationship with the intensity of training, where *Prevotella* levels increased with higher training intensities. In fact, Petersen could effectively predict whether or not an athlete finished in the 25th percentile of downhill racers merely by the presence of *Prevotella* in the gut (that is, if you didn't have *Prevotella*, you were lucky to finish in the middle of the pack). What was the dietary profile of these elite racers? They ate a lot more vegetables, fruit, and nuts than the recreational cyclists and controls, as well as far less white bread in favor of more whole grains (protein and fat intake was relatively similar). Of course, Petersen acknowledged you don't have to have *Prevotella* to be a World Cup racer, and cautioned against falling into the reductionist trap of trying to eat more of one specific food to increase a particular bacteria species as it's not likely to yield much benefit.

How do these findings in endurance athletes compare to strength and team sport? In Ireland, Orla O'Sullivan, PhD, compared the gut microbiome of elite rugby players on the Irish national rugby team to recreationally active and sedentary controls. O'Sullivan and her team found the diversity of gut microbiota of the elite national team players was *double* that of healthy controls.[33] They also had much higher levels of creatine kinase, a recognized biomarker of intense exercise; however, they still had significantly lower inflammatory status. Interestingly, the researchers also noted a strong association between protein intake and exercise intensity as key drivers of a healthy athlete microbiome. Dr. O'Sullivan's group even suggested microbial diversity could become a new biomarker of health status in elite athletes.

Research into a potential "athlete microbiome signature" is very interesting, but it doesn't yet answer the million-dollar question: Are the bacteria driving these changes or are they merely along for the ride? Before addressing this question, let's review some of the top roadblocks to a high-diversity athlete gut.

## Roadblocks to Maximizing the Athlete Microbiome

If athletes have much better gut diversity than the general population, identifying athletes with low diversity could serve as a red flag for poor health. Among endurance athletes, the incidence of gut-related distress is particularly high during competition and can limit performance. You don't have to be an Ironman or marathoner to experience GI disturbances. Strength and team sport athletes are also prone to gut problems such as gas, bloating, constipation, and the like. So what factors most commonly sabotage a healthy athlete gut? Let's review.

### OVERTRAINING

Training produces a positive hormetic stress via increased reactive oxygen species (ROS), stimulation of mitochondrial biogenesis, and fatty acid oxidation.[34] But if you get your training plan wrong and push into harmful overreaching or overtraining syndrome due to too much volume or intensity (or both), a dramatic rise in pro-inflammatory cytokines like TNF-alpha, IL-1, IL-6, and macrophages occurs in a dose-response relationship.[35] At a deeper genetic level, your genome accumulates mutations that eventually compromise the efficiency of aerobic energy production.[36] It is well established that harmful overreaching or overtraining is strongly associated with a rapid onset of fatigue, and the inability to maintain speed and intensity of effort.[37] Studies of elite triathletes reveal four weeks of overtraining was enough to overwhelm the glutathione-dependent antioxidant defense due to high levels of damage to cell membranes.[38] This is also seen when someone engages in as little as 30 minutes of acute, high-intensity, anaerobic training bouts. Does this mean you shouldn't perform intense training? Of course not. But it means you better get your training plan right (more on this in Part Three: Recover). For elite athletes looking to maximize longevity, it's important to consider that overtraining-induced oxidative damage also reduces telomere length, a potential longevity roadblock. Longer telomeres are a recognized biomarker for healthy aging.[39]

### PROLONGED EXERCISE BOUTS

Your tissues have a high demand for oxygen, and the excessive release of stress hormones from prolonged intense exercises produces a tremendous amount of ROS and oxidative stress in your gut. As blood is shunted away from your digestive organs toward your working muscle, your intestinal cell tissues undergo ischemia (lack of blood flow) triggering intestinal hyper-permeability (leaky gut).[40] Incredibly, exercising at only 70 percent maximal oxygen consumption reduces the blood supply to your gut by at least 50 percent, and a recent study of ultramarathon runners found 87 percent had occult blood in their stool post-race.[41] It appears that intense bouts of prolonged exercise can significantly damage the gut. Endurance athletes and coaches should note that athletes who trained 20–30 hours per week had lower ROS production and better antioxidant defense mechanisms.

## Too Many Sport Drinks

Endurance athletes typically consume a lot of simple sugars over the course of a training block and during competition, but over the long-term this practice takes a heavy toll on the gut. Too many simple sugars feed renegade "bad" gut bacteria, leading to inflammation and elevated levels of oxygen levels in the gut lumen, triggering the growth of potential renegade pathogen "blooms" like *E. coli, Klebsiella spp.*, and *Proteus.*[42] Bad bacteria like E. coli can have negative trickle-down effects on your mitochondria and energy metabolism by degrading sulfur amino acids to produce hydrogen sulfide ($H_2S$) in your colon. Large quantities of $H_2S$ can compromise a key component of your mitochondria's aerobic energy system by penetrating cell membranes and inhibiting energy production and anti-inflammatory activity. In short, too many simple sugars is bad news for your gut.

## Too Many Acellular Carbs

Acellular carbs are grains that have been pulverized so that their cell walls are broken open. The research of Ian Spreadbury, PhD, from Queen's University in Canada has discovered that acellular carbs found in packaged and processed foods trigger an inflammatory response, altering gut microbiota signaling and leading to increased visceral body fat, impaired leptin (satiety) and insulin signaling, and potentially adding to the chronic inflammatory load.[43] This is bad news for the athlete gut. If you eat processed cereal for breakfast, processed bread on sandwiches for lunch, processed granola bars for snacks, and processed pasta for dinner — common in high school and collegiate athletes — and you're experiencing GI distress, then reducing acellular carb intake is a good place to start. The constant stream of processed foods, and the acellular carbs they contain, makes it difficult to put the brakes on a bad gut. For perspective, traditional diets before the industrialization of food rarely consisted of more than 20 g per 100 g of acellular carbs, whereas today's modern processed diet consists of a whopping 80 g per 100 g. It's wise to avoid processed foods and dramatically reduce your intake of acellular carbs.

## FAT BOMBS

If you're a keto or low-carb athlete, you might enjoy the occasional (or frequent) fat bomb in your morning coffee or in an afternoon sweet snack. While this might not be a problem for some, for others it can lead to significant problems. Tommy Wood, MD, from Oxford University highlights evidence that shows high-fat feedings can increase the permeability of the gut wall, and worse yet, increase the translocation of harmful LPS from your gut into your bloodstream. Animal studies show elevated levels of LPS can result in a partial uncoupling of mitochondrial oxidative phosphorylation (your aerobic energy system) and a 40 percent reduction of anti-inflammatory cyclooxygenase (COX) enzyme activity.[44] This can kick off a cascade of harmful effects that might compromise your health, recovery, and performance. To put it simply: Don't go crazy on the fat bombs.

## CHRONIC STRESS

One of the most overlooked areas of gut health is a person's *stress* level. Most athletes rate their stress level as low, yet also describe themselves as type-A personalities, characterized by a mind that is always active. What is referred to as general "life stress" silently accumulates below the surface and is a strong contributor to digestive dysfunction. The work of Monika Fleshner, PhD, at the University of Colorado reveals stressors alter gut bacteria signaling in animal models, leading to increased learned helplessness behaviors such as exaggerated fears and social aversion.[45] Incredibly, her research shows early-life exercise increases mood-altering and butyrate-producing bacteria, which rapidly and persistently change the gut microbiota. In humans, low levels of *Lactobacillus* and *Bifidobacterium* species are more common in patients with anxiety and depression, and supplementation has been shown to reduce anxiety and the adverse effects of stress. Many of my clients overcome chronic gut dysfunction after years of strict dietary and supplement protocols by simply adding more relaxing activities into their lives: breath work, light stretching, meditation, float tanks, and the like. Anything to increase parasympathetic activity can help address the root cause of sympathetic dominance and yield impressive results for a dysfunctional gut.

## ANTIBIOTICS

If you push yourself hard to be the best, you've no doubt succumbed to colds and flus along the way. Lauren Petersen, PhD, shared some insights from the athletes in her lab who took recurring rounds of antibiotics and the impacts the antibiotics had on the gut. Dr. Petersen says, "Athletes taking amoxicillin had the most shocking change, a catastrophic 95 percent eradication of gut diversity." Petersen also notes that after each round of antibiotics the gut microbiota were less and less likely to bounce back to health. In fact, in sedentary people with poor diets, the gut microbiota didn't return to normal even one year after taking the round of antibiotics. On the other hand, the good news for athletes taking probiotics is that eating fermented foods and fiber-rich diets can help them bounce back within a few weeks. Petersen also found athletes who took the strong broad-spectrum antibiotic clindamycin had multiple "blooms" of dysbiotic *Clostridia* renegades in the gut, as well as lowered levels of SCFAs. Building a diverse athlete microbiome will help increase your gut resiliency, prevent the need for medications, and in the case you do need a prescription, help you bounce back more quickly so that you can get on with your training.

## NSAIDs AND PPIs

Nonsteroidal anti-inflammatory drugs (NSAIDs) present a major roadblock to a healthy gut. If you use them regularly after exercise to offset pain and muscular discomfort, you'll likely be causing yourself a bigger problem in the long term. NSAIDs have been shown to damage the lining of the gut wall, compromising gut integrity and causing a leaky gut. This is a perfect recipe for chronic and systemic inflammation that can worsen joint pain, increase the likelihood of autoimmune conditions, and hamper the ability to recover. Finally, heartburn medications — a class of drugs called proton-pump inhibitors (PPIs) — also have a major negative impact on the microbiome. A recent study by the Mayo Clinic found regular heartburn drug users had significantly less gut diversity, which put them at a much greater risk of *C. difficile* infections, pneumonia, vitamin deficiencies, and bone fractures.[46]

TRAVEL

One of the most overlooked stressors on your gut microbiome is travel. Whether it's long-haul flights or bus journeys to competitions or the day-to-day travel during your season, changing time zones has a deep impact on your gut microbiome. Long-haul flights have been shown to cause blood sugar dysregulation, dysbiosis, and subsequent intestinal permeability.[47] While you can't change the nature of your travel schedule, upgrading your athlete microbiome is a great way to ensure this roadblock doesn't derail your training, performance, or recovery.

## Digestion Solutions:
## How to Build the Athlete Microbiome

The approach I outline in this book is rooted in the philosophy that you must first be a healthy human in order to truly maximize your performance and sustain it into the long term. A lot of athletes struggle with digestive problems; some seek help, some just put up with it, and many others don't even realize it's a problem. If you struggle with constipation, gas or bloating, frequent colds and flu, discomfort during exercise, or a digestive condition, know that it might be compromising both your health and performance. Regardless, your gut microbiota act as an interface between you, the food you eat, and the outside world, and therefore ultimately influence your physical and mental health. What can you do to promote a healthy athlete gut? Let's review the fundamentals.

THE FUNDAMENTALS OF A HEALTHY ATHLETE MICROBIOME

Your primary goal is to build a robust and resilient athlete microbiome by maximizing your gut microbiota diversity. How can you do it? First, the best way to build a diverse gut microbiota, based on the research, is to eat a *diverse* diet. Gut expert Miguel Toribio-Mateas, PhD(c), from Spain suggests a "50-Food Challenge", encouraging clients to eat a wide array of different types of foods from all colors of the rainbow — regardless if they're carbs, veggies, leafy greens, fruits, beans, legumes, or animal proteins — to support the broadest network of gut microbiota diversity. The rationale is to motivate clients to vary the foods they eat daily with this simple, light-hearted strategy. The soil is also an important factor. Where your food grows plays a massive role in shaping your gut microbiome. Unfortunately, modern industrialized farming practices have stripped the soil of many of its beneficial microorganisms at the expense of our health. To get more dirt in your diet, pick up some leafy greens at your local farmers market, or better yet, grow some in your backyard.

Next, ensure adequate intake of prebiotics and fiber. The standard American diet (SAD) contains a paltry 15 g of fiber per day, which is insufficient compared to the US government recommendations of 25–35 g per day, and woefully inadequate in contrast to the 80–150 g of fiber found in the traditional diets of our ancestors. This doesn't mean you need to eat as much fiber as the Hadza, but you do need to provide some support to your athlete gut. The simplest way to increase your fiber intake is to eat more "real food," rather than packaged and processed foods. How much fiber is enough? Bowel frequency is a pretty good barometer; in general, aim for at least once per day. If you're missing days, up your fiber intake to gut tolerance. If you're still struggling with gut motility issues, know that dehydration and dysbiosis are common root causes. Increase water intake and think about adding a probiotic supplementation (in the short term) to address the problem. If you follow a low-carb or ketogenic diet, your fiber intake can drop (often without you even realizing it) and you might begin to starve out good gut bacteria (not just the bad). This is problematic because the "bad" gut bacteria then shift over to feeding off the protective mucous layer of your gut lining that is responsible for maintaining strong gut integrity. This thinning of the mucous layer compromises your gut barrier and increases the likelihood of intestinal hyper-permeability. A leaky gut can lead to hyperactive immune responses and chronic inflammation, creating persistent inflammatory noise that can limit your capacity to recover, limit your ability to fight off colds and flu, and limit your ability to stay healthy throughout training season.

When you strive for food diversity you typically end up with a good dose of fiber as well as prebiotics, the nondigestible parts of the fruits, vegetables, and starchy carbohydrates that stimulate the growth beneficial *Eubacterium* and *Roseburia* species. Fructooligosaccharides and inulin are common prebiotics found in foods and supplements that help promote the growth of a healthy gut biome. Consult table 2.1 for a list of prebiotic-rich foods you can add to your nutritional arsenal.

**TABLE 2.1.** Prebiotic-Rich Foods

| FOOD TYPE | EXAMPLE OF PREBIOTIC-RICH FOODS |
| --- | --- |
| Vegetables | Onions, leeks, dandelion greens, peas, Jerusalem artichoke |
| Fruit | Apples, bananas, kiwis |
| Starchy carbs | Lentils and oats |
| Seeds and herbs | Garlic, chicory, seaweed, burdock root |

### FERMENTED FOODS AND RESISTANT STARCHES

Fermented foods are naturally rich in the *Bacillus* strain. This anaerobic bacteria naturally ferments foods. In so doing, it extracts energy from otherwise indigestible fibers and resistant starches, producing SCFAs such as acetate for energy, butyrate for metabolic health, and propionate for optimal gut signaling.[48] Why are SCFAs so key to a healthy gut? They're powerful inhibitors of inflammation by way of mediating nitric oxide (NO), IL-6, IL-12 activity and activating immune system macrophages. SCFAs also help regulate AMPK, a key cellular energy-signaling molecule (I'll discuss this in more detail in Part Two: Fuel), and they also dampen LPS-induced damage in the gut. A healthy gut makes its own SCFAs, so you don't need to hammer back copious amounts of MCT or coconut oil, to achieve these benefits. *Bacillus* also promotes the health of your gut cells via stimulation of heat shock proteins and inhibition of pathogens. Common fermented foods include yogurt, kefir, sauerkraut (or any fermented veggies), kimchi, natto, miso, kombucha, and more. A common mistake that doctors, practitioners, and athletes make is thinking that "more is better" when it comes to ferments. Regardless of whether you're referring to fiber or fermented foods, it's less about getting as *much* as you can and more about finding the right *dose* for you. You might just need a small pinch of sauerkraut daily or a serving of fermented veggies a few times per week to prime your gut. (Note: if you add fermented foods and immediately experience discomfort, then you should discontinue. This is likely a sign of dysbiosis or imbalance of the good to bad gut bacteria. Such conditions must first be addressed by your health practitioner before you resume eating fermented foods.)

Resistant starches also play a fundamental role in a healthy gut. Resistant starches (RS) are "resistant" to digestion in your gut and so provide a fuel source to the "good" gut bacteria, which in turn increase beneficial SCFA levels. Many resistant starches are destroyed in the cooking process; however, when the food cools down, the benefit is restored. Common foods high in resistant starches include cooked and cooled white potatoes, oats, lentils, and rice. They're simple to prepare and can be easily added to your raw or preprepared meals to be eaten the next day. If you're following a low carb or keto approach, including regular portions of these foods is a great way to keep your athlete microbiome happy.

### GUT TESTING AND RESOLVING DYSFUNCTION

Gut testing is a controversial space. It can be a powerful tool for understanding the puzzle of your athlete's overall picture, but it can also be easily misinterpreted (even by clinicians and practitioners). The only thing experts can firmly agree on, based on the research, is that *gut diversity* is the most reliable biomarker of healthy gut (and, potentially, overall health). What test can you use to identify this diversity? The uBiome test currently provides a great 30,000-foot snapshot view of the ecosystem in your gut. It's important to note you're not trying to "fix" imbalances or dysfunctions with a reductionist approach; rather, you're trying to collect information in order to to see the picture of athletic health. For example, an athlete who gets sick frequently or one who eats a diet with lots of highly processed foods will likely show low diversity. There are many limitations with such a general test, but overall such a test provides a good general picture of the gut microbiota diversity and athlete microbiome. If an athlete is struggling with a chronic gut problem, then more exhaustive testing of the gut, such as a Comprehensive Stool Analysis (CSA), might be appropriate. These tests can help identify dysbiotic bacteria and yeasts, chronic inflammation, immune suppression or over-activation, as well as SCFA markers like butyrate that reflect good gut health. That said, the gut is still a bit of a "black box," so results need to be interpreted cautiously.

## Resolving Gut Problems

The common advice from experts is to eat more fiber and prebiotics to cure digestive ailments. Unfortunately, if you're struggling with a chronic digestive problem, adding more fiber often leads to more bloating, more pain, and more adverse symptoms (in the initial stages). There is a lot more

## Probiotics: Personalized
## Support for Athlete Microbiome

Do probiotics actually confer any performance benefits to athletes? Do athletes need to supplement with probiotics to offset the demands of intense training? Probiotic supplementation is an exploding area of research, with experts and companies making all sorts of claims. Expert exercise immunologists Nic West, PhD, from Griffith University and David Pyne, PhD, from the University of Canberra in Australia suggests the evidence currently supports two areas of potential benefit for probiotic supplementation in athletes: preventing or reversing chronic upper-respiratory tract infections (URTI) like colds and flu.[49] Dr. West and Dr. Pyne believe these benefits are mediated via changes to the athlete gut microbiota and via enhanced gut barrier function. This is a view shared by other experts in the field. Their suggestions for the application of probiotic supplementation for athletes are as follows:

### How to Apply Probiotics

- Probiotic supplementation should be trialed during the preseason phase, or during the early- to mid-stages of a competitive season so that the athlete can get familiar with taking the supplements.
- Probiotic supplementation should start *at least 14 days before* overseas travel, an intense training block, or competition to allow adequate time for colonization of bacterial species in the gut.
- Note: It's not unusual for athletes to experience changes in bowel quality or frequency of movements in the short term (stomach rumbles, increased flatulence, and so forth), and therefore athletes should be informed that mild side effects for a few days are not uncommon.

This doesn't mean you need to give every athlete a probiotic supplement. Athletes more susceptible to colds and flu, those who struggle with frequent URTI, or athletes who are constantly run-down might want to explore probiotics during intense training blocks, travel, or competition. Look for multi-strain formulas containing *L. rhamnosus*, *L. fermentum*, *L. casei* and/or *Bifidobacterium*. Although the research suggests doses of $10^{50}$ per capsule, a wide variety of doses also show benefits. In other words, don't think more billions per capsule is better than less. It's the strains that count.

nuance to the story, particularly if you suffer from IBS (irritable bowel syndrome) or an autoimmune condition. Let's review how to resolve a problematic gut and rebuild a healthy athlete microbiome.

### STEP #1: RESTRICT YOUR DIET

What you eat has the biggest impact on your gut microbiota. In clinical practice, trimming the diet of fiber is the best strategy — in the short term — to get clients struggling with digestive issues like IBS back on track. In fact, the highest degree of evidence-based research (meta-analysis of randomized control trials) shows restrictive diets perform much better than high-fiber, high-prebiotic diets for improving a dysbiotic gut. The most practical way is to *reduce* your intake of carbohydrates, fiber, and prebiotics (don't worry, it's not forever). Nutrition strategies like the low-FODMAP diet (fermentable oligo-, di-, and monosaccharides, and polyols), the elimination diet, the low-carb diet, and the like can all be very helpful for persistent gut problems in the short term. By adopting these strategies, you starve out "bad" renegade bacteria, reduce chronic levels of inflammation, and restore gut barrier integrity. Subsequently, this system allows you to quickly experience improvements in GI symptoms, which translates to minimizing gas, bloating, discomfort, constipation, or loose stool. Remember, the microbiome is merely the interface between you and the environment, either amplifying or buffering your response to it.

## Step #2: Weed Out the Renegades

In a complex ecosystem, it takes a multifaceted approach to restore balance and order. General therapies that impact multiple systems are the most powerful approaches; thus, modifying your diet with a restrictive approach is critical for your success. However, as described throughout this chapter, certain persistent renegades might be difficult to kick out of the system. Renegade bacteria and yeasts can make biofilms, which are protective fortresses that allow them to avoid your immune system army. Herbal antimicrobials have antibacterial, antiviral, antiparasitic, antifungal, and antibiofilm properties, making them highly effective at trimming the dysbiotic renegades without destroying the entire ecosystem like antibiotics do. Recall Dr. Petersen's findings: The more rounds of antibiotics you take, the more difficult it is for your microbiome to bounce back. Antimicrobial supplements provide a broad range of antimicrobial herbs — berberine, boswelia, goldenseal, wormwood, wild indigo, skullcap, garlic, and more — that can knock out the renegade bacteria and reclaim your gut health. The research shows herbal microbials can be just as effective as general antibiotics if applied over the course of four weeks.

## Step #3: Prime the System

Renegade bacteria are opportunistic. They take advantage of an imbalance in the ecosystem to set up shop, prioritizing their survival at your expense. You can think of the balance of "good" to "bad" gut bacteria like seats on a bus. Once the renegade bacteria find a seat, they're incredibly difficult to kick off the bus, thus the need for a restrictive diet and antimicrobial weeding support. Once you've kicked them out, you need to ensure the good bacteria are present and ready to fill in the spot. In the short term, probiotic supplementation provides this added support. Contrary to popular belief, probiotic supplements do not permanently recolonize your gut, but rather provide a key signal to trigger the growth of beneficial "good" bacterial strains as they pass transiently through the gut. In clients with chronic gut dysfunction, priming the system with beneficial strains of bacteria can help restore gut diversity; look for a multistrain probiotic containing keystone species *Bifidobacteria longum, B. infantis,* and *Lactobacillus rhamnosus. Bifidobacterium longum* supports both arms of your immune system: the "first line of defense" innate immune system by enhancing sIgA levels, and your "seek and destroy" adaptive immune system by knocking out pathogenic *E. coli*

## Learn to Relax to Improve Gut Health

Your thoughts and state of mind have a big impact on your gut microbiome. As noted in this chapter, your gut communicates with your brain and your brain communicates with your gut; it's a two-way street. Gut microbiome expert Miguel Toribio-Mateas, PhD(c), highlights the many routes of communication between the gut and brain, such as the vagus nerve, the immune system, short-chain fatty acids (SCFA), and tryptophan.[51] These channels of communication between the brain and gut are influenced by many factors: the diversity of your gut microbiota; hormones, neurotransmitters, immune- and neuropeptides in the gut; and the integrity of the gut wall. Many athletes, in particular endurance athletes, are classic type-A personalities who have an inherently strong sympathetic drive. While this sympathetic dominance can be highly beneficial during hard training blocks and intense competition, it can place a heavy burden on your gut microbiota diversity, SCFA output, and gut wall integrity. Dialing down your sympathetic drive, particularly away from exercise, will naturally help to restore a healthier gut ecosystem. Add relaxation practices into your regime — such as breathwork, meditation, gentle stretching, walking in nature, and float tanks — to accomplish this relaxation. Such practices are often difficult for "work hard, train hard" types, but if you're struggling with chronic digestive problems that improve but never quite get fully resolved, learning to relax can make all the difference.

and *clostridia*. It also helps to cool chronic inflammation that compromises gut wall integrity. Low levels of the keystone species are common in those with poor health, or in athletes who do not regularly consume dairy products. (Note: if your gut testing revealed renegade *H. pylori* infection, talk to your doctor or practitioner about using *Saccharomyces boulardii*, a beneficial yeast, to eradicate the harmful overgrowth).

Once you've reversed your adverse GI symptoms, embrace the fundamentals of a healthy athlete microbiome as described in this chapter to maintain the healthy gut ecosystem in the long term. This will be time to loosen the reins on your restrictive diet and test out what your new gut ecosystem can tolerate. It's also time to feed the good bacteria by ramping up real food sources of fiber, prebiotics, and resistant starches to help keep your digestive engine running strong.

# CHAPTER 3

# Blood Sugars and Longevity

Today, more than 50 percent of the food bought by American and British households is classified as being "ultra-processed." The tsunami of processed food production over the last four decades has finally reached a tipping point. Processed food is now the norm. Comparably, in Mediterranean countries, where citizens are often touted as having one of the healthiest dietary patterns on earth, the percentages of household purchases on ultra-processed food are as low as 20.3 percent in Spain, a paltry 14.2 percent in France, and 13.4 percent in Italy.[1] These statistics from Mediterranean countries notwithstanding, the implications are that, for those who follow a typical Western diet, processed foods are not good for human health — which, not surprisingly, has taken a dramatic turn for the worse. Today, we're in the midst of obesity, type 2 diabetes, and cardiovascular disease epidemics. The levels have skyrocketed since the 1970s, alongside the unprecedented increase in processed foods. Alarmingly, over 450 million people worldwide have been diagnosed with type 2 diabetes, and the World Health Organization (WHO) predicts by the year 2050 one-third of the population worldwide will either have prediabetes or diabetes. Perhaps even more troubling, prediabetes and diabetes are strongly associated with virtually all other chronic lifestyle diseases. For the first time in human history, chronic lifestyle diseases kill more people than infectious diseases, and our children will fail to live longer than we do. It is no wonder health care systems across the globe are buckling under the tremendous weight (and cost) of managing chronic disease.

The definition of ultra-processed foods is, "Formulations made mostly or entirely from substances derived from foods and additives," which was written by Carlos Monteiro, professor of nutrition and public health, and his team at the University of Sao Paulo, Brazil. Their classification system, called NOVA, places food into four groups: raw or minimally processed food (for example, fruit, seeds, eggs, milk), processed culinary ingredients (oils and butter, for example), processed foods (for instance, canned foods like vegetables and fish, as well as cheeses), and ultra-processed foods (cereals, packaged breads, french fries, soft drinks, pizza, and the like). Incredibly, despite ultra-processed foods having only been around for less than half a century — an infinitesimal 0.004–0.008 percent of our time on earth — the mismatch between these hyper-palatable, calorie-dense, nutrient-poor foods and our evolution-hardwired brains designed to seek out calories to survive is the perfect recipe for this tsunami of chronic diseases. Over the last 84,000 generations, we've been hunting, gathering, and scavenging for food. Calories were hard to come by, you had to work hard to get them, and you had to spend a lot of energy in order to eat. Our early ancestors would have gone extended periods of time without food as the seasons changed, during periods of conflict or war, or simply when searching for their next meal. During this time, evolution hardwired our brains to seek out calorie-dense foods to ensure survival and achieve the ultimate goal of all species — to pass on our genes to the next generation. This period accounts for over 99.5 percent of our time on earth. Just 10,000 years ago, the agricultural revolution began. Small communities formed because the practice of farming land provided stable and reliable food sources for its members. Up until a few hundred years ago, that's pretty much how we ate. The industrial revolution that began in the mid-nineteenth century promoted the idea of eating breakfast every morning to laborers on the assembly lines as a means of sustaining energy throughout the day and to ensure productivity. The first commercially available refrigerator was sold around the 1920s (we've only had fridges for 100 years!) and advances in food processing soon thereafter allowed more shelf-stable foods, ensuring better access to food for people in hard-to-reach corners of the country. In the beginning, food processing was a major win for science and health. Then in the 1970s things started shifting dramatically with the industrialization of the food supply, the ability to make artificial flavors, and customers with more disposable income. These factors gave birth to the processed food boom, which has exploded over the last five decades to include more than 50,000 different options that now line grocery and convenience store shelves. As the processed food boom raged into the 1980s and 90s, promotions for it began dominating the airwaves. Media outlets, advertising, and marketers promoted snacking as a healthy strategy to maintain energy levels through the day. In less than half a century, our food environment completely changed.

So what does the history of processed foods and the modern chronic disease epidemic have to do with athletic performance? Athletes must first be healthy to achieve their potential and maximize their performance. If you want to excel at your sport for the longest possible time, it pays to be healthy (even literally, in the form of renewed and better contracts!). If you're an older athlete, this means better performance into your golden years. But how can you be healthy when the environment around you is intent on making you sick? If you simply go with the flow, you'll consume foods that aggravate blood glucose control, trigger excessive inflammation, devastate gut diversity, compromise sleep quality, and harm your overall health.

Blood glucose control is a keystone in maintaining human health. If you're a coach, trainer, or practitioner it's important to understand that healthy blood sugar control is intimately connected with quality sleep and a healthy gut, and ultimately these factors can significantly impact an athlete's ability to train, recover, and perform. Athletes can seemingly get away with poor nutrition as teens and young adults, but look closely and you'll see that an undercurrent of poor health is present. If you are an athlete who struggles to dial in your diet as you age, you'll likely find yourself battling chronic joint pain and stiffness, excess body fat, nagging inflammation, increased susceptibility to cold and flu, fatigue, low mood, and sleep disturbances, just to name a few. In this chapter, I'll make the case that supporting healthy blood glucose control could be the single best way to improve your athlete health and support longevity.

## Longevity, Blood Sugars, and Chronic Lifestyle Diseases

The scientific study of longevity is a curious one. In science, long-lived species are defined as those that live at least twice as long as expected based on their body size. Based on this definition, bats, the naked mole-rat, and humans stand out as exceptionally long-lived. Why us? To understand longevity (and thus health), we need to first understand the aging process. In the 1950s, one of the first researchers to explore aging was Denham Harman, PhD, professor emeritus at the University of Nebraska Medical Center. He hypothesized that oxidative stress was the principle driver of aging. For decades this was the prevailing view. However, after years of observation the evidence didn't exactly match up. Lots of long-lived animal species have high levels of oxidative stress (reptiles, bats, and birds in particular). They all have long lives despite high levels of oxidative damage. While experts are still in agreement that oxidative stress plays a part in aging — particularly in certain chronic disease states — it's not the whole story. If it's not the absolute amount of oxidative stress that matters, scientists began exploring other concepts, including the resiliency of the cells. It turns out there is a strong relationship between species longevity and cellular resistance to oxidative stress across a wide variety of animals. If certain species are able to augment their cellular resistance to oxidative stress to live longer, it raises the question of how they do it. Before diving into this subject further, let's explore the connection between poor blood glucose control and poor health.

Today, sedentary living and the overconsumption of highly processed foods have resulted in about two-thirds of the American population being classified as overweight or obese (and most Western countries have similar rates). This has had massive ripple effects on health. By the time Americans reach middle age, a whopping 90 percent will struggle with hypertension and 40 percent will suffer from metabolic syndrome, a cluster of symptoms including high blood pressure, high blood sugars, excess body fat around the belly, and abnormal cholesterol or triglyceride levels.[2] After the age of 60, the rate of metabolic syndrome jumps to 50 percent! Obesity and type 2 diabetes are tightly connected and as the American waistline increases at seemingly centripetal force so too do the rates of type 2 diabetes. It's estimated half of the American population is either prediabetic or diabetic (type 2), and diabetes is strongly associated with an increased risk of heart attack and stroke.[3] Heart disease is currently the number one cause of death — accounting for 41 percent of all fatalities — and the worse your blood glucose control, the greater your risk of cardiovascular disease.[4] How does this affect you if you're not overweight or diabetic? Incredibly, even when your blood glucose levels are consistently too high after a meal it predisposes you to cardiovascular disease and mortality, regardless if you're a type 2 diabetic or not. This becomes even more important as you age because blood sugar control, blood pressure, resting heart rate, cholesterol, and triglycerides all typically rise as you get older.

This relationship was first identified in a 22-year study that found when fasting blood glucose exceeded 85 mg/dl (4.3 mmol/L) it was associated with a 40 percent increased risk of cardiovascular disease (after correcting for all variables that skew the number even further).[5] The Whitehall study, another investigation into fasting blood glucose and health, also found an increased risk of cardiovascular disease with the highest fasting glucose values, and it increased in a step-wise fashion as fasting blood glucose worsened (the association was strongest in men aged 40–49).[6] These findings have been replicated by other researchers and hold true once again after correcting for age, cholesterol, systolic blood pressure, obesity, and smoking.[7] With almost 70 percent of the population overweight and 50 percent prediabetic or diabetic, it's not surprising heart disease rates are expected to double in the next 50 years. Despite all the advances in drugs, surgery, and technology, the problem is only getting worse.

It's important to remember that blood glucose dysfunction is a spectrum, with optimal health at one extreme and insulin resistance at the other. Insulin resistance leads to type 2 diabetes and strongly predicts your risk of cardiovascular disease as well as other age-related diseases like hypertension, stroke, coronary heart disease, cancer, cognitive decline, dementia, and overall mortality. In the early 2000s, groundbreaking research by Gerald Reaven, MD, professor emeritus in medicine, and his team at the Stanford University School of Medicine used the direct measurement of insulin sensitivity in lean and overweight individuals — who did *not* suffer from diabetes or diagnosed for cardiovascular disease — to attempt to predict their risk of developing chronic diseases. Over the subsequent half-decade, they observed which individuals were more (or less) likely to have a clinical event or condition. What did they find? The most insulin-sensitive group (the best glucose control) did not have any participants develop a chronic disease or die, while the least insulin-sensitive group (worst glucose control) were 36 percent more likely to develop and die from chronic diseases such as coronary heart disease and hypertension, stroke, type 2 diabetes, and cancer.[8] Dr. Reaven noted, "The fact age-related clinical events developed in approximately 1 out of 3 healthy individuals in the upper tertile of insulin resistance at baseline . . . should serve as a strong stimulus to define the role of insulin resistance in the genesis of age-related diseases." This staggering result highlights how poor blood glucose control plays a fundamental role in the development of modern chronic diseases. It's also interesting to note the characteristics shared by the most insulin sensitive people. Here's a quick snapshot: They typically had lower body fat percentages, exercised more frequently, had lower blood pressure, and had higher levels of protective HDL cholesterol. Reaven's study concluded, "Only insulin resistance was an *independent predictor* of the age-related clinical events." To sum up, blood glucose control is a keystone to longevity and fighting off chronic lifestyle diseases.

A major roadblock to optimal glucose control is the troubling fact that our current standards for healthy blood glucose levels are pretty poor and "quite arbitrarily chosen," with prediabetes loosely defined as a fasting blood glucose level greater than 100–110 mg/dL.[9] A recent prospective cohort study in the journal *Diabetes Care* — examining 12.8 million people and the relationship between fasting blood glucose and mortality — found that fasting glucose levels between 80–94 mg/dL were associated with the lowest mortality, regardless of age and sex.[10] They also found glucose levels 100 mg/dL and above were clearly associated with higher mortality. It appears fasting glucose might be a pretty good proxy for health status and longevity.

Unfortunately, our current food environment seems at odds with healthy glucose control. The evolutionary mismatch between our brain's desire for calorie-dense foods to ensure survival and the ultra-processed food, sedentary living, and stressful lifestyle in our modern culture creates the perfect storm for constant cravings, weight gain, blood glucose dysfunction, and poor health. Throughout human history, the consumption of food (calories in) has been deeply interwoven with food acquisition, be it hunting, gathering, or scavenging for food (calories out). In biology, the optimal foraging theory is a model that helps to predict how an animal will behave when searching for food. Animals attempt to gain the most benefit (food) for the lowest cost (energy expended) during hunting and scavenging to maximize survival. You're not going to spend hours and hours running after a squirrel if it doesn't provide you much sustenance, when the alternative is to wait for a much larger animal that will provide a much greater yield. Throughout evolution, if you didn't move, you didn't eat. Today, we've turned this almost completely upside down. You don't have to move at all, and if you use Uber Eats (or your favorite food delivery app) someone will literally bring you as many calories as you like! Our food environment is a cornucopia of processed convenience snacks and calorie-dense foods. There are numerous benefits to our modern convenience society (don't get me wrong, I love Netflix as much as the next person), but unfortunately a major pitfall for health is that we've completely severed the connection between energy expenditure and food acquisition. Convenience is nice, but it's coming at a high health cost. In our modern environment, sugary and processed snacks light up areas of the brain that trigger the dopamine reward system, driving us to consume more and more, an evolutionary hangover from our past that leads to constant snacking, caloric excess, and worsening health. It's not just a game of willpower. Willpower is finite; the processed-food environment is seemingly infinite.

Another problem is that processed food is literally everywhere. You can't go to a school, hospital, sports complex, or office without running into processed foods. Senior investigator at the National Institute of Diabetes and Digestive and Kidney Diseases in the United States Kevin Hall, PhD, is currently investigating how processed foods impact health, rates of obesity, and type 2 diabetes. It's a really interesting question — did our food environment cause the obesity epidemic? Dr. Hall has started to dissect this dilemma from many different angles. Did a specific macronutrient lead to the obesity epidemic? Is it really all about carbohydrates? Probably not, says Dr. Hall. He highlights food availability in the US per capita has increased approximately two- to threefold over the past few decades — more than enough to explain the obesity epidemic — and that the increased energy availability in today's food environment occured in step with the industrialization of the food supply that mass produced convenient, highly processed food from inexpensive ingredients.[11] Ultra-processed foods contain just the right mix of salt, sugar, fat, and flavor additives to drive our brains crazy and make us crave them. This didn't happen by accident. Food companies hire teams of scientists to ensure their products are highly palatable, and therefore more likely to be purchased again and again. Processed food is also incredibly cheap to purchase and highly accessible, driving more and more people to snack (consciously or not) and eat outside the home. This is a relatively new phenomenon, as 40 years ago almost all meals were eaten in the home. Many people just don't cook their own food or eat at home anymore. The trouble for scientists like Dr. Hall is that it's incredibly difficult to isolate and manipulate variables in complex "population-based" studies to determine *the* cause of obesity. It's much simpler to rule out explanations, like carbohydrates being solely responsible for the current obesity crisis.

Sugar is another polarizing topic. Most people would agree the excessive consumption of sugar in processed food is a big factor in the obesity and type 2 diabetes epidemics. While it's no doubt a strong contributor, the problem with the "sugar causes obesity" argument is that sugar intake has been falling over the past half-decade and yet the incidence of obesity continues to accelerate upward. People are consuming less sugar, but they are still getting fatter. If you look at the problem from 30,000 feet, the energy balance equation tells us these folks are still eating too many calories. But where are these calories coming from if not sugar? A recent study by Emma Stinson and colleagues at the National Institutes of Health in the United States found that high-fat combined with high-sugar foods *independently predicted* overeating and weight gain.[12] In short, processed food consumption predicts excess caloric intake and weight gain. The combination of fat and sugar, virtually unheard of in nature, creates a strong response by the brain to seek out more of this calorie-bomb panacea. Hyper-palatable processed foods have been expertly engineered by food scientists to have just the right amount of sugar, fat, and "crunch" to cue our appetites and cravings. This is probably not surprising to research scientists, because the best known diet to fatten up mice for experimental studies is called the "supermarket diet," which effectively means feeding mice processed foods such as cereals, cookies, cakes, and the like. It's something we already know intuitively — junk food makes you crave more junk food.

All right, all right . . . you're probably wondering how this affects you as the athlete or coach. If you're a trainer or practitioner working with folks in the general population, then improving their blood glucose control is a fundamental way to improve their health. It's also fundamental to weight loss: exercise and nutrition are two of the biggest hammers for improving blood sugar control. To put it simply, supporting athlete health is good for performance. Unfortunately, most athletes assume they have good blood glucose control because they exercise a lot. While this is often true, you might be surprised to learn many athletes wake up with fasting glucose levels above the 100 mg/dl (5.5 mmol/L) threshold, which is in the "not so good" prediabetic range. What gives? (I'll explore this phenomenon throughout this chapter.) Another interesting aspect for the high-level athlete is the application of new technology — continuous glucose monitoring systems (CGMs) — that gives you a snapshot into your individual glucose response to specific foods, 24 hours a day. This technology allows you to better inform your nutrition choices. Before I dive into these areas, let's continue down the longevity road. Chronically high blood sugar levels might increase your risk of chronic disease, but does improving poor blood glucose control actually translate to improved longevity as an athlete? Let's take a look.

## Aging, AMPK, and French Lilacs

Aging is the single most important factor for predicting worsening of blood glucose control. Not surprisingly, aging is also the largest risk factor for a wide variety of chronic diseases: type 2 diabetes and neurodegenerative conditions such as Alzheimer's and Parkinson's disease, cancer, heart disease, and stroke.[13] Unlike smoking or a poor diet, aging is not considered a modifiable risk factor (you can't reverse the aging process). You might, however, be able to slow the accumulation of age-related damage to your cells and tissues.[14] The question is more about extending *healthspan* — the number of years you live in good health — than it is about increasing *lifespan*, the number of years you're actually alive. Tragically, most people spend the majority of the last decade of life in poor health, chronic pain, and requiring medical assistance. Aside from aging, type 2 diabetes is perhaps the greatest risk factor for most all of the other age-related diseases, be it cardiovascular, neurodegenerative, cancer, or kidney disease.[15] In fact, a common feature of accelerated aging is the presence of metabolic dysfunction, encompassing both impaired glucose and mitochondrial function. As a result, better glucose control could potentially slow the aging process and increase your healthspan. If this were the case, then drugs that improve glucose control would surely be beneficial, right? Let's look at insulin and metformin, the two most commonly prescribed drugs to treat diabetes. High blood glucose levels are typically the result of insufficient insulin production and/or increased insulin resistance by the tissues.[16] Type 2 diabetics are given insulin injections to cope with their elevated blood sugars, but a nasty side effect of regular insulin use is weight gain and the resulting downward spiral of requiring larger and larger doses of insulin to cope. Diabetes expert Jason Fung, MD, from Canada says, "The easiest way to make my patients gain weight is to inject them with insulin; . . . it quickly leads to greater and greater weight gain." Insulin is anti-catabolic and blocks the liver's ability to burn hepatic triglycerides (liver fat stores) for fuel, perpetuating the cycle of weight gain and worsening health. Strike insulin off the longevity list.

The most common medication used by type 2 diabetics to control blood sugar levels is metformin. Metformin is a *biguanide*, a synthetic derivative drug from the guanide phytochemical compound found in the French lilac plant. It's used as a first-line antidiabetic agent — in Europe since the 1960s and America since the 1990s — because of its ability to reduce liver glucose production and improve insulin sensitivity.[17] Metformin helps to lower blood glucose levels by activating AMPK (AMP-activated protein kinase), an enzyme inside your cells that triggers energy utilization. AMPK doesn't just lower blood sugar levels; it's also very sensitive to levels of oxidative stress and reactive oxygen species (ROS). So if improving glucose control is associated with slowing of the aging process, then surely there must be some evidence of the effects of metformin and longevity, right? Indeed, reactive oxygen species, poor mitochondrial health, DNA damage, and chronic inflammation have all been shown to play a role in the aging process and metformin has a demonstrated ability to improve all of these key areas.[18] It's no wonder metformin is being touted as the first ever antiaging drug. Studies in animals show promise: Roundworms given metformin have increased AMPK activity and live 20 percent longer, while mice given metformin live 6 percent longer than controls.[19] But what about humans? Perhaps the best evidence to date is that type 2 diabetic patients given metformin live 15 percent longer than age-matched folks in the general population.[20] Does that mean you should start taking metformin? It's not so simple, and there are some important factors to consider. First, metformin has a black box warning. This is the most serious drug warning from the Food and Drug Administration (FDA). This particular warning alerts patients to a rare but dangerous side effect of metformin use called *lactic acidosis*. Metformin increases plasma lactate levels by inhibiting mitochondrial respiration, mainly in the liver. When lactic acid builds up excessively in your blood, it becomes a medical emergency that's fatal in 50 percent of sufferers. Symptoms of lactic acidosis include unusual muscle pain, difficulty breathing, unusual sleepiness, and slow or irregular heart rate along with tiredness and weakness. A client taking metformin would typically need a secondary factor impacting their ability to clear plasma lactate, such as liver disease, moderate to severe kidney dysfunction, or regular alcohol intake. Although it affects fewer than 10 people per 100,000, fatalities occur in 30–50 percent of those sufferers.[21] More common but far less serious side effects include stomach pain, diarrhea, nausea, heartburn, and gas. Regular metformin use can also lead to drug-nutrient interactions that cause deficiency, such as low vitamin $B_{12}$ levels since it requires activation (via intrinsic factor) in the stomach. $B_{12}$ deficiencies and anemias are commonly seen in people taking metformin. Calcium is also depleted with metformin use, and patients are often prescribed 1,200 mg of calcium to take alongside the drug to avoid deficiency. Finally, many women are prescribed metformin when diagnosed with polycystic ovary syndrome (PCOS), so it's important to note there is a drug-nutrient interaction with folic acid as well.

To sum up, metformin helps to extend life and reduce the incidence of illness in people with significant blood glucose dysfunction, such as those with type 2 diabetes. However, metformin is not really appropriate for healthy people or athletes looking for longevity benefits. If we circle back to how metformin works — exerting its beneficial effects via the actions of the cellular energy sensor AMPK — we might find some answers in our quest for longevity benefits. For example, what else activates AMPK? Lots of things, such as hypoxia (that is, exercise or training at altitude), environmental toxins, and depleted cellular energy levels (such as during a caloric deficit or fasting).[22]

## The Glycemic Index: Myth or Reality?

Achieving a caloric deficit is a fundamental, evidence-based principle for achieving weight loss (and thus improve health as well). One of the most popular nutrition strategies over the past few decades, particularly in medical circles, is to follow a low-glycemic diet. The glycemic index (GI) is a relative ranking of how quickly carbohydrates are absorbed into the bloodstream. High-GI foods rush in quickly, low-GI foods are slow and steady, and moderate-GI foods are somewhere in between. (The glycemic load (GL) takes into account the quality of the carbs, along with the quantity.) Choosing foods based on the GI or GL index is a strategy used by medical and nutrition professionals to maintain healthy glucose levels in clients. In theory, this translates to better food choices, fewer cravings and blowout meals, and thus successful weight loss and better health. Does the research back up these claims? Let's review.

One must ask first if a low-GI diet helps with weight loss. In the *Canadian Journal of Diabetes* a recent meta-analysis investigated over 1,500 overweight and obese individuals following low-GI/GL diets and found it did not lead to greater weight loss than higher-GI/GL diets over a six-month period.[23] Strike one. What about low-GI diets and heart disease risk? A recent Cochrane Review meta-analysis of 21 randomized control trials concluded there is currently no evidence regarding the effects of low-GI diets on cardiovascular disease events.[24] Strike two. How about for combating chronic inflammation? Another large meta-analysis of 28 randomized control trials found no significant effect of low-GI/GL diets on inflammatory cyotkines.[25] Strike three. So while following a low-glycemic diet sounds good in practice, and perhaps a nice heuristic to steer you toward whole foods, in and of itself it doesn't produce results. In the real-world scenarios, however, things are much more complex. The trouble with the theory is once you start adding other foods to the meals — as you would do in any normal meal — the added protein, fiber, and other nutrients makes it incredibly difficult to determine the true GI/GL effect.[26] One study found that despite doubling carbohydrates, there was no difference in glycemic response between a large potato (technically high GI, high GL) and a bowl of pasta (low GI, high GL).[27] There is too much complexity in the matrix of nutrients and other constituents that make up our food. The biggest problem with proposed low GI and GL foods is they can actually be very energy-dense, containing substantial amounts of sugars and bad fats that contribute to lowering the glycemic response. The researchers sum things up by stating, "A low glycemic response alone does not necessarily justify a health claim."

Your blood glucose response doesn't necessarily lead to greater weight gain, but it does lead to more blood sugar highs and lows, and thus greater likelihood of cravings for sugars and snacks (that is, increased caloric intake). It appears there is a large degree of variability between what is "healthy" for me and what is "healthy" for you. Recall the groundbreaking study regarding the use of continuous glucose monitoring (CGM) technology to assess the individual glucose responses to meals and the large variability they found among individuals.[28] This line of research might help explain why many people struggle to lose weight despite eating a so-called "healthy" diet. If blood glucose control is a key pillar of human health, how does glucose control impact an athlete's fueling strategy? New CGM technology is allowing us to peer in more closely and assess an individual athlete's response to different nutritional fueling strategies.

## Sensors, CGMs, and Twenty-First-Century Monitoring

Blood glucose monitoring technology is shedding new light in areas never before measurable, and it might potentially change the face of sport nutrition. The use of continuous glucose monitoring (CGM), for example, allows researchers to assess your blood glucose levels 24 hours a day, without a blood draw or finger-prick test. The CGM device is inserted in the back of your arm and passively collects your blood glucose levels, taking snapshots every 1–5 minutes or so, by measuring concentrations in your subcutaneous tissue. The devices were designed to assess glucose control in type 1 and type 2 diabetics, but today they are being used by a growing number of researchers, sport scientists, and recreational athletes to assess the individual responses of their nutrition.[29] Stress also impacts blood glucose levels, and CGM devices not only provide a glimpse of how you're responding to your fueling strategy, but also how other factors impact your blood sugars, like mental-emotional stress, lack of sleep, inflammation, travel, and more. Moreover, the ability to test athletes under "free-living" conditions is a game changer, providing a true snapshot of their day. No longer do they have to solely rely on lab-testing measures, which can often have poor transfer to real-world living.

So what is a normal blood glucose response? The standard for health is defined as a fasting glucose of less than 6.1 mmol/L. This is a pretty generous range when you consider the body of research highlighting a strong association between fasted morning glucose and all-cause mortality starts to increase past a waking level of 100 mg/dl (5.5 mmol/L). Of course, it's not just fasting measures that matter. How do you respond to the food you eat? The World Health Organization (WHO) also recommends your glucose levels fall back down below 140 mg/dL (7.8 mmol/L) 2 hours after ingesting a 75 g bolus of glucose from an oral glucose tolerance test (OGTT). If your levels are above this general threshold, the American Diabetes Association (ADA) would consider you at increased risk of type 2 diabetes.[30]

How does this translate to the athlete specifically? In elite sport, carbs are king on race day; as a result, athletes have always been encouraged to consume a diet high in carbohydrates to support training, glycogen stores, and ultimately performance.[31] A recent study of ten sub-elite athletes found markedly different blood glucose responses to carbohydrates and exercise. Four out of ten participants spent 70 percent of the total monitoring period above 108 mg/dL (6.0 mmol/L), and perhaps more alarmingly, their levels were consistently in ranges classified as prediabetic by the ADA.[32] You wouldn't expect athletes to struggle with glycemic control, but intense training and fueling for performance can be highly stressful on the body. It's especially troubling when levels remain elevated after a taper or extended rest period, when you would expect them to return to baseline.

Elevated morning fasted glucose levels is something Paul Laursen, PhD, a professor and expert physiologist with almost two decades of work in elite Olympic sport, began noticing in himself and other elite athletes. In a recent paper Dr. Laursen coauthored with renowned endurance coach Phil Maffetone titled "Athletes: Fit but Unhealthy," he highlights how "physical, biochemical, and mental-emotional injuries are not normal outcomes from endurance sport participation, yet the incidence of these in athletes is alarmingly high."[33] It seems like a paradox: How can athletes be unhealthy if exercise is so good for you? Laursen explains the terms "fitness" and "health" are often used interchangeably, yet they're not the same thing. Fitness is defined as "the ability to perform a specific exercise task," whereas health is defined as "your state of well-being, where physiological systems work in harmony." This is an important distinction, says Laursen, and a common incongruence he sees in practice. High-level athletes push themselves to the limit — past the fork in the road where health and performance split off — heavily stressing all systems of the body. Is overtraining simply the outcome of an athlete in poor health? (I'll explore Laursen's thoughts further in chapter 5.)

It's not just fueling that impacts fasting blood glucose levels — the intensity of exercise also plays a role, kicking up catecholamines like adrenaline and noradrenaline, resulting in hyperglycemia and hyperinsulinemia post-exercise.[34] Genetics and age play key roles as well. In short, if you're an athlete struggling with traditional fueling strategies, you might be compromising your health (and ultimately performance) by adhering to one-size-fits-all nutrition advice. Even amongst the small group in this study, the wide range of glucose responses to meals suggests a widely varying ability to tolerate carbohydrates. In terms of health applications, the use of CGM devices in diabetic patients was associated with weight loss, increased physical activity, and a reduction of calorie intake alongside a favorable impact on clients' HbA1c levels (a three-month average of glucose control).[35] Sedentary folks with type 2 diabetes using CGM devices during continuous aerobic exercise saw improved glycemic control over the next 24 hours. Thanks to these devices we know that in people with prediabetes even a single lifting session in the gym can significantly improve glycemic control.[36] Moreover, observational studies show a clear relationship between the number of times a person checks their blood glucose status via

CGM and successful blood sugar control (as measured by HbA1c). Just like nutritional interventions, compliance is a major determinant of success with the use of CGM devices. Type 2 diabetics who used their CGM device for greater than 48 days improved their HbA1c twice as much as those who did not.[37] Exercise is generally a great strategy for improving insulin sensitivity — both during and after training — and the positive effects on blood sugar control last approximately 5 days before wearing off, highlighting the importance of movement as an integral part of a healthy lifestyle.[38]

## HIIT, Health, and CGM

In sedentary people, the work of expert kinesiologist Martin Gibala, PhD, at McMaster University in Hamilton, Canada, has shown HIIT (high-intensity interval training) sessions to be a time-saving alternative to steady-state training while providing the same benefits of reducing heart disease risk and improving vascular health and metabolic capacity. Why train for an hour when you can get the same results in 15–20 minutes? When you consider the number-one reason most people don't train is lack of time, it seems like a great strategy. How does HIIT impact blood sugar control? In a recent study using CGM technology where exercise was matched for total work, overweight and obese participants experienced superior glycemic control that lasted longer (into the next day) compared to moderate, steady-state aerobic exercise.[39] Even more impressive, this occurred after just a single HIIT session. The experts believe greater muscle recruitment and faster rate of muscle glycogen depletion might be the key factors triggering superior glucose response in the participants. Other studies show HIIT sessions also help reduce elevated triglyceride levels, a common finding in high-risk heart disease and diabetic (type 2) populations. These results suggest HIIT can be a valuable tool for the general population to improve fitness and overall health.

## How Can CGM Devices Impact Athletes?

At this point many athletes and coaches are probably wondering how the use of CGM devices can help to inform their practice. Researchers in Japan used CGM devices in ultramarathon athletes to investigate the relationship between blood glucose profile, running speed, and performance over the course of a 100 km race. Two runners with experience in ultramarathons participated in the study — one elite and the other a high-level recreational — and performed a battery of preliminary running tests such as $VO_2$ max and lactate threshold to determine their baseline fitness before the race. No instructions were provided on what to eat; the athletes were allowed to simply follow their typical nutritional fueling strategies during the race. What did the CGM devices uncover? The elite Runner A completed the 100 km race in 6 hours 51 minutes at a relative intensity of 89.9 percent of lactate threshold, while consuming 249 g of carbs during the event. Comparably, the high-level recreational Runner B completed the 100 km race in 8 hours 56 minutes at a relative intensity of 78.4 percent, while consuming 366 g of carbs[40] (see figure 3.1). It's no surprise the more elite runner was faster and required less fuel, so what else stands out from the data? First, the difference in fasting glucose levels between the two runners. Runner B had levels upon rising well above 100 mg/dL after the overnight fast while Runner A was below 100 mg/dL (the more ideal threshold). Next, Runner A's CGM response to breakfast elicited a big spike; however, it quickly returned to baseline and came close to morning fasting levels within an hour. On the other hand, Runner B's breakfast elicited less of a spike (likely a smaller meal) yet it took over 90 minutes to return to baseline and was still above the 100 mg/dL benchmark.

What about the athletes' fueling strategy during the race? Runner A slowly drip-fed his carb intake throughout the race, keeping his glucose levels relatively steady (between 100–110 mg/dL) until the latter part of the race. The researchers believed enhanced liver output of glucose during the race, commonly seen in elite ultra-runners, might have been supporting his ability to maintain steady glucose levels along with superior central nervous system and hormonal signaling.[41] The story for Runner B was very different. As he started the race, he fueled early and often, leading to blood glucose levels between 120–130 mg/dl that were constantly rising for the first 6 hours of the event. At the 80 km mark, his blood sugar levels dropped and eventually plummeted as Runner B bonked, hitting the proverbial wall, and so was unable to maintain his running velocity.

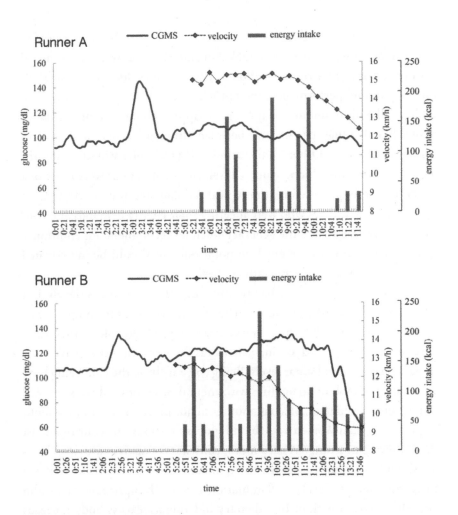

**FIGURE 3.1.** Glucose fluctuation during the race day and running velocity and energy intake during the 100 km race in Runner A and Runner B. The race started at 5 a.m. Abbreviation: CGMS, continuous glucose monitoring system. From Yasuo Sengoku et al., "Continuous Glucose Monitoring during a 100-km Race: A Case Study in an Elite Ultramarathon Runner," *International Journal of Sports Physiology and Performance* 10, no. 1 (2015), https://doi.org/10.1123/ijspp.2013-0493.

The ability to maintain blood glucose plays a key role in performance during ultramarathons. But athletes must be cautious not to over-fuel. The traditional thinking is that athletes who are training hard rarely struggle with hyperglycemia (blood sugar that is too high) and should be more concerned about the performance pitfalls of avoiding hypoglycemia (blood sugar that is too low). But note that the use of CGM technology revealed that Runner B was indeed over-fueled during the race and compromised his performance as a result. Although endurance athletes need carbs on race day to fuel performance, the optimal dose will vary from athlete to athlete. The ideal amount of fueling to support endurance performance is highly individual, particularly between elite and recreational athletes (more in chapter 5). Other studies using CGM technology in sub-elite athletes found that high blood glucose levels (hyperglycemia) were more of a concern than hypoglycemia (the typical red flag amongst coaches), even in recreational athletes who were meeting their energy demands and consuming fewer carbs than the general guidelines recommend for endurance sport.[42] The authors were quick to point out this should be investigated further to assess the impact on athlete health.

Obviously, training has a massive influence on blood glucose levels. But what else in those "other 22 hours" when the athlete is not training impacts blood glucose control the most? First, stress plays a huge role. Cortisol and adrenaline are classified as glucocorticoids for a reason — they have a big impact on your blood sugar levels. Being constantly on the run, being busy at work or school, or struggling with mental or emotional stressors will impact glucose control. Sleep is another major player. Even a single night of poor sleep can worsen your blood glucose response to your breakfast the following morning. What's more, consistently inadequate sleep leads to higher fasting glucose levels. Next, inflammation is also intimately tied to resting glucose levels. Inflammation is actually upstream of insulin and glucose dysfunction. In sedentary individuals, excess body fat leads to the accumulation of pro-inflammatory visceral adipose tissue around the midsection, elevating inflammatory levels and creating a cacophony of inflammatory "noise" that drowns out key signaling pathways. For athletes, exaggerated inflammatory responses can be an early marker of overreaching and overtraining syndrome. Finally, long-haul plane travel crossing time zones not only disrupts your circadian rhythms, but as a result, disrupts your blood glucose control as well. Studies show poorer blood glucose control, exaggerated inflammation, and increased intestinal permeability after long-haul travel. All of these factors can be major stressors that impact blood glucose control. In closing, it's still early days in the application of CGM in athletes, so let's see what the future holds over the next few years.

## Depression and High Blood Sugar

Let's circle back to the importance of blood glucose control. Mental and emotional health is a cornerstone of the new science around peak performance. As we've been discussing in this part of the book, various areas of health are tightly interconnected. If you don't sleep well, your mood is affected. If you struggle with gut dysfunction, your mood is affected. And if you don't have good blood glucose control, your mood is also affected. In fact, there is a growing body of literature highlighting a strong connection between high blood sugar levels (and insulin dysfunction) and depression. Research from Scandinavia has uncovered a clear association between elevated HbA1c and insulin levels with increased risk of depression. They also found young men with insulin resistance were *three times* more likely to suffer from severe depression.[43] Another study in *Diabetes Care* of over 4,000 people showed depressive symptoms were highly associated with higher fasting and 30-minute insulin levels.[44] The authors specifically noted that antidepressant medications did not alter this association because the medications target neurotransmitters (serotonin and dopamine, for instance) and did not address blood sugar and insulin dysfunction.

Another factor impacting blood sugar levels is inflammation. Low-grade systemic inflammation leads to the overproduction of pro-inflammatory cytokines that are also strongly associated with depression.[45] The prestigious *New England Journal of Medicine* recently published a review of findings that show the growing connection between chronic inflammation and the development of today's most common chronic diseases, including depression.[46] The current medical literature tells us that if you are overweight or obese, you likely have low-grade systemic inflammation. But such inflammation is also common at the other end of the spectrum, with athletes who are pushing their bodies to the limit.

Athletes are not immune to depression. Take for example DeMar DeRozan, who seems to have the world in the palm of his hand — he's a perennial NBA All-Star, is adored by fans, and recently signed a contract for over $130 million. For a young kid from Compton in Los Angeles, DeRozan is the ultimate success story. But it's also not so simple. Last year, DeRozan shared with fans that he struggles with bouts of depression. But how could someone with such high professional and financial success struggle with such low mood? Depression, defined as low mood for a 12-month period, affects approximately 7 percent of the adult population.[47] Higher percentages are seen in young adults, and the rates of depression in collegiate athletes is two- to threefold greater than the national average, with female collegiate athletes being the most at risk.[48] Injury, performance, and end-of-career realities are common reasons for athletes to experience depression. Another often-overlooked root cause contributing to low mood and depression is blood glucose dysfunction. As detailed in this chapter, training takes a heavy toll on blood sugar levels. Achieving the right diet to support ideal blood glucose control is an important first step toward reducing the risk of low mood and depression.

## Time-Restricted Feeding, Circadian Rhythms, and Longevity

Nutritionists and doctors will always debate the best diet for human health. However, it's not only what you eat, but *when* you eat that counts. Satchin Panda, PhD, professor and circadian rhythm researcher at the Salk Institute in California, has found that people improve their metabolic health when they restrict their food intake to an 8–10 hour window. In fact, an emerging body of literature shows that eating late at night disrupts our circadian rhythms. This in turn disturbs blood glucose control and triggers a disruptive inflammatory response. Today, Panda's research reveals the typical person eats for 15 hours a day. It starts with an early breakfast of toast or cereal after rising and finishes with a snack or glass of wine on the couch late at night before bed. Avoiding late-night eating is a simple strategy Dr. Panda advocates to improve blood glucose control and fight off obesity, type 2 diabetes, and adverse metabolic conditions. In his book *The Circadian Code*, Panda observes that for hundreds of thousands of years there has always been one constant — the sun rises every morning and falls every night. This means our hormones, organs, and every single cell in the body run on a 24-hour internal clock.[49] Studies show that delaying bedtime in healthy adults for as few as 10 days throws circadian rhythms out of sync and disrupts eating patterns, resulting in increased blood glucose, insulin, and blood pressure.[50] In fact, when researchers force people to stay up late for only a few nights in a row, it leads to reduced insulin sensitivity and weight gain. Nighttime shiftwork is strongly associated with obesity, type 2 diabetes, heart disease, and certain cancers. In 2012, Panda's breakthrough study used genetically identical mice and divided them into two groups. One group had access to high-fat, high-sugar food 24/7 (the equivalent of processed food), and the other group ate the same food but in an 8-hour window. Both sets of mice ate the same number of total calories; however, the mice that snacked as much as they liked got fatter and sicker compared to the time-restricted feeding (TRF) mice that did not.[51] In humans, constant grazing in prediabetic men over a 12-hour eating window worsened insulin function and increased oxidative stress, blood pressure, and cravings compared to when the men who ate the same meals in a 6-hour time frame.[52] Today's food environment, loaded with hyper-palatable processed food that's available 24/7, is no doubt contributing to people's predisposition to eating at all hours. The results are increased disease risk and shorter health-span. Of course, folks in the general population are not athletes who require a significant amount of calories and frequent feedings to support training and performance. That said, this research does reinforce the notion that midnight snacks are likely not the best option for athletes. It also appears to confirm the common heuristic: Eat breakfast like a king, lunch like a prince, and dinner like a pauper.

## Plants, Polyphenols, and Longevity

At the opening of this chapter, I highlighted the strong relationship between a species' lifespan and their cellular resistance to oxidative stress. If an animal is capable of augmenting their cellular resistance to oxidative stress (and by proxy extend life), it raises the question of how they do it. If you're overweight or in poor metabolic health, achieving a caloric deficit and eating in sync with your circadian rhythms are effective strategies for improving glycemic control and fighting off chronic obesity and type 2 diabetes. But what if you're already a healthy weight or an athlete? What else might support longevity?

It begins with diet. Vegetables, fruit, and spices contain phytochemicals that elicit a hormetic stress response in the body. Eating low doses of these phytochemical stressors favor beneficial biological responses, the end result being improved physical and mental health. Naturally occurring plant compounds called *polyphenols* activate AMPK and exert beneficial effects on blood glucose control, type 2 diabetes, and metabolic syndrome. Polyphenols such as resveratrol found in grapes (and red wine), quercetin from fruits and veggies such as apples and onions, genistein in soybeans, epigallocatechin (EGCG) from green tea, berberine from the *Coptis chinensis* plant, and curcumin from the Indian spice turmeric are all great examples of foods, drinks, and spices that activate AMPK.[53] Other foods such as organ meats, broccoli, and spinach are rich in alpha-lipoic acid (ALA) — considered a universal antioxidant for its ability to quench ROS in both water and fat-soluble mediums — also activate AMPK and exert positive effects on metabolic syndrome, heart, and vascular disease.[54] (Interestingly, AMPK also plays a role in the regulation of appetite in the hypothalamus.)[55] Polyphenols appear to be key signals to the body to promote cellular resistance and health. But does increasing your daily intake of them actually make you live longer? A recent study in the *Journal of Nutrition* of 807 Italian men and women over the age of 65 (after a 12-year followup) found overall mortality was reduced by 30 percent in participants who had high-polyphenol diets (>650 mg/day) compared to the low-polyphenol intakes (less than 500 mg/day).[56]

What else impacts longevity? There are hundreds of key protective signaling pathways, but the Nrf2 (pronounced *nerf-two*) pathway appears to play an important role as a master regulator of more than 200 protective genes that shield your cells against toxins and harmful agents.[57] These protective genes encode proteins that neutralize and detoxify both internal and environmental toxins, regulate important factors in cell cycle and growth, and help maintain a high-quality proteome (which is the complete set of proteins in your genome that are present or can be expressed at a certain time).[58] Researchers have also found the Nrf2 pathway is emerging as a critical factor in the protection against cancer, neurodegeneration, and inflammation.[59] In short, the Nrf2 pathway protects your cells from stressors, regardless if they're inside or outside the body.

For athletes, perhaps one of the biggest benefits of Nrf2 is how it protects against inflammation. If you're pushing yourself hard in training, you'll be treading the line between helpful and harmful levels of inflammation. How can you boost your anti-inflammatory Nrf2 activity? Your nutrition is the first place to start. A wide variety of bioactive nutrients in a whole food diet are capable of activating Nrf2 signaling pathways. For example, cruciferous veggies are packed full of isothiocyanates and sulphoraphanes that trigger the Nrf2 cascade of reactions. The organosulphur compounds found in garlic and onions do this as well. Soybeans contain high levels of isoflavones, which are potent Nrf2 activators; one isoflavone in particular, genistein, displays profound neuroprotection, antioxidant, and cognitive function preservation effects. The polyphenols in green tea and turmeric also activate Nrf2 specific pathways. But it's not just food that signals the

Nrf2 pathway. Acute aerobic exercise also triggers Nfr2 signaling, enhancing the body's antioxidant defense. The greater the intensity of the aerobic sessions, the greater the stimulus of Nfr2.[60] This is further evidence that movement is medicine (and is crucial for longevity)! Due to its prominence in a wide variety of age-associated diseases and processes, experts in longevity have stated that "Nrf2 plays a pivotal role in longevity and in the determination of healthspan." It goes to show you, if you provide your body with the right signals and reduce the amount of background inflammatory noise, you can achieve health and performance.

## Blood Glucose Solutions: Test, Don't Guess

There is no one perfect diet for everyone. Because human physiology is robust and adaptable, assessing blood glucose control is a good method to learn whether an athlete's preferred dietary strategy is working for them to support health and performance. When establishing baseline measures, it's important to have athletes tested in the preseason when they're in a rested state. I'll go into some brief detail about the applicable tests.

### HbA1c

Hemoglobin A1c is a blood test that provides a snapshot of your estimated three-month average of blood glucose control. It's a great baseline to assess client health. Aim for levels at 5.5 percent or lower. Remember, HbA1c has a time dependency, which means it more closely reflects your more recent levels of blood glucose.[61]

### HOMA-IR

HOMA-IR is a calculated measure of your level of insulin resistance. Your HOMA-IR score can give you a snapshot of your state of health. It is a particularly useful tool for assessing the general public and recreational athletes who are trying to improve health while training. Ideally, aim for levels between 0.5–1.4. If your levels exceed 1.9, it likely indicates early insulin resistance, while a level above 2.9 is a red flag for significant insulin resistance.

### FRUCTOSAMINE

The fructosamine blood test measures glycated albumin (effectively most all serum proteins) and not just hemoglobin like HbA1c. Since albumin turns over every two weeks or so, fructosamine provides an estimated two-to-three week average of your blood sugar levels.[62] This test, which is typically run on clients or athletes who are struggling with glucose control, is used to get timely feedback on an individual's progress (compared to the longer HbA1c measure). The desired range is 180–223 umol/L.

## GGT (Liver Enzyme)
GGT is a liver enzyme associated with blood sugar dysfunction, insulin resistance, and fatty liver disease. It's often one of the earliest red flags for poor metabolic health. The desired range for GGT is less than 30 U/L.

## CRP-hs
CRP (C-reactive protein) is a measure of overall systemic inflammation. Typically, the more overweight or out of shape you are, the greater your inflammatory levels. The desired range is less than 0.8 mg/L.

———

An athlete's health is pivotal to their ability to train, perform, and recover optimally. This is the essence of the Human First paradigm, and elite performance staff in professional sport across the world now understand this deep connection. As Hippocrates, the "Father of Medicine," once said: "Health is the greatest of human blessings." We often don't appreciate our good health until we don't have it, athletes included. Ensuring adequate sleep, gut diversity, and ideal glucose control are all strategies to support athlete health. And now that you've dialed into your foundational health, you're ready to train and compete.

# PART TWO

# Fuel

*It's not the will to win that matters.*
*It's the will to prepare to win that matters.*

— PAUL "BEAR" BRYANT

# CHAPTER 4

# Physique Nutrition

I t was 2015, the middle of a hot and humid summer in Toronto, Canada. Phil Kessel, NHL All-Star of the Toronto Maple Leafs, was busy doing his favorite summer off-season activities: golfing and fishing. On this occasion, a picture of Kessel eating hot dogs at a charity golf event kicked off a media frenzy. Why? Analysts had been highly critical of their team captain's apparent lack of concern for his nutrition and preparation, calling out Kessel for being "too fat," "eating too many hot dogs," and "not being tough enough." It was the off-season, the Maple Leafs were attempting to rebuild the team with young players, and the press was openly questioning Kessel's leadership abilities and the perceived negative influence of his habits on the young Leafs squad. It opened the door to an interesting question: Does an elevated body fat percentage directly impact athletic performance? Phil Kessel's situation was an interesting one because what was conveniently omitted from the story was that despite Phil's perceived elevated body-fatness, he consistently tested as one of the fastest and strongest players in camp. Kessel topped the charts on all of the Maple Leafs performance metrics. Moreover, Kessel had never missed a game due to injury over the previous eight seasons, five with the Toronto Maple Leafs and three with the Pittsburgh Penguins (where he's won two Stanley Cup championships, considered to be the hardest trophy to conquer in sports). In the rough-and-tumble world of ice hockey, that's saying something. If an athlete is the strongest, fastest, and experiences the fewest injuries, does it matter if their body fat is a little high? Could it *even* be advantageous? It's a complex question with a lot of nuance, so let's explore.

Do team sport athletes really need to be lean to perform? Does it actually help their performance or is being lean merely a by-product of optimal training, nutrition, and good genes? Shawn Arent, PhD, the director of the Health and Human Performance Lab at Rutgers University, says there are two main reasons he tests the body composition of his athletes throughout the playing season: to assess the risk of injury and to monitor in-season losses of lean muscle mass, which can compromise performance. But at what point are there diminishing returns when athletes are too lean? And at what point does being lean hinder an athete's ability to recover and maintain health?

Body composition is particularly important for athletes in aesthetic sports like gymnastics, figure skating, and dance, and in weight-making sports such as Olympic lifting, mixed martial arts, boxing, and others. Elite sport is enamoured with appearances. Every year at the NFL combine, coaches and scouts gather for what's been dubbed the "underwear Olympics" with shirtless players showing off their incredible athletic talents. There is the famous quote from the baseball movie *Moneyball* when actor Brad Pitt, playing the role of Billy Bean, says bluntly, "Do you want to date him or pick him in the draft?" Similarly, in the NBA how "cut" a player looks can influence (consciously or not) their draft stock or whether they make the team. There is a wealth of research highlighting general body composition ranges for athletes specific to their sport. Of course, these are general observations. The important questions are these: Does an athlete need more muscle to perform better? Do they need to get leaner to beat the competition and reach the top of the podium? Maybe, but maybe not. Context matters.

In strength- and power-based sports, size and strength are massive contributors to athletic success, often at the expense of being lean. In this case, performance is more important than body composition. There is currently no evidence in the research that says you can predict athletic performance by body composition alone.[1] (The example of Kessel is a case in point.) There are certainly ranges to shoot for, but no exact numbers. In today's world of relentless social media, athletes often want to look lean and ripped, but often they don't fully understand the degree to which it might negatively affect performance. Having clarity in your goals is crucial. If you're a bodybuilder or physique-focused athlete, then you can live with performance drops because focusing on physique gets you closer to your ultimate goal. But if you are a performance-driven athlete, it's a nonnegotiable. In team sports there is a line between gaining more size at the expense of agility that cannot be crossed or performance *will* suffer. If you're bigger but you've sacrificed your technical, tactical, or psychological factors in the bargain, then you probably won't play your best. That said, in many endurance sports, such as cycling and long-distance running, an athlete's power-to-weight ratio is crucial for performance. Therefore, greater pressure to stay lean is placed on these athletes. It's all about context.

There is yet another layer to this story: athletes who need to make weight for competition. Those who fail to hit their competition weight can't compete. This can be a harsh punishment for boxers, MMA fighters, and others who need to achieve a goal weight just to enter the competition. Unfortunately, the vast majority of these athletes still use unproven, risky, and sometimes deadly old-school strategies to cut weight before a fight.[2] Health risks aside, if you lose weight too quickly, you'll compromise performance via loss of muscle mass, subpar glycogen status, and dehydration, all of which regularly occur during rapid cuts. In short, old-school strategies compromise your ability to perform. And in the fight game, you don't often get a second chance for your one big fight.

In this chapter, I review the fundamentals of energy balance, discuss the key nutrition principles of hypertrophy, outline a systematic approach to leaning out and achieving your desired body fat level, and examine how expert sport scientists are bringing evidence-based nutrition approaches to "making weight" in the fight game. Then I review the various assessment tools you can use to test athlete body composition to inform your practice. You'll learn what world experts are doing to propel their athletes to the top of their game.

## The Energy Equation: It's All about Balance

A calorie, as defined in nutrition, is the measure of the amount of energy required to raise the temperature of 1 kg of water by 1 degree Celsius. In the research to date, it's a highly effective and proven method for measuring the "energy" in the food you eat, and thus how much or how little you should incorporate into your nutrition plan. However, the term "calorie" seems like a dirty word these days. Claims that "calories don't matter" or "the calorie myth has been debunked" rage in the online blogosphere and social media posts, even among seemingly evidence-based and respectable doctors and practitioners. No wonder athletes and the general public are confused.

When it comes to changing body composition, it still comes down to calories in versus calories out. Calories are by far the biggest lever signaling your body to build or break down. It's all about energy balance, and calories do matter (whether you choose to count them or not). However, the further down the rabbit hole you go, the more complex the story gets. Let's review the key factors to consider when it comes to the energy balance equation (see figure 4.1).

## ENERGY IN: FACTORS TO CONSIDER

Appetite plays a pivotal role in conserving bodyweight. From an evolutionary perspective, you're driven to survive and pass on your genes, and to effectively do that you need to maintain a healthy weight. Our ancestors spent 99.5 percent of their time on this planet rarely knowing where their next meal would come from. Appetite and hunger cues were essential for survival. During this time, it was an evolutionary advantage to store body fat more easily, thus passing on this thrifty gene to future generations to promote survival.[3] Today, our *food environment* has massively changed. Over the past half-century, the food landscape has been completely transformed with the ever-increasing availability of processed foods. As Stephan Guyenet, PhD, highlights in his terrific book *The Hungry Brain*, our brains are biologically driven to seek out high-calorie foods in order to favor weight gain, reproduction, and survival. Today, our environment is loaded with hyper-palatable processed foods — available everywhere and all of the time — engineered by teams of scientists to make us want to eat more. Your brain gets a little hit of the dopamine reward signal from these processed foods that are purposefully designed to contain just the right amount of salt, fat, and sugar. In fact, snacking is a recent phenomenon created by the processed food boom. The work of Kevin Hall, PhD, at theNational Institute of Diabetes and Digestive and Kidney Diseases in the United States highlights the daily caloric excess from snacking alone, over the past 40 years, has risen to approximately 425 kcal per day.[4] This calorie surplus is enough to account for our current obesity epidemic. The food environment can get pretty complex, and it plays a massive role in weight control.

Finally, psychology is another important factor on the "energy in" side of the equation. Do you feel like you're being forced to follow a restrictive or bland diet? Is your sport dominated by coaches and athletes who obsess over weight and body image? Are you suffering mentally or emotionally and using food as comfort? Mindset is huge when it comes to controlling food intake. Dieting can be incredibly difficult, and that's why using an evidence-based approach is so crucial.

## ENERGY OUT: FACTORS TO CONSIDER

Your resting metabolic rate (RMR) is the amount of calories required to keep you alive. It's typically measured in a lab with a metabolic cart, as close to first thing in the morning as possible, while you lie still in a dark room. Your heart and kidneys are the biggest RMR energy hogs in the body, gobbling up 400 kcal per kilogram daily, while your brain and liver also use up a decent amount (240 and 200 kcal respectively).[5] If you think about this from the perspective of a general weight loss client (overweight, obese, or sedentary) their resting metabolic rate (RMR) accounts for 60–70 percent of the total calories they burn on a day-to-day basis. (That's massive!) To put things into perspective, hitting the gym and building muscle only contributes about 13 kcal/kg/day to your RMR. It's a small drop in the energy expenditure bucket. This is important because when you lose weight, your metabolic rate will also drop. If you drop the calories too quickly, the RMR will soon bottom out as well. Furthermore, if you attack weight loss too aggressively, you'll burn off precious muscle mass. You must strategically navigate the inevitable drop in metabolism, which can slow weight loss progress down to a crawl, leaving you stuck or regressing backward. That said, rapid initial weight loss in obese clients shows better outcomes in the long term, so if you're a practitioner, you must take your client's context into consideration. If you're an athlete, RMR accounts for less of your total daily energy expenditure (EE), which makes sense when you consider how much you train. For elite endurance athletes, RMR accounts for only 38–47 percent of total daily EE while strength and team sport athletes land around 50 percent or so. Rapid weight loss is highly problematic for athletes due to the dramatic losses in lean muscle mass, which will likely compromise performance.[6]

Realistically, most coaches and practitioners don't have access to lab equipment like a metabolic cart to accurately assess a client's RMR. That's no problem, as there are RMR population-specific equations you can use, the most common being the Cunningham equation for women and the Harris-Benedict equation for men. In practice, seeing the difference between an athlete's "predicted" RMR and the actual score in a lab-based test can reveal if the athlete is rundown and overtraining (more on this in Part Three: Recovery). Ultimately, the biggest problem with calculating RMR is that it's constantly changing. As you lose weight, your RMR decreases. How much? Nobody knows for sure and it varies markedly between individuals. Your RMR changes based on how much (or little) you eat, how much (or little) you train, how much (or little) you sleep, how lean or fat you are, your age, sex, as well as mental and emotional stressors (see table 4.1).[7] In short, you're chasing a constantly moving target. As your client loses weight, their metabolism will change. As they restrict calories, their

**TABLE 4.1.** Factors Influencing Metabolism

| FACTORS THAT INCREASE METABOLISM | FACTORS THAT DECREASE METABOLISM |
|---|---|
| Exposure to hot | Aging |
| Exposure to cold | Reducing training volume |
| Acute stress | Reducing training intensity |
| Fear | Loss of muscle (or fat-free mass) |
| High-altitude exposure | Menstrual cycle: 1st phase (*estrogen-dominant phase*) |
| Injury | Chronic stress |
| Caffeine | |
| Medications | |
| Increase in lean muscle | |
| Menstrual cycle: 2nd phase (*progesterone-dominant phase*) | |

*Source:* M. M. Manore and J. L. Thompson, "Energy Requirements of the Athlete: Assessment and Evidence of Energy Efficiency," in *Clinical Sports Nutrition*, 5th ed, eds. Louise Burke and Vicki Deakin (Sydney, Australia: McGraw-Hill, 2015), 114–39.

metabolism will change. As they train more frequently and get fitter, their metabolism will change. The goalposts are always moving, which can make nailing down the caloric intake a challenge in practice.

Once you've nailed down your resting metabolic rate, you need to determine your energy expenditure from daily *activity*. How much energy do you expend just going about your daily routine at work? Are you sedentary all day, or does your job require you to stand? Do you work manual labor? You'll need to take all of these questions into account. Next, the sport you play contributes heavily to your energy expenditure. Even though a bodybuilder might hit the gym six times per week, doing so costs far less energy than a basketball, soccer, or hockey player sweating through 2-hour practices (and then hitting the gym on top of that). Using a metabolic equivalents (METs) chart online, an objective measure of the energy expended by an individual performing a specific physical activity, you can nail down how much energy you'll likely be spending during your sessions.[8]

Nonexercise activity thermogenesis (NEAT) is the scientific term for all the calories you burn getting up and going about your day. Walking, pacing, taking the stairs, carrying your groceries, stressing over your to-do list, playing with your kids, or chatting with friends all increase NEAT and are a key component of the fat-loss equation. It accounts for up to up to 50 percent of daily energy expenditure in fit folks, but only a paltry 15 percent in sedentary folks, so you can see how getting overweight clients moving is crucial for weight-loss success.[9] Busy work schedules and kids at home can force a lot of people into sedentary lifestyles, and so carving out more movement in the day is a great way for them to support health and weight loss.

Finally, the macronutrient breakdown of the food on your plate impacts not only your calories in but also your calories out. It costs your body more energy to metabolize certain foods over others, which is called the thermic effect of food (TEF). Protein has far and away the biggest TEF, costing your body 25–30 percent of its calories to process compared to a paltry 6–8 percent for carbs and 2–3 percent for fat.[10] One of the reasons "hard-gainers" need to add so many more calories to their diet is because as they eat more, they also burn more energy via the thermic effect of food. The thermic effect is also influenced by food processing and refining. Research shows eating whole foods versus processed foods doubles TEF, the amount of calories it costs your body to process them. When you eat a diet high in processed foods, the TEF plummets. Therefore, it is best to minimize the amount of processed foods in your diet if body composition is your primary goal.[11] That said, a key X factor that helps to buffer this effect in packaged foods is protein content. If protein is included in the processed food, it performs just as well (sometimes better) than whole food options.[12]

Calculating your energy balance is incredibly complex: Food labels have a 30 percent error range; client food logs are often inaccurate; weight loss drops energy expenditure; you weigh less, and therefore in training you're moving less weight; you have less ATP for the same level of movement; and on and on. The overarching name for all these dynamic changes is *adaptive thermogenesis*. Incredibly, if you lose 10 pounds, you'll burn 15 percent less calories at the given bodyweight. If you include the majority of the population in this assessment, some people will only burn two-thirds of the predicted calories.[13] Experts believe increased fight-or-flight (sympathetic) drive and reduced thyroid activity play key roles in these dynamic differences. Energy expenditure is complex, but you need a starting point and a

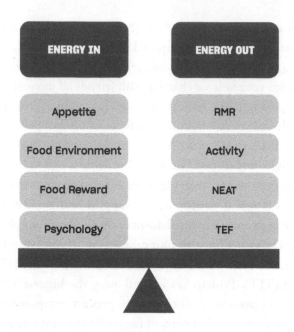

**FIGURE 4.1.** The Energy Balance Equation.

roadmap. The higher the level of your athlete, the more exact you'll need to be with your calculations and estimations. So how does this evidence-based research inform what you do in your practice to get athletes bigger, leaner, or make weight for competition? Before we dig in to the insights from world-leading experts, let's make sure you're clear on your goals.

## GOALS: CLARITY AND SACRIFICE

Clearly defining your goals is the first and most important step toward achieving your desired outcome. You must have clarity in your goals. Health, body composition, and performance are three distinct destinations, and the more intensely you pursue one the higher the chances you'll sacrifice gains in the others. Many clients and athletes think they can maximize all three, but unfortunately this is not the case. If you want to be among the elite, you must make some sacrifices. For example, if performance is your goal, you'll likely — but not always — be moving further away from health and body composition (see figure 4.2). There is a tipping point where chasing body composition gains or prioritizing ideal health will limit your ability to push performance. Similarly, if aesthetics and six-pack abs are your goal, then you're likely going to sacrifice performance in the gym. You won't be able to lift as much weight or maintain

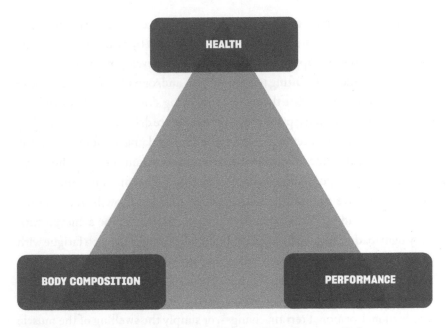

**FIGURE 4.2.** The Body Composition, Health, and Performance Dilemma.

intensity, and you might also be compromising your health if you get too lean. Poor athlete health often leads to more illness and subsequently missed training days, which is incompatible with elite performance. It's a fine balance. In short, to truly achieve elite levels you will likely have to sacrifice in other areas (and that's okay). If you take the time to identify your primary goal, your journey will be that much more efficient.

## The Physiology of Mass Building

Stress is essential for growth. Regardless if you're in the gym, classroom, or office, stress provides the stimulus to improve. Stress is what allows you to get stronger, fitter, leaner, and smarter. Brad Schoenfeld, PhD, a legend in the science of strength and hypertrophy research, is the director of the human performance lab at Lehman College and the performance nutritionist for the NHL's New Jersey Devils. Dr. Schoenfeld emphasizes how important it is for practitioners to have a "foundational knowledge of how the body reacts and adapts to exercise stress." Let's do a quick review. The early adaptations to training are mainly driven by the nervous system, resulting from increased muscular activation due to greater muscle recruitment, rate coding, and synchronization.[14] Muscle fiber recruitment follows Henneman's size principle, which states the capacity of a muscle to produce force is directly related to its size. Muscle fiber recruitment is mainly influenced by two key factors: the amount of force you apply and the rate of force development you achieve. This can be achieved by lifting heavier weights and/or with the intent to move the weight quickly (despite the bar velocity being slow with higher loads).

Training adaptations specific to hypertrophy are driven by three main factors: muscle tension, metabolic stress, and muscle damage. But which is the most important factor to consider when it comes to training? Dr. Schoenfeld says the evidence points to mechanical tension.[15] Receptors in your muscle cells are sensitive to both the magnitude of the load (how heavy) and the duration of loading. This explains why hypertrophy can be achieved with very light loads if trained to failure.[16] It just takes longer to reach fatigue with lighter loads, so it is not ideal for athletes (but great for older populations!). Metabolic stress and the metabolites produced during exercise also play a role in increasing muscle, which researchers believe is likely due to myokine production, hormonal terrain changes, or simply the swelling of the muscle from training. Myokines are signaling molecules from the cytokine family (more in chapter 8) that are produced inside muscle cells when you lift. They have unique effects on your ability to build or break down muscle.[17] Finally, muscle damage is often a misunderstood area of hypertrophy. While exercise-induced muscle damage does enhance muscular adaptation, Dr. Schoenfeld is quick to point out the evidence also shows excessive damage has negative effects on hypertrophy.[18] In short, more damage isn't better — you need to find the sweet spot. Now that you've freshened up your muscle physiology, let's tackle the nutrition fundamentals for hypertrophy.

## Nutrition for Hypertrophy: Hardgainers, mTOR, and MPS

Calories are king when it comes to hypertrophy, and your muscular adaptations are heavily influenced by your caloric intake. As an athlete, you must be in a positive energy balance to add mass and achieve your goals, because if you're underconsuming energy your body quickly sends out signals to favor catabolism (breaking down muscle) over anabolism (building muscle). For instance, caloric restriction initiates a reduction in muscle protein synthesis and increases key survival-signaling pathways.[19] A caloric deficit also activates AMPK (a fuel sensing enzyme in cells) thereby blunting mTOR (the mammalian target of rapamycin-signaling pathway that acts as a central regulator of cell growth) activity and increasing the rate of protein turnover, which is bad news for your lean muscle gains.[20] In fact, even if you're in a eucaloric state (which means you're matching your total caloric intake to your energy expenditure), it's still not an ideal state to be in to *maximize* your hypertrophy gains. Why? Your body will still be breaking down protein to fuel your resting metabolic rate (RMR) and vital organs to keep you alive (sorry, but your brain prioritizes survival over having a beach body!). To maximize hypertrophy, you must be in a caloric excess. This makes sense from an evolutionary perspective: your body can adapt to different fuel sources so long as you provide the total fuel required. Schoenfeld drives home the importance of total fuel when he states that "the ratio of carbs to fats means *virtually nothing* so long as your protein and calories are met." Achieving a positive energy intake is by far the biggest stimulus telling your body to build muscle.[21] Dr. Schoenfeld suggests a good ballpark to start with is a 200–400 calorie surplus daily and notes that naturally lean athletes, also known as "hardgainers," should aim for the upper end of this range (and sometimes higher).

Once you've nailed down your total caloric intake, you need to set your protein intake. Your ability to build muscle is also dictated by your net protein balance over time. But how much do you need if you're in a caloric excess to build muscle? World-renowned protein expert and researcher Stuart Phillips, PhD, and his team from McMaster University in Canada have found strength-based athletes should get a minimum of 1.6 g/kg/day of protein to meet their requirements.[22] If you're in a caloric excess, a recent meta-analysis by Dr. Phillips found that protein intake *above* 1.6 g/kg bodyweight — double the RDA's recommendation — did not produce further resistance training-induced gains in fat free mass.[23] It looks like 1.6 g/kg/day is the sweet spot for protein intake when calories are in surplus. Naturally lean athletes who struggle to build lean muscle mass often have higher protein requirements than other athletes. The International Society of Sports Nutrition recommends a protein range of 1.6–2.0 g/kg when you're in a caloric excess, though some studies show a benefit up to a daily dose of 2.2 g/kg/day (this is consistent with the heuristic of one gram of protein per pound bodyweight).[24] Whatever dose you pick, be consistent and make sure you hit it every day. For older athletes, hitting the 1.6 g/kg/day target for protein is also very important. Phillips's research found older adults require more protein to reach the same muscle protein synthesis (MPS) threshold compared to younger individuals.[25] (Master athletes take note!)

Now that you've determined your daily calorie and protein needs, let's talk carbs. For physique-focused athletes looking to *maximize* gains, getting enough carbs is crucial to their training performance. Carbs provide as much as 80 percent of the energy to working muscles, and low-carb diets with less than 25 percent of total caloric intake coming from carbs have been shown to reduce time to exhaustion during training.[26] That said, the ideal carb intake is highly individual. A recent study comparing a diet made up of 65 percent carbs versus only 40 percent found no difference in lower-body lifting performance.[27] In general, the more elite the athlete, the more intense the training and thus the greater the benefit of including more carbs (particularly around the time of exercise). If your carb intake is insufficient to top up glycogen status, you'll likely struggle to maintain work output during high-volume training.[28] Carbs also play a key role in keeping your immune system robust during intense training blocks (I'll discuss this in more detail in chapter 8).

Achieving the sweet spot for carb intake takes a bit of trial and error. It's highly dependent on your training phase and whether you're competing in-season, training in the off-season, or resting. In general, the recommendations for carb intake in strength-based athletes is 4–7 g/kg/day.[29] Research in elite male and female bodybuilders by nutrition expert and five-time British bodybuilding champion Andrew Chappell, PhD, found the top men bodybuilders consumed approximately 5 g/kg/day of carbohydrates (women approximately 4 g/kg/day), which was more than the competitors who failed to "place" in competition. They also consumed an average of six meals per day and approximately 38 kcal/kg bodyweight.[30] Of course, bodybuilders or physique-focused clients don't expend the same amount of energy as team sport athletes — an hour lifting in the gym expends nowhere near the same amount of energy as running up and down a basketball court or skating multiple shifts in a hockey game. Moreover, the consumption of carbs during training can vary as much as fourfold from one athlete to the next. Dr. Schoenfeld says a good starting point for carbs in recreational athletes who are looking to add more lean muscle is 3–4 g/kg/day, then titrating up the dose to meet individual training and genetic requirements.

The majority of your carbohydrates should come from whole foods: rice, oats, tubers (yams, sweet and white potatoes, and similar), root vegetables (carrots, beets, parsnips, and the like), beans and legumes, and pasta and freshly made breads. (According to the NOVA food groups, breakfast cereals and industrialized packaged breads are classified as ultra-processed foods. If you notice your diet is chock-full of these types of carbs, aim to replace them with more of the whole food options.) Your minimum intake should ensure a sufficient amount of carbohydrates to top up glycogen stores. Of course, don't get confused by the broscience of "spiking insulin" post-training, which has been thoroughly debunked in the research. Even if you consume three meals a day, you'll double your resting levels of insulin, which is sufficient to support your gains. Contrary to popular belief, insulin is not an anabolic hormone but rather anti-catabolic, which prevents the breakdown of muscle and other tissues (rather than increasing MPS).

Finally, the remaining calories make up your daily fat intake. Dietary fat provides a great source of energy to meet your daily requirements at 9 kcal/gram and brings along with it important fat-soluble vitamins. There is not a lot of high-quality research on the dietary fat intake for hypertrophy, but Schoenfeld suggests a *minimum* intake of at least 1.0 g/kg for hypertrophy athletes. If your total fat intake falls below 15 percent of total calories, testosterone levels will also start to fall pretty quickly.[31] This highlights why it's crucial to achieve high carb (and energy) intake, as calorie- and fat-matched diets revealed the group consuming more carbohydrates had higher testosterone and lower cortisol levels.[32] This hormonal milieu is more beneficial for athletes looking to add mass. The story changes if you're cutting mass, which I'll discuss in a following section.

Ensure the majority of your fat intake comes from real food. Too many saturated fats from *aggressive* addition of butter or MCT oils (keto folks, I'm talking to you) can decrease cellular signaling markers and potentially limit hypertrophy. Polyunsaturated fats play an important role in keeping your cell membranes happy and healthy. This increased fluidity allows for superior passage of nutrients, hormones, and chemical messengers into and out of cells, which is important for supporting muscle growth. In particular, a diet rich in omega-3 fats has been shown to have beneficial impacts on membrane fluidity, increasing mTOR response, as well as providing anti-inflammatory benefits.[33] Aim for approximately 1,600 mg of omega-3 per day for men and 1,100 mg for women.

Whether you choose to achieve your target energy intake with a low-fat, low-carb, or mixed diet is entirely up to you. Dr. Schoenfeld is quick to point out that "you can definitely build muscle on a ketogenic diet, but you won't maximize your gains." There is evidence to show this. After eight weeks of hypertrophy training of a keto group (5 percent carbs) versus a mixed diet group (55 percent carbs), the results were comparable *if* you allowed the keto group to "carb-up" for a week afterward.[34] For elites looking to maximize performance and hypertrophy, there still isn't enough evidence among elite bodybuilders to suggest a keto nutrition strategy can win championships. However, if you're looking to get leaner or you're struggling with poor blood sugar control or a metabolic dysfunction, then keto or low-carb nutrition strategies might be a great fit for you.

## Supplements for Hypertrophy

When it comes to evidence-based supplements that truly make a difference in your lean muscle gains, there aren't very many on the list. The International Olympic Committee recently commissioned a group of experts to analyze all the data around supplements for performance. The goal was to determine what really works and what doesn't. Here's a breakdown of three top evidence-based supplements for hypertrophy.

### 1. CREATINE

The research on creatine is robust. It's easily the most proven strategy to support training, performance, and lean mass gains. Research has consistently shown creatine supplementation increases intramuscular creatine concentrations, improving adaptations to intense exercise.[35] Creatine has been shown to boost the expression of proteins and growth factors that support muscle remodeling and rebuilding, as well as accelerating creatine resynthesis and glycogen uptake — big wins during intense training sessions or if you're doing multiple sessions in 1 day. In addition, creatine supplementation might also enhance recovery, injury prevention, thermoregulation, rehabilitation, and concussion neuroprotection. Creatine is head and shoulders above other supplements when it comes to hypertrophy and athletic support.

### 2. PROTEIN

It's not always easy to eat enough protein. Cooking at home can be a serious challenge for athletes who have little extra time in their schedule. Adding supplemental protein is a time-efficient, convenient, and tasty strategy for achieving daily protein needs in order to stimulate muscle protein synthesis (MPS) and put the brakes on muscle breakdown. A high-quality supplement with at least 3 g leucine or 10 g of essential amino acids (EAA) is key to trigger MPS, so if you're adding a whey protein supplement you're all set.[36] If you opt for a vegan version or prefer it due to digestive or immune concerns, be sure to choose high-quality supplements with adequate leucine content. The recent International Olympic Committee consensus statement notes that "evidence-based reviews conclude protein is effective at promoting lean mass gains when combined with resistance exercise." Aim for 20–40 g per serving with higher doses for bigger athletes.

### 3. Caffeine

The role of caffeine in building muscle is not as clear as its role in endurance performance. The impact of caffeine on strength and power gains is still unclear. The research shows the best strength and hypertrophy gains are seen at the 5–6 g/kg dose. However, this is definitely pushing the upper end of tolerable levels for most athletes, and not all studies show benefits.[37] A real-world limitation is that these studies are only performed over a short duration (2–4 weeks), and thus don't provide a true reflection of the potential negative effects of high caffeine intake on sleep or anxietylike symptoms in the long term. New research in nutrigenomics highlights different genetic responders to caffeine — fast, slow, and ultraslow — and therefore it's prudent to start at the lower effective dose and then work your way up (more on this in the next chapter). A good general heuristic is not to

**TABLE 4.2.** Evidence-Based Supplements for Athletic Performance

| Supplement | Dose |
| --- | --- |
| Creatine | 5 g daily or loading phase (5 g × 4 for 5–7 days), then 5 g daily |
| Caffeine | 3 mg/kg or up to 5–6 mg/kg (caution at this dose) |
| Whey protein | 20–40 g per dose |
| Beta-alanine | 65 mg/kg/day (divide doses to reduce symptoms of paresthesia) |
| Dietary nitrates | 310–560 mg, 2–3 hours prior to training |
| Sodium bicarbonate | 0.2–0.4 g/kg, 60–150 min. before training (divide doses if have GI problems) |

*Source:* Ronald J. Maughan et al., "IOC Consensus Statement: Dietary Supplements and the High-Performance Athlete," in *British Journal of Sports Medicine*, April 2018, 52(7):439-55, doi: 10.1136/bjsports-2018-099027.

**TABLE 4.3.** Nutrition and Supplementation for Hypertrophy

| MACRONUTRIENTS | LOWER END | UPPER END |
|---|---|---|
| Protein | 1.6 g/kg/day | 2.2 g/kg/day |
| Carbs | 3 g/kg/day | 7 g/kg/day |
| Fats | 1 g/kg/day | 80% of daily calories |
| Supplements | Creatine: 5 g daily<br>Protein: 20 g<br>Caffeine: 2 mg/kg | Creatine loading<br>Protein: 40 g<br>Caffeine: 4 mg/kg |

*Source:* Brad J. Schoenfeld, *Science and Development of Muscle Hypertrophy* (Champaign, IL: Human Kinetics, 2016).

exceed 6 mg/kg of caffeine — the upper tolerable limit — on any given day. If you are pushing the top end to get performance gains, then do your best to train in the morning rather than late afternoon or evening to limit the impact on sleep quality. Caffeine supplements provide the most accurate way to obtain and adjust caffeine dosing, but care is required. Ian Dunican, PhD, with the Western Force, an Australian professional rugby union team, found that most players didn't realize their pre-workout formula contained caffeine and that it was indeed having a negative effect on sleep quality.[38] This finding reminds practitioners and coaches to always ask their clients if they're taking preworkout supplements. Don't assume anything.

Table 4.2 summarizes the top six evidence-based supplements that have the biggest impact on athlete performance as listed by the International Olympic Committee on their consensus statement on supplements.

### ASSESSING HYPERTROPHY PROGRESS

Building muscle takes time. You need to monitor progress over months, rather than just days and weeks. A good rule of thumb is to aim for a 1–2 percent increase in total body weight per month. If you've gained more than 2 percent body weight (and too much fat), dial back your total calorie and/or dietary fat intake. If you've not made progress, then you'll need to ratchet up your total energy intake. Aim for an additional 250 kcal per day. As the subsequent months progress, continue monitoring for the minimum weight gain of 1 to 2 percent body weight. (See table 4.3 for a summary of nutrition and supplementation for hypertrophy.)

## Lessons in Leanness: Bodybuilders, Nutrient Timing, and the Big 3

You've learned the fundamentals of hypertrophy nutrition from world-leading experts. But how do the rules of the game change when you're trying to get leaner? This is where you can learn a few lessons from the bodybuilding community. Competitive bodybuilders typically allow for a three-month period to achieve a high degree of leanness (more elite athletes allow for up to six months). For most athletes, this means the typical off-season gives them plenty of time to get leaner, especially when you consider that they are not aiming to get as ripped as a bodybuilder or figure competitor. Of course, the objective here is to learn the principles bodybuilders use to consistently and successfully achieve fat loss and gain an impressive physique. (If you're reading this book because you want to look good naked, pay attention here!) Depending on whether your goal is body composition, performance, or health, you might have to adjust accordingly. The work of Eric Helms, PhD, an expert hypertrophy and nutrition researcher at the Sport Performance Research Institute New Zealand (SPRINZ), and his team helps shed some evidence-based light on the ideal approach to getting leaner.

First off, how many calories should you trim to reach your goals? The general textbook recommendation is approximately 500 kcal per day to achieve a 3,500 kcal weekly deficit to lose one pound of fat mass. Of course, as you lose weight it becomes increasingly harder to lose more as time goes on (especially in the general population), meaning that this old-school generalization actually tends to over-promise weight loss. New research by senior investigator Kevin Hall, PhD, at the National Institute of Diabetes and Digestive and Kidney Diseases in the United States, has uncovered that aiming for a caloric reduction of 55 kcal/pound/day for the general population "reimagines a dynamic relationship between dietary calories and weight loss and presents a more realistic view of the challenges experienced by patients with obesity."[39] In athletes, the rules are a little different. One key reason to lose weight slowly and steadily is to minimize the loss of lean muscle mass. This means the greater the caloric deficit when an athlete is trimming to get leaner, the greater the losses of lean muscle mass.[40] Studies show if you lose 1 kg of weight per week, compared to only 0.5 kg per week, you'll sacrifice 5 percent of your bench press strength and experience a 30 percent reduction in testosterone levels over a 4-week period.[41] On the other hand, if you take a slow and steady approach, you minimize the risk of losing lean muscle.

What should you aim for when trying to shed fat mass and maintain or increase size? Dr. Helms suggests 0.5 kg per week is ideal for bodybuilders or physique-focused clients — assuming the majority of weight loss is fat mass. If you're an athlete engaging in a 12-week off-season program, this could translate into shedding 6 kg (13 pounds) of fat mass. Of course, the bigger the athlete the more weight they can lose, but just be mindful that accelerated weight loss will compromise an athlete's muscle mass. If you try to lose weight too quickly, such as within a two-to-four-week time frame, you're really putting yourself as an athlete at risk. If you're a practitioner training a client who is looking to get ripped for their next holiday or for summer, 12 weeks is a good time frame to aim for. Okay, so while this theory sounds great, how do you actually apply it in practice to get leaner? Here's a quick breakdown of Dr. Helms's systematic approach for getting leaner.

## 1. Set Your Protein Intake

The rules of the game for protein intake change during a "lean-out" phase. Why? Because you're in a caloric deficit. (Remember, context matters.) Recall that research by Professor Stuart Phillips and his team found 1.6 g/kg/day of protein was adequate for athletes getting sufficient calories. If you're in a caloric deficit, Helms has found a protein intake between 2.3–3.1 g/kg/day of fat-free mass (not bodyweight) is effective for limiting lean muscle losses when trying to trim body fat and get leaner.[42] If you're a team sport athlete, it's important to take into account the effects of your sport-specific training. Studies show that athletes who consume 2 g/kg of protein and run 5–10 miles per day during a caloric deficit were still in a negative protein balance.[43] (This highlights the importance of ramping up protein during a cutting-phase.) Also, if you're a hardgainer or a naturally leaner individual, your protein intake might be higher compared to other athletes with higher body fat.[44]

It's not only about the amount of protein, but also how you *pace* your protein intake. Protein pacing, as defined by Paul Arciero, PhD, professor at Skidmore College in the United States, consists of spreading out your protein intake over the course of four to six meals throughout the day. Arciero found this method was superior to less-frequent protein feedings for improving body composition in overweight individuals when they were in a hypocaloric state.[45] If you're an athlete who is trying to get leaner, protein pacing can also be a highly effective strategy. How much protein in one

## The Irrational Fears about Protein and Kidney Health

The myth that protein intake harms your kidneys sadly still persists today in medical circles and the media. Unfortunately, this fake news is still put forth by some dietitians and doctors who aren't up to speed on the latest evidence-based research. Studies conducted by Jose Antonio, PhD, reveal protein intakes of up to 3.0 g/kg in active people, for an entire year, had no adverse impacts on kidney function.[47] The state of the research is also well summed up by Professor Stuart Phillips who states that "high protein intake is not damaging to healthy kidneys." Case closed.

serving? Aim for a protein dose of 0.3–0.5 g/kg per meal to maximize MPS (approximately 20–40 g), spread out over 4–6 meals every 3–5 hours.

Lastly, protein is incredibly difficult to convert into body fat. Jose Antonio, PhD, cofounder of the International Society of Sports Nutrition (ISSN) and the director of the exercise and sports science program at Nova Southeastern University, studied protein overfeeding in bodybuilders. Study participants jacked up their protein intake to 4.4 g/kg/day for 8 weeks (compared to 1.8 g/kg/day). Despite the additional 800 calories, there was no effect on the body composition of the athletes.[46] In general, calories really do matter, but this is the exception. Therefore, if you're cutting and struggling with cravings, then ensuring a high protein intake can be a great strategy.

## 2. ADJUST YOUR FAT INTAKE

When the goal is to get leaner, Eric Helms, PhD, says the next macro to address is your dietary fat intake. Athletes and bodybuilders should consider different factors. First, research shows that reducing your dietary fat intake from 40 percent down to 20 percent can result in significant reductions in testosterone levels.[48] While this might not be as much of a concern for physique-focused athletes (when performance is not prioritized), free testosterone is one of several biomarkers that might help flag overtraining or overreaching in athletes (more in Part Three: Recovery).

Therefore, Dr. Helms recommends bodybuilders only consider reducing fat intake lower than 20 percent during contest prep periods. Ensuring you get enough saturated fat in your diet might help buffer those declines in testosterone, but as Helms highlighted in our recent interview, "If you're preparing for a competition, your testosterone levels are going to be low, and lowered for several months post-event, simply due to the reductions in total caloric intake." If you aim to cut too quickly, your testosterone levels can drop even more dramatically. Athletes losing 1 kg (2.2 lb.) weight loss per week experienced a 30 percent drop in testosterone levels compared to those aiming for 0.5 kg (1.1 lb.) per week.[49] If you're aiming to prep for a competition, your testosterone levels will fall for three months straight and take another three months to return to your normal baseline. That should highlight how powerfully calories impact testosterone levels. Helms is also quick to point out that lower testosterone doesn't mean lower muscle mass. Aim for 20–30 percent of calories from fat and no lower than 0.5 g/kg of daily fat intake.

### 3. The Rest Is Carbohydrate

Once you've set your protein and fat intake during your cutting phase, the remaining calories will come from carbohydrates. Typically, when athletes drop their carb intake and increase protein, they enhance their body's ability to burn fat and preserve muscle. They also tend to see an improvement in satiety (up to a certain point).[50] However, there is another side of the coin. If you keep cutting out carbs, eventually you'll start to impair workout performance, which will compromise your strength and deplete your glycogen stores. These are critical for being able to train at intensity in the gym or on the playing field. When you lift, you burn glycogen as your main fuel, so carbs are important. If you play a sport or you're an endurance athlete, your fueling demands will be much higher. The carb intake recommendations for team and strength sport athletes is 4–7 g/kg/day, so you'll need to tailor the dose to suit you. If you're a bodybuilder or physique-focused athlete, the recommendation is 3–5 g/kg/day of carbs, depending on your age, fitness level, and how much weight you have to lose. Of course, when you need to continually drop calories, carbohydrate intake might also drop to 1–2 g/kg/day as you aim to achieve your body composition goal. A study of athletes where protein intake was kept the same showed that the lower-carb group experienced decreases in workout

## Expert Weight-Loss Heuristic

If your client is struggling to lose weight, Dr. Eric Helms has some advice. He uses a simple method with bodybuilders and physique-focused athletes to help determine the right diet for them. In the off-season, over eight weeks he has them adopt a higher-fat (40 percent) and lower-carb diet while keeping protein intake stable. After a short washout period, Helms has the client flip the nutrition strategy — adopting a higher-carb, lower-fat (20 percent) diet — for another eight weeks. At the end of the experiment, Helms compares how they looked, felt, and performed on the two different diets. After years of practice and coaching, Helms finds this to be an extremely helpful method for determining what side of the coin will generally benefit an individual. From there, Helms can tweak and adjust the total intake of fats and carbs — like turning the dials on a DJ mixing table — to determine the right breakdown of macros and calories from day to day. Remember, this tends to fluctuate daily, depending on the demands of your training and where you are in your preparation (hypertrophy versus leaning out).

performance while the low-fat group did not. Contrary to many social media posts, leaning out is not just about lowering carbs!

### Nutrient Timing

What about nutrient timing? How does *when* you eat your macros or take your supplements impact the bottom line for leaning out? The latest research confirms there are gains to be made in this area, but they're only *marginal* gains. For high-level bodybuilders or physique-focused athletes, this can be the difference between making the podium or not. For novice trainees, their tendency is to prioritize the small buckets — supplements, nutrient timing, micronutrients — over the big buckets like calories and macros. When is nutrient timing most important? If you're training in

**TABLE 4.4.** Nutrient Timing: When Is It Important?

| Minimum Importance | Maximum Importance |
|---|---|
| One session in the day | Multiple training sessions |
| Training in fed state | Training in fasted state (nothing eaten in 4 hours) |
| Supplement: creatine | Supplements: caffeine, carbs, electrolytes |

Source: Eric R. Helms, Alan A. Aragon, and Peter J. Fitschen, "Evidence-Based Recommendations for Natural Bodybuilding Contest Preparation: Nutrition and Supplementation," Journal of the International Society Sports Nutrition 11, no. 1, (2014), https://doi.org/10.1186/1550-2783-11-20.

the fasted state (in relation to both carbs and protein), if you're training multiple times in 1 day, or if you're training for more than 2–3 hours in a single session like many endurance athletes (see table 4.4). When it comes to supplements, nutrient timing is much more important with respect to caffeine, carbohydrates, and electrolytes (and less so for creatine). In terms of overall benefit from supplements during a cutting phase, Dr. Helms's Big 3 are creatine, whey protein, and caffeine. He also reveals his three most overrated supplements that don't hold up to the evidence: BCAAs, arginine, and glutamine (for more details, check out *Dr. Bubbs Performance Podcast*, Season 2, Episode 7). If your supplement budget is bulging out of control, stick to the most impactful and evidence-based products.

## Monitoring Progress

Once you've developed your nutrition plan, how do you progress the nutrition strategy? Dr. Helms suggests aiming for a weekly weight loss of 0.5–1.0 percent (total bodyweight), adjusting caloric intake accordingly. For example, a 100 kg football player would aim to lose 0.5–1 kg of body fat per week in order to minimize muscle loss. If he isn't losing at least 0.5 kg per week, then a reduction in calories of 250 kcal per day is a good place to start (see table 4.5). Remember, the key principles of all successful weight-loss diets are achieving a caloric deficit, supporting client satiety (so they're not hungry all the time), and finding a plan they can adhere to. Adherence is the best predictor of successful weight loss, regardless of the diet method. At the end of the day, you're either there, or you're not there yet. Be nimble and adjust as needed.

**TABLE 4.5.** Nutrition Summary for Weight-Cutting Phase

| Macronutrient | Dose | Notes |
| --- | --- | --- |
| Protein | 2.3–3.1 g/kg/FFM | Calculate on fat-free mass, not bodyweight |
| Fat (% total calories) | 15–30% | % of total calories |
| Carbs (% total calories) | Remaining | Once protein and fat intake are set, the remaining calories are consumed as carbohydrates |
| Weekly weight loss (% of total weight) | 0.5–1.0% | % of bodyweight |

*Source:* Eric R. Helms, Alan A. Aragon, and Peter J. Fitschen, "Evidence-Based Recommendations for Natural Bodybuilding Contest Preparation: Nutrition and Supplementation," *Journal of the International Society of Sports Nutrition* 11, no. 1 (2014), https://doi.org/10.1186/1550-2783-11-20.

## Bodybuilders and Fat Loss: Why Not HIIT?

The nature of physique-based training is that it requires a high volume of work. Oftentimes, more high-level trainees work out multiple times a day. This means recovery and nervous system stress are important factors to consider. Helms prefers that bodybuilders do slow, steady-state cardio to prioritize fat burning and because it's not too taxing on the nervous system. In his experience, combining High-Intensity Interval Training (HIIT) with bodybuilding can be a recipe for disaster because it puts too much stress on the nervous system and thus negatively influences recovery time. Bottom line: Keep cardio slow and steady for bodybuilders and high-level, physique-focused clients.

## Making Weight: Saunas, Starvation, and Going Old-School

In 2017, Mizuto Hirota was swaying badly from side to side, barely able to maintain his balance. The world-class UFC featherweight MMA fighter was not in the octagon, but was simply trying to walk across a stage to weigh in before his upcoming match in Tokyo, Japan. Stumbling over to the scale with eyes glazed over in a zombielike state, Hirota weighed in at 150 pounds. Notwithstanding his obvious poor health, Hirota's result was disastrous: He was four pounds over the cutoff and was disqualified from his match. Hirota had failed to make weight. Unfortunately, the bad news didn't end there for him. Not only did Hirota get pulled from the fight, he lost 30 percent of his paycheck. As he stepped off the scale, he stumbled badly and appeared to pass out, but luckily UFC staff were there to catch him before he hit the floor. It was a tough lesson to learn after months of dedicated training for the fight.

Getting leaner is one thing, but "making weight" is altogether a different animal. In the following weeks, MMA fighter Ray Borg got pulled from a championship fight due to complications from weight-cutting, and MMA star Paige VanZant admitted she'd changed weight classes after passing out trying to make weight. In certain sports, if you can't make weight, you can't compete. With their livelihoods on the line, athletes will go to extremes to get the job done. Old-school rapid weight-loss techniques are still commonly used in boxing and mixed martial arts today, putting the athlete's health (and performance) at serious risk. In 2013, a Brazilian MMA athlete died in a sauna while attempting to lose weight before his upcoming fight.[51] In 2015, a Chinese MMA athlete died of a heart attack as a result of the extreme dehydration strategy to make weight for competition.[52] Expert Dr. Doug Kalman, PhD, performance nutritionist to elite professional fighters says countless MMA athletes and boxers put themselves at serious health risk following old-school advice of water loading, hot saunas, training in "sweat suits," restricting fluids, skipping meals, aggressively cutting calories, or fasting for 24–48 hours in order to dramatically cut weight in the final days and hours before a prefight weigh-in. While clearly there are tremendous health risks, these old-school approaches also harm a fighter's ability to perform, compromising a fighter's ability to retain muscle mass and reducing punching peak force.[53] The dramatic reduction in hydration can also impair immunity, leaving the athlete more exposed to cold or flu and lower mood during the crucial period leading up to the competition.

It's the dark underbelly of combat sports, but thankfully the tides are starting to change.

Expert sport scientists are now teaming up with fighters to guide them through the weight-making process in an attempt to discover how making weight can be achieved without compromising health and performance. Recently, an elite super featherweight fighter had grown tired of the dehydration and fasting leading up to weigh-ins — and the impact it had on his training and health — so he consulted with a performance team at Liverpool John Moores University in England to develop a plan for a 12-week training camp leading up to his next fight. The sport scientists were confident they could achieve the weight-loss target, but they were slightly concerned it might compromise too much lean muscle. How could they achieve his weight-making goal of 59 kilos (130 pounds) without any extreme weight-cutting strategies? They laid out a plan to gradually cut calories from his diet while also increasing the amount of energy he burned during training. Here's how they did it.

First, they calculated his resting metabolic rate (RMR) and energy expenditure for the running, training, and weight-lifting sessions the fighter would undertake, in order to determine his daily energy intake. The goal was to consistently lose 0.5–1.0 kilos per week (1.1–2.2 lb.) to make weight. To minimize the impacts of this caloric deficit on the fighter's lean muscle mass, they increased his daily protein intake to 2.0 g/kg (0.9 g/lb.) bodyweight.[54] The calorie cut would come from a combined reduction of both fat and carbs, and they aimed to keep his carb intake at 2.0–2.5 g/kg (0.9–1.14 g/lb.) daily to provide enough fuel for him to train effectively. The performance team acknowledged they might need to use a dehydration protocol to shed the last 1–2 kilos (2.2–4.4 lb.) to make weight, and if they did have to resort to it, they were confident he could recoup the lost hydration in the 30 hours before his fight.

How did the fighter respond to the new evidence-based regime? His initial reaction was worry — it was far more food than he was used to eating. As a result, he was regularly failing to finish all the food on his plate because this program was so different from his old regime and he was afraid the new approach wouldn't work. What happened over the next 12 weeks? The fighter steadily and consistently lost weight over the 12 weeks, shedding fat mass and maintaining a good deal of lean muscle as well. His outcome highlights the major gap between evidence-based and old-school nutrition approaches. An evidence-based approach to making weight resulted in a slow and steady loss of bodyweight over the 12-week period and the fighter successfully weighed in below 59 kg (130 lb.) before the fight (without using any harmful, old-school strategies). Scott Robinson, PhD, from England, a performance nutritionist to multiple world champion boxers, highlights the importance of evidence-based practices for fighters, stating that "using nutrition smartly enables fighters to be in the best possible condition throughout camp, and gain all of the possible advantages over their opposition before they step foot in the ring."

Of course, once the fighter makes weight, the job isn't done: the fighter still needs to fight! His fight weight is over 5 kg (10 lb.) heavier than his weight-making weight. This was achieved by dramatically ramping up his carb intake to 12 g/kg/day (5.45 g/lb.) from 2.5 g/kg (1.14 g/lb.) in the 30 hours before the fight, in order to replenish glycogen and bring on threefold the amount of water. The nutrition strategy evolves again post-weigh-in: You can't just eat as much food as possible. After a prolonged cutting phase, gut absorption rates are limited, and so fighters need a strategic approach. Traditionally, old-school refueling strategies would have fighters eating high-fat foods like ice cream, bacon, and sausages to ramp up their calories. Today, nutrition strategies are more evidence-informed. Post-weigh-in, liquid nutrition is implemented immediately. It typically consists of 20–30 g of protein, 50–60 g of simple carbs (for rapid absorption), and an electrolyte solution (to replace losses). Next, the athlete will continue to eat a low-fiber diet to avoid gastrointestinal aggravation, dramatically ramp up carbohydrate intake, and keep fats to a modest level. To rapidly replenish glycogen, fighters consume anywhere from 7–12 g/kg/day of carbs in the 24–32 hours before a fight. To achieve this intake, you need to rely on highly palatable, easily digested simple carbs. In this context, it's all about the fuel. A fighter will struggle to eat 10–12 cups of rice or oats to hit their carb targets, but this target is much easier to reach with processed and simple carbs, which is hard for many practitioners to wrap their heads around. Maximizing glycogen status is crucial for performance in combat sports because it's the primary fuel source during competition. Carbohydrates also confer performance benefits in addition to their impact on glycogen, such as buffering perception of fatigue.[55]

The elite super featherweight fighter also successfully weighed in without any dehydration protocols, the first time he has ever not had to rely on such a last-minute strategy. This has potentially huge implications for fight-night performance. A recent study in MMA fighters evaluated athlete hydration

## The Dangers of Old-School Water Loading

Old-school strategies die hard. Unfortunately, too many MMA fighters, boxers, jockeys, gymnasts, and others in aesthetic sports still use dangerous rapid weight-loss practices to make weight for competition.[57] A commonly used dehydration strategy is called water loading. Four days before a fight, the athlete consumes about 10 percent of their bodyweight in water. For example, an 80 kg (176 lb.) male would drink 8 liters (approximately 17 pints) of water in a day (an unimaginable amount!) and transition to a low-salt diet (1,000–1,500 mg/day). Next, 2 days out from the weigh-in, the fighter would then dramatically restrict water consumption down to about 1 liter (about 2 pints). Then, the day before the weigh-in, the athlete ramps water intake back up to a ridiculous 8 liters (17 pints) per day, combined with a high salt intake of about 4,000 mg. Finally, on the actual day of the weigh-in, the athlete consumes little to no fluids for 12+ hours. How does this lead to weight loss? When you drink too much water, your hypothalamus detects water levels in the blood rising too high and triggers the pituitary gland to reduce antidiuretic hormone (ADH) output, signaling your kidneys to increase your urine output. This is done in an attempt to restore balance to hydration status. This water-loading strategy effectively hijacks your brain's evolutionary drive to conserve water, meaning you begin to pee out large amounts of stored body water. It's not uncommon for a fighter to lose up to 7.5 kg in the week before a fight, a level so extreme that it can result in death. In fact, three collegiate wrestlers died attempting to make weight in the 1990s (the NCAA since changed the weigh-in rules around competition). Unfortunately, the practice still remains. It also creates an unfair playing field. Some athletes regain so much weight that they end up being 2–3 weight classes heavier than the opposition. Not only is this poor sporting spirit, but in a contact sport like MMA it creates a high-risk situation for head trauma and injury.

Changes are being made to safeguard athletes. The ONE Championship MMA organization has changed its rules to prevent athletes from dropping weight classes when they are 8 weeks out from competition, and the final weigh-in is performed 3 hours before the actual fight (encouraging safe practice). Also, both the NCAA and ONE require athletes to pass a urine-specific gravity test at the weigh-in so as to prevent them from using dehydration techniques to achieve their fighting weight. These are massive steps in the right direction and we can only hope they're more widely adopted by larger organizations like the UFC.

before competition — 32 hours after weighing in — using urine osmolality testing via a portable device called a refractive index osmometer (a fancy piece of lab equipment where you place a few drops of urine into it to assess hydration). When urine osmolality is between 250–700 mOsmol/kg the athlete is assumed to be hydrated. If the athlete is drinking too much water and is hyper-hydrated, the urine osmolality falls below 249 mOsmol/kg. If the athlete is dehydrated, the urine osmolality climbs to between 701–1080, and when severely dehydrated it is between 1081–1500 mOsmol/kg. What did researchers find in elite MMA fighters? Fifty-seven percent were still dehydrated going into the fight, and incredibly, the remaining 43 percent were severely dehydrated.[56] Dehydration has significant repercussions on their ability to perform. The evidence-based weight-making strategy used by the fighter involved no sweat suits, no water-loading protocols, and no ridiculous sauna regimens. By ramping up carb intake (with a high priority on total amount and a lower priority on quality), ensuring adequate protein and electrolyte intake, and minimizing fiber and fats in the 24–30 hours before the event, the fighter made weight and was in peak condition for his match. He had used an evidence-based nutrition program tailored to his needs. This is a revolution in weight-making nutrition.

## Assessing Body Composition: Pinching, Prodding, and Pulsing

If you're trying to get leaner, obtaining objective data via a body composition assessment can be highly valuable. Shawn Arent, PhD, from Rutgers

University highlights two key reasons why monitoring athlete body composition is important. The first is injury prevention (for example, heavier athletes put more strain on their joints). Second, assessing lean muscle mass helps to track losses during the athlete's season, which could compromise performance. How does an expert like Dr. Arent assess his athletes? There are several options. The most commonly used tools are dual-energy X-ray absorptiometry (DEXA), Bod Pod, skinfold calipers, and bioelectrical impedance (BIA). Each method has its pros and cons.

Let's start with DEXA. Often considered the closest to a gold standard today, its benefits include accuracy and its ability to assess bone density, fat-free mass, and fat mass (this is referred to as a three-compartment model). It's also really easy to use: athletes just lie down and get scanned. However, like all testing methods, there are still drawbacks with DEXA. It's costly, not easily accessible for most people, and it exposes clients to low doses of radiation (not ideal for regular monitoring). Despite what many practitioners might think, DEXA is not an infallible test and is still subject to confounders like client hydration status, glycogen, and muscle creatine status.[58]

Next, the options include the more commonly used two-compartment models that assess fat mass and fat-free mass: the Bod Pod, skinfold caliper testing, and BIA. Air displacement plethysmography, known simply as the Bod Pod, is used in high-performance clinics and is Dr. Arent's top choice to assess and monitor his athletes at Rutgers. It's quick, reliable, and emits no radiation, but it's important to note that it can underestimate body fat by 2–3 percent in athletes.[59] Most professional sports teams use DEXA or Bod Pod measurements throughout the year, as well as specialty medical or performance clinics.

Not everyone has access to these devices, and these lab-based methods aren't always practical when you work in the field. For coaches, trainers, and practitioners, skinfold calipers and BIA might be better tools. Skinfold calipers are relatively easy to use and give you a good idea of your client's lean mass and fat mass. Research in collegiate athletes shows calipers are a reliable method compared to Bod Pod and DEXA; however, there is an error rate of about +/-5 percent.[60] Also, the skill of the practitioner is very important. You need to control as many variables as possible when caliper testing: time of day, time away from recent training (8–12 hours), hydration status, and the like. If you're looking to add this tool to your toolbox, the International Society for the Advancement of Kinanthropometry (ISAK) is an international organization aimed at developing international standards for skinfold testing and anthropometric assessments, and it offers courses with accreditation.

Bioelectrical impedance (BIA) is another commonly used tool. BIA works by sending a current through the body and uses a mathematical equation to calculate FFM and FM based on the speed of the current. The error in body fat percent calculation can be quite high, up to 8 percent. The more expensive versions tend to be more reliable.[61] An interesting application of BIA currently being investigated by Dr. Arent and his team is the use of BIA to detect hydration status in different areas of the body. Depending on your sport, this could have important implications.

With so many tools to choose from, what method should you use? There is no universally superior method for body composition assessment.[62] Arent highlights it depends on you, your clients, and your environment. If you can only run a DEXA scan once a year and your client is trying to get leaner in 8–12 weeks, is it really going to help inform your strategy? Probably not. However, if you see a client every year and they're struggling with bone density concerns, then performing an annual DEXA might be a highly informative tool for monitoring progress. Arent emphasizes that *relative changes* (rather than achieving an absolute goal) via consistent monitoring is where you'll find the most practical data to inform your decision-making and nutrition plan. How does your athlete's result compare to last month or last year? How do they compare to other athletes in their sport or at their position? Answers to these questions can help flag clients who are not keeping up with the competition and also inform how you can modify an athlete nutrition and training plan to achieve their goals.

So do athletes need to be lean to perform? The answer to this question is all in the context. If you're a team sport athlete, being lean is not the be-all and end-all. If you're a bodybuilder, it's the ultimate goal. If you're a fighter or participate in a weight-making sport, achieving leanness while mitigating losses in muscle mass and performance is the delicate balance you try to achieve.

———

You've now learned the evidence-based fundamental principles of adding lean muscle, improving body composition, and making weight from leading world experts. In the next chapter, I'll discuss how to tailor nutrition strategies specific to endurance performance.

# CHAPTER 5

# Endurance Nutrition

F our eggs, smoked salmon, and a full avocado. It was the picture of breakfast, but not just anybody's breakfast, that sent the Twittersphere into a total frenzy. On July 19, 2016, Tour de France champion Chris Froome posted a picture of his breakfast on Twitter after completing stage 16 of the Tour. It wasn't what was on Froome's plate that created such a stir, it was what was noticeably absent — carbohydrates. The online blogosphere blew up with "Froome is low-carb, I told you so!"; "Not a lot of those energy-driving carbs"; and "Carbs are for suckers!" Incredibly, a single photo of a champion cyclist's breakfast — a snapshot in time — and the verdict was in (on the internet anyway). Was Chris Froome really following a low-carb diet during the Tour de France, where the average rider is consuming over 6,000 kcal per day? (That's a lot of avocados.) Was it a ruse to throw off the competition? Or perhaps was it part of a planned nutrition strategy to promote specific recovery adaptations? The revolution of endurance nutrition was underway. (Oh, by the way, Froome won the Tour de France title that year, and he won again in 2017.)

More than a century ago, sport scientists made an important discovery: Carbohydrates were a key fuel for exercise.[1] In 1939, researchers found carbohydrate utilization during exercise could improve your tolerance to training and be influenced by what you ate. By the 1960s, muscle glycogen's role as a key influencer during exercise was identified, and in the 1980s the first-ever studies emerged that concluded that carbs consumed during exercise improved performance.[2] This is a quick snapshot of what became the birth of nutritional sport science in the twentieth century, and which eventually led to a boom in the focus carbohydrates played in the 1980s and '90s to enhance endurance training. Endurance athletes began eating high-carb all the time, and supplemented this diet with carbs to optimize recovery and performance.

Today, the general nutrition recommendations from the American College of Sports Medicine (ACSM), the Academy of Nutrition and Dietetics, and the Dietitians of Canada is for endurance athletes to consume daily 1.2–2.0 g/kg of protein (divided evenly throughout the day), approximately 30 percent of total calories of fat, and 6–10 g of carbs for high-level endurance athletes.[3] This last recommendation, the amount of carbohydrate a high-level endurance athlete should consume, has been fueling a battle on social media between low-carb and high-carb (low-fat) advocates. (If you think people can get passionate about politics, nutrition isn't too far behind!) The low-carb proponents cite plenty of anecdotal evidence stating that limiting starches augments fat burning, delays glycogen usage, keeps blood sugars stable, and prevents bonking in the late stages of a competition (not to mention the often-cited improvements in digestive problems). While there are indeed benefits emerging in the research from deliberate periods of reduced carbohydrate availability to support positive endurance performance adaptations — such as mitochondrial biogenesis, increased lipid peroxidation, and superior resistance to fatigue — the battle cry in the blogosphere seems to be that carbs are for suckers.[4]

Ironically, in academia and high-performance circles the view is almost completely the opposite. Over 100 years of research in endurance sports has confirmed that carbs before training fuel performance, carbs during training improve performance, and carbs post-training support recovery by buffering exercise-induced increases in stress hormones and inflammatory markers, maintaining immune status, and replenishing muscle glycogen stores.[5] The foundations of sports nutrition have been cemented in the principle that adequate carbohydrate availability fuels winning in competition. Overwhelmingly, the last four decades of endurance sport research has confirmed without a doubt that high glycogen stores in muscle before a competition improve performance.[6] But how else do carbs fuel endurance performance? For one thing, carbohydrates consumed during exercise improve physical performance, cognitive function, and the technical elements of sport.[7] Carbs consumed during training spare muscle glycogen, liver glycogen, maintain blood glucose levels, and keep carbohydrate oxidation rates stable.[8] The research is clear that carbs are definitely highly effective after 60–90 minutes of intense exercise, but it also reveals benefits in bouts of less than 60 minutes via direct effects on the nervous system.[9] Incredibly, just rinsing your mouth with a liquid form of carbohydrates immediately (5–10 minutes) before exercise also elicits a performance boost.[10] Interestingly, this effect is even more pronounced if you follow a low-carb or keto approach, meaning it is not simply the result of sweetness or glycogen status.[11] For all of these reasons, elite endurance athletes are advised to eat 6–12 g/kg bodyweight in the 24–36 hours before a competition to maximize performance and therefore the odds of winning.[12] So the research is clear: Athletes need carbs to push the pedal to the metal on race day, as without it they sacrifice their top gear in competition. But should we take this as the last word? Maybe not. In the last decade, a growing body of research has highlighted the role of altering macronutrient availability around exercise and the impact it has on cellular-signaling pathways that control muscular adaptations to exercise.[13] Let's explore.

## Periodized Endurance Nutrition

In the early 2000s, a series of breakthroughs were made by sport scientists that marked the beginning of a new era in endurance nutrition research and application. Experts were discovering the concept of periodized nutrition, which is the strategic combination of exercise plus nutrition, or nutrition alone, to improve performance. Ironically, this wasn't even a new concept. World-leading expert endurance and nutrition researcher Asker Jeukendrup, PhD, from the Netherlands points out that in the 1800s, the term "training" encompassed both exercise and nutrition, and was defined as "the act of undertaking a course of exercise and diet in preparation for a sporting event." The research had come full circle (albeit today with a lot more depth and technology at its disposal). Jeukendrup describes periodized nutrition as a structured and planned process designed to enhance and maximize training adaptions. The quality and quantity of your food choices around exercise can make a difference when it comes to achieving your performance potential. Every athlete is accustomed to periodizing their training to maximize performance. Endurance coaches and sport scientists all apply the concept of periodization to achieve specific training outcomes, be it manipulating training intensity, types of exercise, duration, frequency, and so forth. This long-term progressive approach is designed to improve and optimize athletic performance by systematically altering training throughout the year. However, until recently not many were consciously and purposefully adjusting their endurance nutrition to amplify these training adaptations. The rules of the game are changing.

Once again, carbohydrates in particular are at center stage. They seem to be playing a pivotal role in influencing muscular and metabolic adaptations to exercise. But this is not an absolute high-carb or low-carb approach, which is what you almost exclusively read about online. This is about nuance. Amateurs talk low-carb or low-fat around exercise; experts talk carbohydrate availability around exercise. It might sound like the same thing, but it's very different. Altering carbohydrate availability triggers significant positive adaptations in athletes, and it was a potent trigger in Froome's championship performances. Let's take a closer look.

## Carbohydrate Availability: The Glycogen Training Regulator

Nutrition should be periodized and altered to support an athlete's individual goals, their training level, and their in-season versus off-season training requirements. This is the revolution in sports nutrition. James Morton, PhD, sport nutritionist for Team SKY (and four-time Tour de France champion Chris Froome), has been studying carbohydrate in athletes for over a decade. His recent work highlights new advances in cutting-edge molecular biology techniques that have kicked off a new era of "nutrient-gene" insights. One of the major findings is that muscle glycogen levels play a key role in adaptations to training, acting like a "training regulator," says Morton. In short, if you deliberately engage in training sessions with inadequate glycogen fuel stores, it can activate molecular pathways that promote muscle adaptations. This new "Train Low, Compete High" paradigm (more recently dubbed "carb periodization") has researchers giddy at the prospect of the plethora of potential training strategies for inducing adaptations that might elicit tangible performance gains.

Morton's work has been pivotal in Chris Froome's remarkable winning performances at the Tour de France. A common refrain used by Dr. Morton and his colleagues is to "fuel for the work required." Rather than always maximizing carb and glycogen stores 100 percent of the time, as was common practice (and still is for many), athletes and coaches manipulate the availability of carb around *specific* training sessions to enhance adaptations. Just like a strength coach altering the sets, reps, or cadence of a lift to exert a desired effect, practitioners can manipulate nutrition before, during, or after training sessions to potentially amplify gains. Dr. Morton's work suggests endurance athletes should periodically undergo training sessions (30–50 percent of the time) with reduced carbohydrate availability to trigger acute cell-signaling pathways that yield positive adaptations in skeletal muscle, and in some cases, improved exercise performance.[14] Interestingly, the evidence is accumulating so quickly that the recent Position Stand by the ACSM and Dietitians of Canada gives the same suggestion as an evidence-based strategy for supporting endurance performance. We know high-carb works, but the evidence is clear that altering carbohydrates can also enhance training effects. It's about *training day* nutrition strategies versus *race day* nutrition strategies; they aren't always the same thing.

How does training with reduced carbohydrate availability improve training adaptations? Let's take a look at a few of the most relevant pathways. (Take a deep breath, we're going down the rabbit hole.) When your muscle glycogen levels fall, it increases the internal cellular energy sensor AMPK, activating PGC-1 alpha that then enters the nucleus of the muscle cell and stimulates key mitochondrial proteins in the electron transport chain. In short, this is good news for your fitness. Also, low-carb availability acts as a "training regulator" when you exercise: it ramps up intramuscular fat usage as well as breaks down stored body fat via the increased production of adrenaline. This increases free fatty acids in your bloodstream and activates another signal in the nucleus of your cell called PPARs, increasing your ability to use fat as a fuel source (another win for endurance athletes). In fact, even a high-fat meal can alter PPAR signaling and upregulate genes with that enhanced fat breakdown. If you always start your slow, steady-state aerobic sessions with higher-carb meals, you'll downregulate AMPK and blunt the PPAR signaling effect. Periodizing carbs allows you to enhance training gains, regardless if you're recreational or elite.

Restricting carb availability to achieve these benefits comes in many different flavors. Let's look at three simple strategies used by top-level endurance athletes that the expert-generalist can add to their toolbox to help augment training adaptations. Remember, Train Low is defined as when an athlete trains with low-carb availability during or after exercise, or trains with low muscle glycogen or low liver glycogen (or some combination of the above).

### "Two-a-Day" Training

If you want to dip your toe into carb periodization and the impacts of manipulating your glycogen stores, performing two training sessions in 1 day is a great place to start (a common practice for triathletes and Ironman athletes). In this Train Low version, you perform an intense morning training session to strategically deplete glycogen, then purposefully restrict carb intake post-training and during the afternoon. Therefore, when you engage in your second training session in the afternoon, you'll begin the session with low muscle glycogen. Studies comparing training twice a day (performed every second day) versus training once daily found athletes experienced an increased utilization of both intramuscular and body fat for fuel, superior exercise capacity, and improved performance.[15] You then finish the day with a higher-carb dinner — adding rice, tubers, root vegetables, pasta, and the like — to top up glycogen stores. In this scenario, your glycogen status is lowered for 3–8 hours.

## Fasted Training

Fifty years ago, top-level French cyclists would commonly wake up, grab a quick espresso, and hit the road (after probably having a cigarette, too!). Today, researchers are uncovering some of the potential benefits — without the cigarette — of this training approach. Fasted training is another simple Train Low strategy you can add to your routine. After your dinner or last meal of the day (around 7–10 p.m.), wake up the next morning and train in the fasted state before you eat breakfast (caffeine, however, is allowed). In this scenario, your muscle glycogen will still be high but your liver glycogen levels will be low after the overnight fasting during sleep. In this scenario, free fatty acids and fat burning ramp up quickly, making it a nice potential strategy for morning aerobic sessions (a normal breakfast with carbohydrates is consumed post-training). Fasted exercise increases AMPK and post-exercise gene expression, and the really cool part is researchers have now found that consuming 20 g of whey (before or during) fasted training still allows for high-fat breakdown while improving muscle protein balance.[16] Win-win!

## Sleep Low, Train Low

In this periodized carb strategy, you perform an evening training session and then deliberately restrict carbohydrates in your post-training evening meal and overnight during sleep (this is the Sleep Low part). The following morning, you perform *another* fasted-exercise session, typically at an aerobic exercise pace to facilitate fat oxidation for fueling.[17] A recent study of elite triathletes and cyclists found that a Sleep Low fueling strategy improved overall cycling efficiency (3.1 percent), 20-km cycling time trial performance (3.2 percent), and 10-km running performance compared with traditional high-carb (all the time) approaches.[18] Sport scientists are still trying to define the Sleep Low, Train Low strategy more specifically, but in general, athletes who restrict carbs completely after the evening session (still eating protein and fat) typically have the best outcomes.

―――――――

In real-world scenarios, athletes are going to mix and match and likely incorporate multiple strategies, rather than just doing one in isolation. That said, if you're new to these Train Low strategies, it's recommended trialing them one at a time and seeing how you perform. If you're training for an Ironman or marathon, you might be training for 20–30 hours per week, and unfortunately, the studies to date have used programs of 10 hours or less per week. Endurance athletes also engage in different nutrition strategies (to induce a caloric deficit) to improve body composition in prep for a race. The Train Low strategies can be a nice method to help support these goals, as well as to promote helpful training adaptations. To date, experts can't yet say for certain whether carb periodization works due, specifically, to carb restriction or to the reduction in total energy intake itself (the two are tightly interconnected and are extremely difficult to tease out in studies). Individualized nutrition is another cornerstone of the new science around peak performance, so do some detective work and test-drive these evidence-based methods to inform your practice. Of course, you need to remember that training nutrition and race day nutrition are not the same thing. This is the notion of "Train Low, Compete High." Before we dive into treading this line, let's look at traditional (and not-so-traditional) fueling strategies during endurance exercise.

## Traditional (and Not-So-Traditional) Fueling During Endurance Exercise

The general recommendation by the American College of Sports Medicine (ACSM) is for endurance athletes to consume between 30–60 g of carbohydrates *during* exercise. This is a pretty wide range, and more important, this recommendation doesn't take into account the type of exercise (high-intensity versus aerobic session), the duration, or the level of the athlete. It's long been known that carbs during exercise can improve exercise capacity and performance.[21] During endurance exercise lasting longer than 2 hours, carbs clearly prevent hypoglycemia, help to maintain high rates of carb

## Can a 100-Percent Keto Diet
## Fuel Winning Performances?

If a ketogenic diet is the secret weapon to elite performance, then the best athletes, sport scientists, and evidence-based research should be loaded with examples of fat-adapted athletes dominating the competition, right? Not quite. The literature on elite athletes who are on keto diets is very sparse. Research by Louise Burke, PhD, head of sports nutrition at the Australian Institute of Sport, recently studied a collection of elite and Olympic racewalkers to determine if a ketogenic diet could improve performance. Twenty-one male racewalkers participated in the study that culminated in an official IAAF (International Association of Athletics Federation) competition. The participants were divided into three groups: high carb, periodized carb, and keto. They lived in residences where all of their meals and training were under strict supervision from the research team. The racewalkers performed precamp testing to assess the effects of the three-week dietary interventions. What did Burke and her team uncover? After three weeks of training, all three groups of racewalkers improved their aerobic fitness levels regardless of the assigned diet.[19] (Not surprising as they were all in a training camp setting.) The keto group did burn fat at higher rates during the competition, averaging approximately 1.5 g/min (on par with Stephen Phinney's early research in the 1980s). Sounds promising, but how did the keto group perform in the race? Did they beat the competition? Unfortunately not. Both the high-carb and the periodized-carb groups improved their race time — by 6.6 percent and 5.3 percent, respectively — while the keto group performed worse than their precamp testing. Another concern among the keto group was the increase in heart rate and perceived exertion.

So why does keto impair race-day performance? Renowned endurance expert Trent Stellingwerff, PhD, of the Canadian Sport

Institute Pacific, has found that chronic high-fat feedings down-regulate the main enzymes (pyruvate dehydrogenase complex, or PDH) responsible for burning carbs as a fuel source.[20] During a race, athletes are burning almost exclusively carbohydrates for fuel due to the intensity of the effort required to win. Therefore, if fat adaptation compromises your ability to burn carbs for fuel, you're going to sacrifice your top-end performance. In Burke's study, she found that exercise economy — the amount of oxygen an athlete uses to maintain a certain training intensity — was also impaired in the elite racewalkers following a high-fat keto diet. If it "costs" you more oxygen to run at the same speed, this is a problem for elite endurance athletes. There is cost-benefit to everything in life. For recreational exercisers, a keto approach can help improve body composition and fitness (typically via the caloric deficit and increased protein intake); however, if elite performance is your ultimate goal, then going exclusively 100 percent keto is not yet a proven winning strategy on race day.

oxidation, and increase exercise capacity (although some experts challenge this notion). It used to be thought that carbs were only good for these longer bouts of training, but this thinking has evolved. Carbs provide a benefit to shorter-duration, high-intensity endurance sessions (less than 1 hour), but via a completely different mechanism.

In order to determine if carbs can improve short-duration endurance performance, sport scientists decided to infuse glucose directly into the athletes' bloodstream to see if it would be absorbed at higher rates. They noticed the glucose was indeed taken into circulation more quickly, but interestingly had no actual impact on performance.[22] It didn't seem to make sense: If the glucose was being absorbed more readily but was not impacting performance, then how were carbs helping athletes during short, intense training sessions? The answer comes from new research that uncovered how the brain, and not just the conventional metabolic advantage, was triggering enhanced signals to working muscles.[23] Incredibly, simply *rinsing your mouth* with carbohydrate before training produces performance gains, and numerous studies have confirmed the benefits of "carb mouth-rinsing" on performance.[24] How does this not-so-traditional fueling strategy work? When you take your first bite of a meal or sip of a drink, about 50–100 taste buds light up to analyze the ingested food. The taste experience in your mouth gets relayed to your brain via a complex interplay of cranial nerves, the medulla, the thalamus, and finally the primary taste cortex of your brain.[25] There is also a link between these complex pathways and your emotional, cognitive, and behavioral response (further proof of the food-mood connection!).[26] Incredibly, the brain areas that get stimulated by carbohydrates are not impacted in any way by artificial sweeteners. (Perhaps this highlights the value of simple carbs throughout evolution, which were scarce.) But how does carb-rinsing impact performance outcomes? If your training session lasts from 30–60 minutes, mouth-rinsing with carbs can provide an amplified neural signal to muscles that might give you a potent performance edge.

Now let's look at the role of carbohydrates in longer bouts of endurance training. For example, if you're training up for an Ironman or ultramarathon, you'll definitely have many long sessions to get through to build up your fitness. Traditionally, it was thought you should only ingest one gram of carb per minute of exercise, up to a maximum dose of 60 g per hour. That was it. Of course, scientists also knew an athlete's ability to burn carbs was a limiting factor for performance, and so they tried to figure out how to get more carbs into the athlete's system. Your gut limits the absorption of carbs, and this effect is independent of body size. Back in 2004, sport scientists *paired* fructose together with glucose during training, and oxidation rates of carbohydrates jumped from 1 g/min. to 1.26 g/min.[27] This was a huge performance win. It didn't matter if it was from a gel, drink, or solid food — it worked every time.[28]

In longer training bouts, sport scientists found athletes could push the boundaries even further, especially during cycling. In one study, athletes who consumed 1.5 g/min. of a glucose-fructose drink (versus glucose alone) over the course of a 5-hour moderate-intensity training session experienced a rate of perceived exertion (RPE) that was much lower, and subsequently they were able to maintain a better cadence at the end of sessions.[29] (This traditional fueling strategy is almost the complete opposite of the Train Low strategies discussed previously.) In this scenario, you're literally trying to cram as much fuel as you possibly can into your system to support performance. Cyclists who performed a 2-hour steady-state bout of training followed by a 60-minute time trial experienced a 9 percent improvement in power by consuming a glucose-only drink, whereas another group ingesting a glucose-fructose mix drink achieved a 17 percent boost in power. This was the first study to show major benefits for glucose-fructose over glucose alone. Although there were definitely performance gains, pushing the ceiling of what the gut can absorb did lead to digestive discomfort among the riders. For endurance athletes, gut problems are common. Unfortunately, they're often thought of as an annoying part of the sport that you must simply learn to deal with. But is this the way it has to be? Or is there an alternative to this approach? (I'll dive deeper into this topic a little later on.)

Of course, researchers weren't finished yet. The big question they wanted to answer had to do with a dose-response relationship for carb intake during exercise. In other words, at what point does adding more carbs stop helping? Surprisingly, there are very few quality studies in endurance athletes. A study in 51 cyclists and triathletes attempted to nail down a more specific dose. They used 12 different combinations of carb drinks, ranging from 10–120 g of carbs per hour (in a 2:1 glucose to fructose ratio). Athletes performed a 2-hour steady-state moderate-intensity ride followed by a 20-km intense time trial. Once again, performance improved along with carbohydrate intake, with the greatest improvements at 60–80 g of carbs per hour (these findings are backed up by recent meta-analysis).[30] What does this look like in real-world competition scenarios? Sport scientists investigating Ironman competitors found that women took in 1 g/kg bodyweight per hour of carbs while men took in a little more at 1.1 g/kg/hour.[31] They also noticed Ironman competitors consumed the most carbs during the bike ride at 1.5 g/kg/hour, which is triple the amount compared to the run portion of the competition. Interestingly, how it impacted the bottom line varied: in men it correlated very highly with performance, while in women not so much.

A common question endurance athletes ask is this: Does my physical size impact my carb dose during training? The research says no. Remember, your gut is the limiting factor when it comes to absorption of simple sugars, and it is largely independent of your bodyweight. As such, the advice to athletes should be in total amounts (30 g of carbs per hour, for example) and not relative amounts based on body size. This is a really important distinction highlighted by the experts.

Of course, these recommendations depend on your ability, training intensity, and duration. If you run a marathon in 4 hours, should you be consuming carbs at the same rate as elite world-class athletes? Do you really need the same nutrition strategy as Kenyan Eliud Kipchoge — who recently smashed the world record for the fastest marathon at 2:01:39 in the 2018 Berlin Marathon — if you're a recreational runner trying to lose 10–20 pounds and improve your general health? Not a chance. Do you really need to fuel your cycling training like Chris Froome — multiple Tour de France champion with 8 percent body fat — while preparing for your next recreational cycling competition despite the fact you're carrying significant belly fat and have sore, achy knees? Not likely. When exercise intensity is low, the carbs you burn in training are also low. Your body burns carbohydrates at about the same rate between exercise intensities of 60–75 percent, which means the amount of carbs you need to ingest should be dialed down (often considerably) if weight loss, health, and longevity are your primary goals. Personalizing your nutrition to match your goals is absolutely crucial.

## Is Unconventional Fueling the Future of Endurance Sport?

In chapter 3, I introduced the work of Professor Paul Laursen and endurance coach Phil Maffetone and the incongruence they see in their practice while working with elite endurance athletes. They want to know how so many endurance athletes can be physically fit and yet still be unhealthy. Recall that the term *fitness* is defined as the ability to perform a specific exercise task, whereas the term *health* describes the state of well-being. High-level endurance athletes experience physical, biochemical, and mental-emotional injuries at alarmingly high rates, and Laursen and other leading sport scientists are studying why this is happening. There are many factors that contribute to health, and Professor Laursen and Coach Maffetone put forward two key areas they believe are heavily influencing the increased incidence of poor health among endurance athletes (and thus the greater likelihood for overtraining syndrome): inappropriate training intensity and the modern processed diet.

Laursen and Maffetone note that diets high in refined sugars and carbs from processed foods quickly lead to chronically high blood sugars and impaired fat oxidation in the body, the end result being a dramatic increase in inflammation, pain, and the production of reactive oxygen species (ROS).[34] They believe the modern processed diet heavily contributes to this pro-inflammatory state and argue this state of chronic inflammation is synonymous with poor health (something endurance athletes are certainly

## Hydration: Should You Drink to Thirst?

Dehydration can impact your performance. Today, experts know fluid deficits as little as 2 percent bodyweight can compromise cognitive function and aerobic exercise, 3–5 percent dehydration can impair sport-specific technical skills and anaerobic output, and severe dehydration at 6–10 percent bodyweight can decrease cardiac output, sweat production, and blood flow to muscles. Rewind back to the 1960s when drinking water during a marathon was seen as a sign of weakness. Your opponent would pounce on the opportunity to up their pace and leave you in the dust. By the late 1970s, the science on hydration had evolved. Then over the next few years something strange started happening: runners were getting sick, sometimes dangerously sick. They were drinking water to excess. The term is *hyponatremia*, and sadly endurance athletes have died in competitions as a result. Meanwhile, renowned South African sport scientist and emeritus professor Tim Noakes of the University of Cape Town was leading the boom in research on the importance of adequate hydration for performance. As Noakes and colleagues scrambled to uncover why this was happening, they discovered that a small group of individuals were genetically predisposed to problems if they drank too much water. For most people, if they drink too much water they begin to urinate much more frequently. Because it's an annoying and undesirable side effect, most people simply adjust their intake unconsciously. In individuals who over-secrete the powerful antidiuretic hormone (ADH), this doesn't happen and they become overly hydrated.[32] Due to the exaggerated output of ADH, their brain acts as if they're dehydrated, pumping out more and more ADH until they eventually stop urinating completely (and if they do urinate, it's dark yellow or brown). These people then assume (mistakenly) that they're dehydrated and decide to drink more water. This is when things turn deadly. Blood levels of sodium start to drop and water moves into the brain, causing swelling and loss of consciousness. They effectively become waterlogged. It's an avoidable situation that only impacts one out of five people. Because the consequences are potentially fatal, the American College of Sports Medicine (ACSM) changed their position in 2007 to recommend recreational athletes "drink to thirst" (and not ahead of thirst) to avoid this tragic outcome. If you want to personalize your hydration strategy, a simple "weigh-in" and "weigh-out" before and after training can help estimate the amount of fluid you should be consuming. Typically, a loss of 1 kg bodyweight (2.2 lb.) represents approximately 1 L (about 2 pints) of fluid loss. Most athletes will consume between 0.4–0.8 L/hour during exercise and will hydrate a little more aggressively post-training or postgame at 1.25–1.5 L for every 1 kg bodyweight lost.[33]

not immune to). Excessive training, high stress levels (physical, mental, or emotional), too many simple sugars, a modern diet high in omega-6 fats, and too much alcohol can all contribute to the chronic inflammatory load.[35]

On the training side of things, while acute inflammation is a necessary and essential signal to trigger positive adaptations to training, if the endurance athlete is engaging in training sessions at inappropriately high intensities or volumes (or both), it can create a terrain of systemic inflammation, increased ROS, and compromised nervous system function. Ultimately, all this inflammatory "noise" drowns out the signals that drive positive adaptation and change, leaving athletes struggling to recover and perform. When combined with a diet high in processed and refined foods, the noise is amplified further, perpetuating maladaptation and poor athlete health.

Laursen and Maffetone also note the wide variety of physical, biochemical, and mental-emotional injuries that endurance athletes experience. Adverse physical effects like persistent fatigue, maximal and submaximal performance decrements, chronic muscle soreness and stiffness, abnormally low resting heart rate, and altered heart rate variability (HRV) are common findings. Disease conditions like asthma, thyroid and adrenal dysfunction, diabetes (type 2), iron deficiency, and hypertension are also seen. Adverse biochemical effects of excessive oxidative stress and damage, compromised immunity, systemic inflammation, and hormone balance are also common signs of overtraining syndrome (OTS), or as Laursen and Maffetone postulate, of an athlete who is in poor health. Finally, mental-emotional symptoms such as depression, anxiety, loss of motivation, impaired concentration, and disrupted mood are also symptoms of OTS, which is seen in much higher rates in endurance athletes compared to strength and team sport athletes (more on this in Part Three: Recovery). Laursen and Maffetone sum things up succinctly: "For optimal performance, athletes must be fit and healthy."

Professor Laursen is part of an emerging group of elite and renowned endurance sport scientists — which includes expert physiologist Daniel Plews, PhD, who over the past decade supported numerous New Zealand athletes who won Olympic medals in the 2012 and 2016 Games — who are challenging the traditional dogma in endurance sport circles that high levels of carbohydrate are required for athletes to perform at their best. Their findings reveal that athletes who fuel many of their training sessions with far less simple sugar while maintaining training performance should experience better health. Laursen and Plews, who have over 150 peer-reviewed scientific publications between them, believe there is a middle ground. In fact, they even go so far as to say that "there is no need to maintain high blood glucose levels during endurance exercise, as we've been told in the past." Typically, the further you aim down the path toward elite performance, the further you get away from health. Laursen and Plews are trying to close that gap.

How did Professor Laursen and Dr. Plews get interested in this type of approach? The balance of health, longevity, and athletic performance was a major driver, but they were also influenced by the observations they made from experimenting with continuous glucose monitors (CGMs) on themselves. It opened Laursen's eyes to the significant interindividual differences in nutritional responses and what the body was capable of doing at supposedly "hypoglycemic" blood glucose states. Laursen was able to maintain performance on rides of 3 hours or more, with power outputs of 250–300 watts, at blood glucose levels below 3 mmol/L (considered hypoglycemic). Remarkably, Laursen felt great during those sessions. He said, "It's amazing how low blood glucose can actually get, and you still maintain performance, once you're better fat-adapted." Laursen has also noticed larger spikes of glucose and longer clearance rates in himself compared to other endurance colleagues, as well as how some "healthy" foods such as fruit can spike glucose levels to the point it looks like he's just eaten a bag of candy.

Stress was another eye-opener for Laursen and Plews. High-intensity training sessions can have lasting effects on blood glucose levels, something Plews noticed in his own training. Early on in his CGM experimentation, after performing a short 14-minute time trial, Plews immediately noticed the reading from his CGM monitor spiked up to 8.9 mmol/L upon completion of the session. For Plews, this was a very high reading. But even more concerning for him was the amount of time it took to return to baseline. His research and experience of coaching elite athletes highlighted the heavy toll high-intensity training inflicts on endurance athletes. It was hard for him not to imagine how other stressors in life — lack of sleep, deadlines at work, family concerns, and the like — coupled with the training could stack up and exacerbate this effect.

Intense training, if not properly periodized and planned, could be a recovery roadblock for endurance athletes. If you want to assess the impact of high-intensity training but don't have access to a CGM device or find it too cost-prohibitive, the next best method is to measure your morning fasted glucose. Dr. Plews says athletes should aim for levels below 90 mg/dL (5.0 mmol/L) daily upon rising. In chapter 3, you learned if longevity is your goal, then a low fasting blood glucose is also a potentially powerful marker for healthspan. General daily targets for average blood glucose range from 90 to 95 mg/dL (5.0–5.3 mmol/L) with a variance of <10 mg/dL (0.5 mmol/L). In short, you're looking for steady levels with as little fluctuation as possible (no rollercoaster-ride blood sugar responses).

Of course, high-intensity interval training plays a big role in the training plan of most endurance athletes. Because carbs are crucial for exercise at high intensity, athletes are wary to limit them before such sessions. New research by Laursen, Plews, and colleagues challenges this premise in recreational cyclists. Initially, when endurance athletes reduce carbohydrate intake, muscle and liver glycogen stores fall in the first few days. The effect of reduced glycogen, without an improved capacity to burn fat, has been shown to impair performance, reducing both prolonged submaximal and high-intensity efforts.[36] It seems obvious, then, that if you reduce carbs, you're going to impair high-intensity performance. However, until recently no long-term studies on carb restriction and HIIT training had been performed. Laursen and Plews recruited 18 moderately trained men who were divided into two dietary groups. One was a keto group and one was a standard mixed-diet group. The participants performed a graded exercise test before and after the study, as well as HIIT sessions — five sets of 3-minute sprints with 90 seconds rests in between — before the intervention. The tests were given again after two and four weeks. How did the keto group hold up against the other group who consumed carbs before the HIIT training sessions? They observed no difference in psychological or physiological response to HIIT. Athletes in the keto group had the same $VO_2$, heart rate, and perceived exertion compared to the other group, who consumed a higher-carb diet.[37] Plews and Laursen found no evidence that high-intensity performance was compromised in the latter stages of the graded exercise test or in the HIIT sessions. This is highly encouraging for recreational cyclists who often are trying to lose weight and improve their health while they train for an event or competition.

In clinical practice, I see a lot of clients in their 40s, 50s, or 60s transition into cycling to ease the pounding on their joints, but have fueling strategies that leave them stuck carrying 10–20 pounds of extra bodyweight (despite being aerobically "fit"). They also often have chronically elevated blood glucose levels (high HbA1c), inflammatory markers (CRP-hs), and low hormone status (free testosterone, free T3, and free cortisol). These trends are commonly accompanied by low energy (particularly in the morning), an inability to lose weight, poor sleep, and strong sugar cravings. Worse yet, increased HbA1c and CRP-hs levels are associated with increased risk of all-cause mortality. Recreational athletes aren't getting paid to perform. They exercise for enjoyment and health. Surely nutrition strategies should support these end goals.

On the other hand, if you're a professional endurance athlete earning a living from your sport or an elite recreational one aiming for a new personal best — and if you don't struggle with GI complaints or experience poor recovery with your current fueling strategies — a low-carb or keto strategy might not be worth the effort. Elite endurance athletes might be interested in this concept, but if it doesn't support elite performance then there is no reason to adopt it. Of course, Laursen and Plews coach world-class endurance athletes such as Kyle Buckingham and Jan van Berkel, who've placed in the top five in the world in Ironman competitions. In fact, being "elite" confers added advantages with this approach, because fat oxidation rates are three times higher in elite versus recreational athletes who adopt more low-carb availability for their training sessions.[38] Elite endurance athletes increased fat oxidation by 75 percent when exercise was performed after a morning bout with a fasted recovery compared to fasting alone (recall the Train Low strategies). The dietary guidelines from the American College of Sports Medicine, the Academy of Nutrition and Dietetics, and the Dietitians of Canada recommend that endurance athletes consume 6–10 g/kg/day when performing 1–3 hours of moderate- to high-intensity training. For endurance athletes who struggle with traditional fueling strategies — whether it's poor blood glucose control, digestive problems, or persistent inflammation — or as athletes get older and glucose control naturally tends to worsen, this new paradigm of endurance nutrition might be a valuable alternative for improvements in health, performance, and longevity.

How long does it take to adapt to a low-carb approach? When recreational athletes are given a full four weeks to transition to a ketogenic diet, for example, they can maintain work outputs at higher intensities.[39] A recent study involving a 12-week adaptation period before a 100-km cycling time trial found improvements in both peak and relative power (during a 6-second sprint and critical power test), while performance was maintained over the 100-km race.[40] Does this mean everyone should adopt a keto or low-carb approach for endurance sports? Of course not. But Laursen is quick to point out the traditional strategy of high-carb fueling doesn't work for everyone, and he believes it's a major root cause of the high incidence of gastrointestinal complaints, maladaptation, and overtraining in endurance athletes. Make no mistake, the research is clear: Traditional endurance fueling strategies work, and elite athletes follow them for a reason — because they want to win! The question for Laursen and Plews is "at what cost" to the athlete. For recreational (as well as elite) endurance athletes, this is very important question to ponder.

All of this said, when it comes to race day the rules of the game change. Again, context matters. While the traditional endurance nutrition and low-carb availability camps disagree on the best strategies to fuel *training* nutrition, they agree that *race day* nutrition requires adequate carbohydrates to maximize performance. Remember, training nutrition and race day nutrition are not the same thing. This is the concept of Train Low, Compete High, which I introduced earlier in the chapter. Competing high refers to your carbohydrate availability on race day, because carbs are crucial for prolonged maximal efforts during competition. As Plews says, "You've got to treat your body like a rental car on race day!" What's his strategy? Three days out from competition he increases his carb intake up to 150 g, then he

## Body Composition Periodization: The Evolution of Endurance Performance

Trent Stellingwerff, PhD, from the Canadian Sport Institute Pacific, has been working in elite endurance sports for well over a decade, supporting elite endurance athletes in numerous Olympic Games, including his wife Hilary. In 2017, Stellingwerff shared data of his wife's body composition fluctuations over her nine-year career as an elite middle-distance runner, during which she competed in two Olympic games.[41] Contrary to popular belief and pictures in magazines, Hilary was not always ultra-lean and in competition shape year-round (see figure 5.1).

As competitions got closer, she got leaner to support performance; as she moved into off-seasons, she didn't chase the same

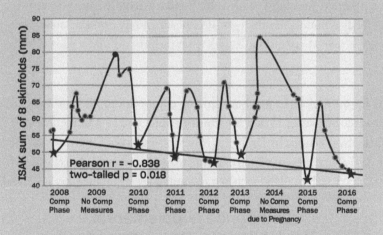

**FIGURE 5.1.** Anthropometric data over a 9-year career. International Society for the Advancement of Kinanthropometry sum of standard 8 skinfolds in mm. Star indicates the lowest sum of 8 during each peak competition season. White zones indicate yearly competition phase (May to August, yearly). Trent Stellingwerff, "Case-study: Body composition periodization in an Olympic-level female middle-distance runner over a 9-year career," *International Journal of Sport Nutrition and Exercise Metabolism* 28, no. 4 (2018), https://doi.org/10.1123/ijsnem.2017-0312.

level of leanness. How did she achieve this periodized body composition success? Stellingwerff implemented a planned and strategic nutrition strategy to support health and optimize performance. Hilary did not dramatically cut calories, but patiently and strategically dropped her caloric intake in the buildup to her big events. This strategy, which included ramping up protein intake as she trimmed calories, allowed Hilary to maintain her muscle mass as she peaked for competition. In a sport like running, where bodyweight accounts for 80 percent of the metabolic cost, maintaining muscle while getting leaner is a big advantage. This enabled her to achieve an ultra-lean physique without compromising health, menstrual function, immunity, and injury risk. Perhaps most interesting of all, her total bodyweight didn't fluctuate very much (always around 152 pounds) over the nine-year span, but her level of leanness dramatically changed. Consistency, patience, and hard work is how Hilary achieved her successful body composition changes. It's not the trendy or "sexy" new diet you read about online, but it's what the pros do, and it works!

aims for 60 g of carbs per hour during competition. He definitely feels it afterward, but says, "When it's winning time, you've gotta go for it!" This philosophy is echoed by Dr. James Morton who says, "Carbs are still king on race day." Regardless of which endurance fueling strategy you choose, ensuring optimal carb availability when the gun goes off on race day is crucial.

## Endurance Supplements: Harder, Better, Faster, Stronger

For athletes pushing the limits of performance, supplements can make the difference between reaching the podium and finishing in the pack. The International Olympic Committee (IOC) recently brought together leading experts from around the globe who subsequently issued a consensus statement regarding supplements. Only six supplements made their list for performance benefit. In this section, let's take a closer look at some evidence-based supplements that support endurance performance, as well as a new kid on the block that has some potential.

## CAFFEINE: YOUR GENES MATTER

The most widely consumed drug on the planet is caffeine. Trimethylxanthine, the chemical name for caffeine, is a naturally occurring compound in plant foods. It has been consumed for many centuries across cultures all over the world to increase alertness, well-being, and work capacity. Today, about 90 percent of adults regularly consume caffeine from coffee, tea, soda pop, or energy drinks. But how does caffeine work to improve endurance performance? Incredibly, experts still aren't totally sure. Stuart Phillips, PhD, from McMaster University in Canada says the old theory centered on caffeine's ability to break down body fat for fuel, thus sparing glycogen. This was thought to be the primary driver of caffeine's ergogenic benefits. Today, research shows caffeine's direct impacts on muscle tissue, and perhaps most important, its impact on the central nervous system. Caffeine can reduce the perception of effort, fatigue, and pain associated with exercise.[42] This is a big win for long, grueling bouts of endurance training. Caffeine might also allow athletes to push harder during key training sessions, thereby enhancing training outcomes.[43] What dose is ideal for endurance athletes? New research shows your genes might hold the answer.

Nanci Guest, PhD, at the University of Toronto recently conducted a study to determine whether the type of CYP1A2 gene you possess — the gene responsible for metabolizing caffeine — impacts performance effects in endurance athletes. More than a hundred male athletes participated in her study. They completed a time trial under three conditions: no caffeine and 2 mg of caffeine and 4 mg of caffeine per kilogram bodyweight.[44] Incredibly, the variation in the CYP1A2 gene could predict performance outcome. For example, the AC genotype showed no impacts of caffeine on endurance performance, whereas the AA genotype showed benefits at both 2 mg and 4 mg doses. But perhaps the most interesting and surprising finding in her study was that at a 4 mg/kg dose, athletes with a CC genotype performed *worse* with the caffeine. This was the first time it had been shown that genes might predict a response to caffeine as it relates to endurance performance. Guest recommends athletes get screened for the CYP1A2 so that they can make a more informed decision about whether caffeine can help their endurance performance.

## BEETS: THE PURPLE POWER

It's been almost a decade since beet juice was first identified as a performance aid. The inorganic nitrates present in beetroots, abundant in all leafy greens as well, get converted in the body to nitrite. When oxygen levels are low in the bloodstream, as during prolonged exercise, nitrites get converted into nitric oxide (NO), which is a potent vasodilator. Supplementation with dietary nitrates like beet juice also reduce the oxygen cost of training during submaximal exercise, potentially enhancing an athlete's exercise tolerance and performance.[45] Thus, the nitrate-nitrite-NO pathway is garnering a lot of interest in sports, nutrition, and medicine. How many dietary nitrates do you get in your food? Spinach, arugula, beetroots, and celery contain about 250 mg of dietary nitrates per 100 g of fresh weight. Acute doses of 500 mg of dietary nitrates taken 2.5 hours before exercise, as well as longer-term daily consumption over the course of 6 days, has been shown to increase plasma nitrite concentrations and ultimately increase the capacity of the nitrate-nitrite-NO pathway to produce nitric oxide (NO).[46] Experts believe enhancing this NO availability is responsible for improved exercise capacity via a number of mechanisms, such as regulation of blood flow, contractility, glucose and calcium balance, and mitochondrial respiration and biogenesis.[47]

How long does it take the beetroots or leafy greens to hit maximum levels in your bloodstream? Dietary nitrates peak after 1–2 hours and the downstream nitrites peak about 2–3 hours before everything returns back to baseline after 24 hours. Dietary nitrates might also be a big win for recreational athletes who need to correct high blood pressure, as the added nitric oxide is a potent vasodilator. Recreational athletes seem to get the biggest bang for their buck with dietary nitrates, as elite athletes appear less responsive to nitrate supplementation protocols. Experts believe this could be due to the greater dietary intake of highly trained athletes, their greater capacity to produce NO, or simply because elite athletes have better genetics and so are better able to enhance oxygen delivery (it's also worth mentioning that there is a very small margin for improvement in truly elite athletes). A shortcoming of many of the beetroot studies is that they're mainly timed-to-exhaustion and incremental tests, which are valuable scientifically (and highlight exercise capacity) but don't tell us much about performance. These studies also make the results look more impressive than they really are. For example, a 15 percent improvement in time-to-exhaustion might only translate to a 1 percent improvement in a time trial performance. That said, a 1 percent improvement could be the difference between winning and losing.

## Sodium Bicarbonate: The Poor Man's Performance Edge

Baking soda. As unlikely as it might seem, the stuff you use to keep your fridge smelling fresh has consistently shown, year after year, to improve endurance performance. When training kicks up into that glycolytic "burning" gear, the accumulation of hydrogen ions build up in the muscle, leading to the burning sensation that makes it very difficult to keep pushing hard through the session. Sustained efforts of 1–7 minutes, repeated sprints, or longer 30–60-minute sustained efforts just below the lactate threshold might all potentially benefit from the addition of sodium bicarbonate.[48] Traditionally, athletes will take 300 mg/kg bodyweight of bicarbonate dissolved in water 1–2 hours before exercise. This dose provides a modest 1–2 percent bump in performance, but at a high level that bump can make all the difference in the world. Sodium bicarbonate is cheap and it works. Just make sure you test it out, as it can cause GI upset, so you need to dial in your personalized dose. Dividing up the doses and consuming it with a snack or small meal seems to help manage the adverse symptoms.[49]

## Vitamin D and Other Supplements to Consider

Professor Graeme Close, PhD, and his team at Liverpool John Moores University were one of the first to investigate the effects of vitamin D on athletic performance. Athletes deficient in vitamin D showed signs of impaired muscle function, impaired muscle regeneration, and impaired immunity. These are important concerns for endurance athletes as well. The Endocrine Society has defined sufficient vitamin D levels as 75 nmol/L (30 ng/mL), insufficient levels between 51–74 nmol/L, and deficiency as less than 50 nmol/L (20 ng/mL). The deficiency states can be further categorized as mild (25–50 nmol/L or 10–20 ng/mL), moderate (12.5–25 nmol/L or 5–10 ng/mL), or severe (less than 12.5 nmol/L or 5 ng/mL). The big question that researchers such as Dr. Close are trying to answer is this: Does vitamin D provide a performance benefit if you're not deficient? Ensuring that vitamin D status is above 75 nmol/L appears to be important for muscular (satellite cell) recovery, while new research shows a potential enhanced effect at vitamin D levels above 120 nmol/L. Because endurance athletes are highly prone to illness, maintaining a higher vitamin D status could be an important factor to consider to prevent illness. The recommendation from Dr. Close and his team is to get your vitamin D from the sun, and in the winter months (or if deficient) aim for a supplement of 2,000–4,000 IU per day.[50]

## Antioxidant Supplements and Problems with Putting Out the Fire

Inflammation and reactive oxygen species (ROS) are essential and necessary signals to trigger adaptations to training — the adaptations you need to get stronger, fitter, and faster. It's now well recognized in research that taking antioxidant supplements post-training reduces ROS levels and blunts exercise adaptations.[52] In short, never take antioxidant supplements after you train. Context is everything. Inflammation and increased ROS are essential for the right signals to be sent so that you can get the most from your training sessions. But taken at the wrong time, antioxidant supplements blunt both training adaptation and some of the health benefits of exercise. For example, resveratrol supplementation after HIIT training in older men not only blunted the increase in maximal oxygen uptake but also reduced the effects of the exercise to reduce LDL and triglyceride concentrations in the blood.[53] Most important, there is no data to date to suggest that eating high-quality fruit and vegetables attenuates adaptations to exercise. The best advice for athletes is to consume a high-quality diet and to avoid a megadosing of antioxidant supplements.[54]

### NICOTINAMIDE RIBOSIDE (NR)

Niacin, commonly known as vitamin $B_3$, is naturally found in meat, poultry, fish, eggs, and green veggies. Niacin is actually a combination of nicotinic acid and nicotinamide. A novel supplement called nicotinamide riboside features a particular form of niacin that contains a pyridine-nucleotide (a ribose bond). You can think of it like a different flavor of niacin. What does this new flavor mean for endurance performance? Nicotinamide riboside is a direct precursor for NAD synthesis in your muscle, and therefore could potentially impact your muscles' mitochondrial function via key signaling pathways (NAD-SIRT1-PGC-1alpha, for those scoring at home).[51] Recall that PGC-1alpha is the master switch for triggering training adaptations. Thus, researchers believe if nicotinamide riboside supplements are capable of altering the amount of NAD in the muscle, then this could increase mitochondria in your muscles as well. More mitochondria, means more oxygen — a big win for endurance athletes! Research is still in the early days — all the studies being done in mice, not humans — but this could be the next wave of supplements.

———

Now you've dialed in your endurance nutrition to help you achieve your personal best or prepare for an upcoming season with personal health as a cornerstone. In the next chapter, I'll dive into team sport athletes and all the different aspects to consider: training camp nutrition, in-season, halftime, and playoffs. Let's do it!

# CHAPTER 6

# Team Sport Nutrition

In 1996, when Arsène Wenger took over as manager of the legendary Arsenal FC, he was dubbed "Mr. Nobody." With his spectacles, the relatively unknown Frenchman looked more like a schoolteacher than a soccer coach. He was attacked by the media for being odd, arrogant, and reclusive. Even his players openly wondered: What does this guy *really* know about soccer? If only they knew what was to come. From the outset, Wenger put his fingerprints on every aspect of the team. He brought in sport scientists, nutrition experts, and highly qualified conditioning personnel — the first of their kind in Arsenal history. He brought in this support staff 20 years before anyone else (they're now a mainstay of every Premier League team). Wenger's training was different, too; sessions were sharper, more organized, and more efficient. Gone were the brutal morning runs and repetitive practice sessions. Everything was timed to the minute. Wenger's take on nutrition was also very different (at the time). Prematch meals, which had previously consisted largely of burgers and french fries, were replaced with fish, small plates of pasta, and steamed vegetables. Vitamin supplements, creatine, cod liver oil, and postgame recovery drinks were added to the players' daily regime. Gone were all the beer and processed snacks in the players' lounge. (Wenger famously banned the Gunners' pregame ritual of Mars chocolate bars in his first year, triggering a revolt that quickly softened as the players won game after game.) Wenger strongly believed "if a player does not have a healthy diet, they will not be able to train as hard, will struggle to improve their play and be more susceptible to tiredness." How did his team fare? Arsenal won the Premier League title in 1997–98, Wenger's second year in charge, along with the FA Cup that same season (known as "The Double"). In 2001–02, they won both the League and FA Cup again before making history in 2003–04 with the first undefeated season in over a century. Arsène

Wenger was two decades ahead of the competition on the team sport nutrition front, and he ushered in a new era of evidence-based science practices.

Sport nutrition has its roots in endurance sport. An athlete training on a stationary bike or treadmill provides the sport scientist with the ideal scenario to test, measure, and assess countless performance and recovery biomarkers. It's a sport scientist's dream. In team sports, things are much more dynamic and unpredictable. There are no direct correlations between an athlete's heart rate, lactate threshold, VO₂ max, and whether they'll be elite in their sport. In the last decade, the emphasis on nutrition in team sports has exploded. Baseball teams, including the Los Angeles Dodgers, are implementing 100 percent organic food policies throughout the organization; NBA teams, including the Philadelphia 76ers, spend millions of dollars on new kitchen facilities and top-flight chefs; NFL teams spare no expenses to ensure all food and supplements are available 24/7 to players; and world-class footballers such as Cristiano Ronaldo not only employ a full-time chef but also a full-time nutritionist to direct the nutrition plan. It's obvious that team sport nutrition has dramatically shifted in the last decade.

The nutrition demands of team sports are very different from the demands of physique and endurance sports. Similarly, you don't often see elite, best-in-the-world team sport athletes with the same muscular development you would see in a bodybuilder. Tom Brady doesn't *need* to have a six pack to be the best quarterback in the world. In fact, you could argue being *too* lean would compromise his ability to take a hit and perform. Clayton Kershaw doesn't need huge biceps to throw the nastiest fastball and cutter in Major League Baseball. The best hockey players in the world look more like lumberjacks than supermodels, because they need to be skillful, to absorb contact, and to initiate it. Differences aside, should an athlete's nutrition be the same in preseason compared to in-season? How about during halftime breaks or in compressed schedules like the playoffs, when athletes are tired after a long, grueling season but need to perform their best? Different context, different goals, different nutrition strategies.

Energy balance is the "biggest rock" when it comes to driving anabolism or catabolism. Therefore, an athlete who tries to get too lean or who simply does not eat enough food is treading a fine line and is at increased risk of fatigue, weakness, illness, and injury (to name only a few). Furthermore, being leaner might not, in fact, provide a physical, technical, tactical, or psychological advantage for the athlete. In order to support a team sport athlete, you need to understand the energy systems used in their specific sport as well as the common fueling strategies athletes follow so as to uncover the gaps or opportunities to support the athlete's performance, recovery, and health.

## Lessons from "The Beautiful Game"

Football is the most popular sport in the world. And I'm not talking about the North American version with helmets and pads, I'm talking about soccer — "the beautiful game" that the rest of the world calls football (and rightfully so!). Soccer is classified as an intermittent and high-intensity skill-based sport — it's got brief sprints, high-intensity running, jumps, and tackles that require high-energy fueling and longer recovery times that potentially expose athletes to exhaustion.[1] (Similar demands are placed on basketball and hockey players, although hockey probably falls somewhere between a skill-based sport and a power-sport, such as American football and rugby.) What energy systems are required to fuel these demands? The rapid and explosive alactic phosphocreatine system is needed so that the player can jump high in the air for a header or dive to make a tackle; the alactic glycolytic system is needed so that the player can sprint and chase attacking players down the field; and the aerobic system is needed so that the player can log all those miles in between games and during the game. In short, all of the energy systems are needed! Team sports call into play all energy systems, though, depending on the game, some systems are emphasized more than others. Skill-based sports like basketball and soccer also require a high demand of technical proficiency that is learned through countless hours of practice.

The physical demands of soccer players vary depending on position, training status, and specific tactical roles.[2] This same theme applies to the big four American sports: football, basketball, hockey, and baseball. An athlete's energy expenditure is largely dictated by their training load: a hard day of sprints is far more taxing on the body than a light day of jogging during a tactical practice. This must be taken into account by the practitioner when planning nutrition strategy for the week.[3] Soccer players are going to require a lot more fuel to get through a 1-hour practice (let alone a 2–3 hour session) compared to a bodybuilder training in the gym for an hour. Explosive movements require rapid ATP turnover, long sprints require clearance of acidic cellular metabolites, and aerobic activity demands high amounts of fatty acids in the bloodstream. Team sport athletes exert a lot of energy running, cutting, and absorbing contact against the opposition.

Maintaining this work output while fighting off fatigue is strongly associated with the depletion of muscle glycogen, making glycogen status in
the lead-up to competition an athlete's top priority. In addition, athletes
must have all the different fuel sources on board so that they can compete
at their best. Unfortunately, there is very little information on what elite
team sport athletes eat throughout the day. For example, despite over 40
years of research in high-level soccer only recently have experts been able
to get a glimpse of what professional players consume on a daily basis in real
time. In 2017, Liam Anderson, PhD, from England and his group attempted
to uncover for the first time the energy intake and expenditure in professional
soccer players in the English Premier League (EPL). Using state-of-the-art
technology like DEXA scans to assess body composition, doubly labeled
water isotopes to assess energy expenditure, remote food photographic
method (RFPM) to assess food intake, and GPS devices to assess training and
game-day load, researchers were able to get a real glimpse into the real-life
demands of elite professional athletes in the field (not just the lab). Here's
what they found. The caloric intake of players was much *lower* throughout
the week compared to game days, approximately 2,950 kcal to 3,800 kcal
respectively[4] (see figure 6.1). Why such a dramatic difference? It wasn't due
to the players' protein and fat intakes, which remained largely unchanged
throughout the week. The big shift was in carb consumption. Pro EPL players
were consuming approximately 4.2 g/kg of carbohydrates on training and
rest days (on the very low end of the suggested carb intake), yet were ramping
up their intake to 6.4 g/kg per day on game days. It was consistent across
all the players, so researchers wanted to know if players were being told by
coaches or training staff to do this. Were they knowingly adjusting their own
intake on competition day? Was it just an unconscious choice? They couldn't
pin down the exact root cause, but interestingly, the same phenomenon was
observed in a similar study of Dutch professional soccer players.[5]

At the highest level, the margin between winning and losing is incredibly
small. These subtle yet significant findings mean a lot when you consider
pro or high-level athletes (including high school, college, and the like) are
playing multiple games in a week over the course of many months. Exercise
intensity and duration is much higher in a competitive game compared to
practice. Incredibly, the research shows athletes consuming even 8 g/kg/
day of carbs couldn't fully replenish glycogen stores in fast-twitch (type
2) muscle fibers 48 hours after training.[6] This has massive implications. If

EPL players are eating 6.4 g of carbs on game days, and it takes 48 hours to recharge top-gear power at 8 g/kg/day, this could have direct effects on the outcome of the game. If athletes aren't consuming enough carbs throughout the practice week and before and after games, they could be impacting their ability to train, compete, and recover.[7] This could easily be the difference between winning and losing. (However, they did observe that the players who logged the most miles in a game — not surprisingly, the midfielders — consumed the highest amount relative to the other players.)

Interestingly, four out of six professional English Premier League players failed to meet the guidelines of 6–10 g/kg for carbs during high-intensity practices, which is crucial for optimizing physical, technical, and cognitive performance.[8] Is this a strategic and purposeful nutrition plan by team nutritionists? Is it the player's unconscious or conscious decision? Are the current guidelines too high? Game-day nutrition isn't the same as training-day nutrition — this is a central theme of a periodized nutrition approach. As Fergus Connolly, PhD, says so well in his book *Game Changer*: "You need to work from the game backwards to support performance." Game day matters most; thus, flagging nutritional habits that might directly or indirectly compromise the outcome in competition is crucial.

Another key aspect of the study was to observe the protein intakes of EPL players. Pro soccer players competing in the English Premier League consume more than 200 g of protein per day, well above the low end of the recommended 1.6–2.2 g/kg/day range for strength and team sport athletes. Compare today's consumption with 20 years ago, when the average pro soccer player was consuming a paltry 108 g of protein per day, evidence of how the evolution of sport science and the advancement of nutrition research has *truly* influenced the game and shifted player mindset. If your message to football players today is to be protein-focused, know that the current evidence suggests most of them have already got their protein foundation covered.

Carbohydrates appear to be the biggest margin for gains in team sport athletes. Although the study was only one week in duration (and none of the players experienced adverse symptoms of overtraining or illness), it's important to wonder about their glycogen status. If it was suboptimal after a week of in-season play, what happens over the course of a month or an entire season? What happens when the competition schedule gets compressed during playoffs or international play? What happens at the start of the season, after players have been training at their highest intensities and volumes in training

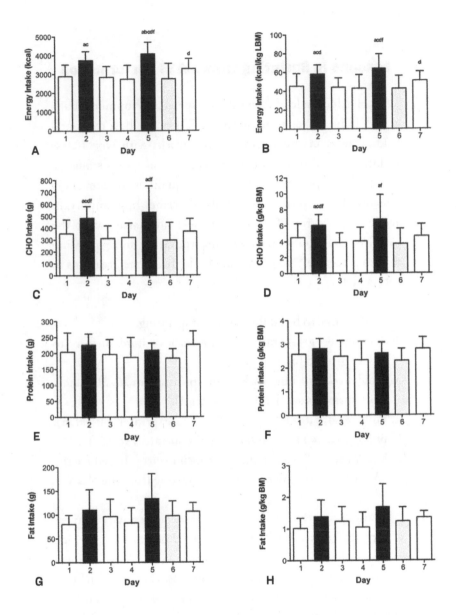

**FIGURE 6.1.** Daily energy and macronutrient intake over the 7-day testing period, showing training days (*white bars*) and match days (*black bars*). *A*, absolute energy expenditure; *B*, absolute carbohydrate; *C*, absolute protein; *D*, absolute fat; *E*, absolute protein; *F*, relative protein; *G*, absolute fat; *H*, relative fat. Liam Anderson et al., "Energy Intake and Expenditure of Professional Soccer Players of the English Premier League: Evidence of Carbohydrate Periodization," *International Journal of Sport Nutrition and Exercise Metabolism*, 27 (2017), https://doi.org/10.1123/ijsnem.2016-0259.

## Lessons in Sprinting from ALTIS Performance

Jason Hettler is a lead strength and speed development coach at ALTIS in Arizona, home to the best of the best track and field athletes in the world. Hettler works with world-class sprinters and also consults with professional sports teams on how to development better sprinting qualities in team sport athletes. The mantra "speed kills" describes how important acceleration is for elite performance, no matter what the sport. What if you want to start incorporating more sprinting into your regime? No problem. Hettler has some great tips to get started.

1. It takes time to build the "skills" of sprinting.
2. Start off on grass, rather than a track or hard surface (to reduce ground force impact).
3. Build *acceleration* by working on sprints from 20–30 meters (elite sprinters accelerate up to 50 m!).
4. Build *speed* at distances of 30–60 m (elite sprinters 50–90 m).
5. Build *speed endurance* at 60 m+ (elite sprinters 90 m+).
6. Use "drop-ins" — a skip into the sprint start — to reduce the force of overcoming the inertia of starting from the blocks.

Hettler points out that drop-ins are ideal for novice runners who typically have much greater ground contact time, which increases the impact and stress on the body. As your form improves, the ground contact time decreases and you can build your capacity for and tolerance to sprints. Sprints provide benefits across all sports: acceleration, speed, and speed endurance are tops on the list, along with nervous system activation and development of proper sprint mechanics, which helps to improve coordination. In Hettler's experience, athletes can make big strides in one off-season (6–12 weeks) of sprint training. But like any skill, the results are compounded when practiced regularly. If you're a recreational high-level athlete, it might take you 6–12 months to build the skill of sprinting. As Hettler has shown countless pro athletes, it's well worth the investment!

camp in preparation for the rigors of the competitive season to come? If they don't fuel adequately, it stands to reason that it will compromise how well the team comes out of the gates to start the season. Let's take a closer look at what happens in preseason training camps as athletes prepare for the season.

## Setting the Stage:
## Preseason and Training Camp Fueling

"Practice. We talking about practice. Not a game, not a game . . . practice!" This famous quote is from NBA all-star Allen Iverson when reporters questioned his dedication to practice sessions (check out the YouTube clip; it's fantastic!). It seems an appropriate reference point to discuss team sport nutrition; does nutrition in training camp really matter? We're only just beginning to learn about the *in-season* fueling strategies of team sport athletes, but what about the preseason? Interestingly, it is during the preseason when training loads and training intensity reach the highest levels.[9] Therefore, it makes sense to ask if players are meeting their nutritional needs during this crucial and grueling training camp period. If athletes aren't achieving their energy (calorie) and macro requirements in the preseason, it can leave them struggling to hit the ground running when the competitive season starts. Preseason training camp is a critical period where physical, technical, tactical, and cognitive demands are all high. Players should be consuming more fuel compared to the relatively lower demands in-season, but are they?

In Brazil, a recent study investigated the nutritional intake of 19 professional soccer players during their daily 90-minute preseason training sessions — including physical, technical, and tactical elements — in the buildup to qualifications for the prestigious Brazil Cup. A typical week in training camp consists of six training sessions in 5 days, with higher training loads and intensities compared to the competitive season. Two-a-day sessions also take place, similar to most American sports. What did the player nutrition look like in this critical period? Similar to the English Premier League soccer players discussed previously, the Brazilian pros easily achieved (and exceeded) the sport nutrition recommendations for protein (and fats) and there were no differences among the different position players in total energy or macronutrient intake.[10] However, once again when it came to carbohydrate intake, the players were falling short. The Brazilian pros were barely meeting the minimum requirement of 5 g/kg of carbs per day. Their intake was higher compared to the English Premier League players in-season, but when you consider the higher demands of training camp, it still fell short of ideal. The physical output data shows players definitely work harder and longer during the preseason training camp period compared to in-season. If players lack adequate energy, their recovery (and potentially adaptation) could be compromised, leaving them dragging their feet coming into a new season or — worse yet, exposing them to an increased risk of illness or injury. This highlights a potential opportunity to increase fueling to better support training and recovery. The preseason period is the time when carb intake should be *highest* — even higher than during the season — in order to support recovery from training and prepare for the demands of the sessions on the following days. Teams that recognize this opportunity can place a focus on this performance gap and, as a result, find tangible gains.

Interestingly, the study also examined the micronutrient status of the players. How did the Brazilian pros manage in terms of meeting their daily micronutrient requirements? Unfortunately, a large percentage failed to meet the Estimated Average Requirement (EAR) for several key micronutrients: 58 percent of players didn't get enough folate, 68 percent had insufficient levels of magnesium and calcium, 74 percent lacked vitamin A, and surprisingly 100 percent failed to get enough vitamin D[11] (see table 6.1). Dietary folate is easy to obtain from vegetables and leafy greens, and if over half the players are lacking this, it's likely a clear sign they're not eating their veggies. Next, and perhaps more surprising, is even in sunny Brazil players struggled to reach adequate levels of vitamin D. Is this due to lack of sun exposure because players were covering up? Genetic difference? Increased utilization in training and recovery? It's difficult to say exactly, but inflammation, oxidative stress, and player health are also likely factors. Calcium is also found in abundance in dairy products, yogurt, cheese, and proteins like clams and in the small bones of sardines. A closer look into the specific foods players are choosing to eat can provide a window into the nutrient density, or lack thereof, in their diet. Processed foods provide fuel to train but are strongly lacking in essential micronutrients (which is

**TABLE 6.1.** Micronutrient Intakes of Brazilian Soccer Pros

| MICRONUTRIENT | ESTIMATED AVG. REQUIREMENT (EAR) | PLAYER INTAKE (% OF EAR) | % BELOW EAR |
|---|---|---|---|
| Vitamin A (ug) | 625.0 | 84.4 | 74 |
| Vitamin C (mg) | 75.0 | 287.0 | 21 |
| Vitamin $B_2$ (mg) | 1.3 | 132.4 | 16 |
| Vitamin $B_6$ (mg) | 1.1 | 199.3 | 0 |
| Folate (mg) | 320.0 | 81.2 | 58 |
| Vitamin $B_{12}$ (ug) | 2.0 | 345.3 | 5 |
| Vitamin D (ug) | 10.0 | 31.0 | 100 |
| Magnesium (mg) | 330.0 | 91.0 | 68 |
| Zinc (mg) | 9.4 | 44.0 | 5 |
| Iron (mg) | 6.0 | 44.5 | 0 |

*Source:* Raquel Raizel et al., "Pre-season Dietary Intake of Professional Soccer Players," *Nutrition and Health* 23, no. 4 (2017), https://doi.org/10.1177/0260106017737014.

why makers of these foods "fortify" them in the first place), meaning that practitioners need to take this into consideration for players with highly processed diets. A diet deficient or insufficient in micronutrients might reflect the player's subpar nutrition choices or increased demands due to training or health concerns. In a real-world scenario, it's likely both.

None of this research even takes into account what players do on the weekends, when their nutrition choices aren't dictated directly by team meals or indirectly by the food choices of their peers. Do they go off the rails? Do they hold strong? Do they eat enough food to support recovery? It's difficult to say, but building a strong team culture around nutrition and fueling is one way to guide players toward making better dietary choices.

What are the consequences of micronutrient deficiencies in athletes? As the season progresses, if players aren't getting enough energy or are lacking in micronutrients, it can impair immunity, recovery, joint and muscle health, physical performance, and possibly delay return to play after injury.[12] The ability of an athlete to optimize training adaptations also depends on the health of the athlete. Although energy balance and macros

## Fueling High-Level Youth Athletes

Should you fuel younger athletes the same way you do adults? Research in elite academy-level soccer players in England found they generally under-consume total calories throughout the week (just like the EPL players), until the rest day before matches when consumption is much higher than expenditure.[14] Red flags for youth athletes include low energy intakes on high-intensity days, a pattern also seen in pro soccer players. This is more concerning in youth athletes because high-intensity efforts require carbohydrate for fuel. If players are cutting themselves short, it could not only hinder their ability to train at a high level but also hamper their natural growth and development if the trend persists. This is an important differentiating factor between adults — where mild deficits in energy balance don't necessarily translate to performance deficits — and youth athletes, where energy balance for health, growth, and maturation is top priority. Athlete and coaching staff education is therefore crucial when working with youth athletes.

are first priority, micronutrients are also important in keeping the athlete healthy. This study on preseason nutrition intake also reveals how changes in body composition can vary significantly depending on a player's role and position. This is an important factor to consider once the season starts, because some players will log heavy minutes while others will come off the bench and play sparingly. Different nutrition and training strategies will be required to maintain athlete body composition, health, and performance.[13] This difference highlights the critical need for an individualized nutrition approach among the various players on the team.

## Contact Sports: The Big, the Bad, and the Ugly

Skilled-based sports with minimal contact like soccer and basketball are one thing, but what about sports with intense physical contact throughout the game such as American football and rugby? How do the nutritional needs of big American football players and badass rugby players, who run into one another for hours throughout an entire game, compare to the more skill-based sports? While there is limited public data on professional NFL football players, the amount of research on rugby players has dramatically increased over the last decade. Analysis of energy expenditure in rugby players comparing the forwards (generally bigger, slower players involved in the scrum) to the backs (who are typically the faster, more skilled players who run greater distances) reveals some compelling differences. The shorter, faster players covering more kilometers burned *fewer* calories (3,359 kcal) compared to the forwards grinding it out in the trenches (3,800 kcal).[15] Seems counterintuitive, right? How can the players who run greater distances be burning less fuel than the bigger brutes plodding along down the field? It's simple: physical contact. It takes a lot of energy to take a hit, to fight off a block, and to battle through physical contact. The effect of impact in contact sports dramatically increases energy demands and is often overlooked, potentially compromising an athlete's ability to recover and ultimately to perform. When you consider these athletes need to maintain their size in order to compete at the highest level, it becomes even more crucial to fuel them for the demands of their sport.

How did the power-based rugby players stack up against the skill-based soccer players in terms of macro intake? A recent study in the *European Journal of Sport Science* investigated the dietary intakes of professional rugby union players over the course of 7 days. Similar to pro soccer players, pro rugby players easily achieved their daily protein intake, averaging 2.7 g/kg/day — well above the recommended intake when athletes are in a caloric deficit.[16] (No surprise there; big athletes love to knock back protein!) How about dietary fat intake? Once again, it was pretty consistent throughout the week at 1.4 g/kg, which makes sense if the majority of fat intake comes from food (not supplements). In terms of carbohydrates, it's a similar refrain to the skill-based sports. Just like the English Premier League pros, rugby players naturally increased their intake in the 2 days out from games, topping out at more than 5 g/kg for the forwards and just under for the backs. And just like the football players, they tended to periodize (consciously or unconsciously) their carbohydrate intake to suit the demands of the day. However, a similar risk of underconsuming on higher-intensity days might limit training adaptations and recovery over the course of an entire season. Circling back to individual player requirements — how did the position differences influence carb intake? The rugby union forwards consumed 3.5 g/kg/day on average throughout the week, compared to 3.4 g/kg/day for the backs. Recall the energy demands of the constant contact and physical demands of the forwards had them burning 400 kcal more per day than the backs. Based on the rugby forwards' current intake, it appears they're underconsuming total carbohydrates and calories. When athletes are underfueled it can lead to poor recovery or maladaptation, which often dovetails into strong cravings for sweets and sugars as well as an increased risk of cold and flu and injury. Keep underfueling on your radar (and remember, athletes lie on their food intake forms too!).

Elite sport is decided by the smallest of margins, and every inch counts. Research in professional athletes reveals that they seem to be self-selecting a periodized carb approach, with lower levels throughout the week and ramping up carb intake as they approach game day. Again, is this the result of instruction from team coaches? Are they being influenced by the current nutrition trend of a lower-carb approach? Is it the player's own initiative, the influence of the nutrition habits of their peers, or simply an unconscious choice? If a periodized carb approach is a purposeful and planned strategy and players are recovering well, it could represent a performance gain. However, if an athlete starts to display the subtle symptoms of acute fatigue, lowered immunity, slower recovery, sleep problems, or altered mood, then it's important to reassess the plan to ensure they've got the fuel they need to train, recover, and compete. Ideally, this would involve establishing sound nutrition fundamentals and an individualized nutrition plan that is tailored to each player. On big teams, it's a difficult task to achieve (seemingly impossible sometimes). Flagging athletes who aren't responding appropriately is a great first step. If you have athletes who will be with your team for many years, then tracking them over time and implementing changes incrementally will be helpful to both player compliance and practitioner success. The revolution in sport nutrition is evidence-based fundamentals combined with an individualized approach, and whoever can uncover the best strategy to achieve it will lead the way.

It's not just preseason and in-season nutrition that matters; research is delving further down the rabbit hole to extract every possible gain. As games are decided by the slightest of margins, a new area of interest is the importance of halftime nutrition (and recovery) modalities to propel athletes in the latter stages of the contest, when most games are ultimately decided. Let's look at how halftime nutrition can impact the final score.

## Halftime Nutrition: Major Outcome Influencer

It's 2005, halftime of the Champions League final. Liverpool FC are licking their wounds after falling behind 3–0 to the favorite, AC Milan. The lead is seemingly insurmountable, and the Italian fans are already celebrating what appears to be the inevitable European Championship trophy. Then coming out of halftime, the tables quickly turn in the first 15 minutes. Liverpool changes tactical formations in an attempt to put pressure on Milan's defense. Six minutes into the half, Liverpool captain Steven Gerrard connects on a crossing pass from the edge of the 6-yard box and scores. Liverpool trails 3–1. Two minutes later, another Liverpool goal from long range goes into the bottom left-hand corner. Liverpool trails 3–2. Incredibly, not even 3 minutes later, Gerrard is taken down in the box and awarded a penalty. He scores, and the game is tied 3–3 after only 11 minutes of play since the start of the second half.

Halftime is a unique break in team sports. Players return to the dressing rooms, decompress, review tactics with team coaches, and then get themselves ready again for play in the second half (or subsequent period) by rehydrating, refueling, and rewarming up. The second half of games is "winning time," and there are marked differences between the start and finish of a contest. First, risk of injury increases significantly in the first 10–20 minutes coming out of halftime.[17] Next, there also appears to be a decline in physical performance in the second half compared to the first half (perhaps not surprisingly). Finally, mental performance can really nosedive in the last 10–15 minutes of a game. This new line of research is confirming what experienced coaches have known for a long time: the start and finish of a half in basketball, football, or soccer (or period in hockey) plays a massive role in determining who wins and who loses. For example, in English Premier League soccer, an overwhelmingly disproportionate number of goals are scored in the final 10–15 minutes of game action.[18] Like a boxing match between two heavyweights, teams feel each other out for the majority of the match, trying to figure out weaknesses in the opposing team's defense. Then in the lead up to the final whistle, there is a flurry of action. A game is often decided in those last 10 minutes. If players could more effectively fight off fatigue or lapses in concentration, could this late-game goal phenomenon be mitigated? In American sports, there seems to be a similar theme. Football games often see two teams with their heels dug in. It's an intense tug-of-war until the second half, when the better teams typically pulls away for the win. Basketball is no different, as the last few minutes of the fourth quarter all too often determine the final outcome of the game.

Halftime nutrition is therefore a key opportunity to fuel athletes effectively for the late-game charge. It can potentially influence the outcome of the game. All teams provide food and snacks for players at the break, but surprisingly, players are typically left to their own whims and cravings. Is it time for more structured support? Is it *really* possible to increase second-half performance via specific nutrition (or therapeutic) strategies? Obviously, team tactics have a major impact, but only recently have researchers looked into the effects of halftime nutrition (and other strategies) to enhance second-half performance.

The work of Mark Russell, PhD, and his team at Northumbria University has focused on the application of different halftime nutrition strategies for performance. Any time athletes have prolonged periods of reduced activity between exercise periods, it can lower their physical performance, reduce cognitive function, and increase injury risk, all of which have been identified as higher-risk for athletes in the second half of team sports.[19] Dr. Russell's interest in the topic began rather serendipitously with an unexpected finding from an earlier study in youth soccer players. While investigating the impact of carbohydrates on skill performance, he noticed something dramatic happened directly after halftime: a rapid decline in blood glucose levels.

The major drop in blood glucose levels, known as *rebound hypoglycemia*, is typically due to excessive or poorly timed intake of simple carbs in the first half of play or before games. Athletes who knocked back a bottle and a half of a sports drink (75 g of glucose, for example) 75 minutes before exercise, compared to 45 and 15 minutes before, revealed the worst hypoglycemic response. That is, when consumed more than an hour before the game, sports drinks sent players into a glucose tailspin. This has massive implications for athletes. Consuming sports drinks far too early before tip-off, kickoff, or puck drop can easily sabotage performance — yet this is still the reality for many elite team sport athletes. It's not always easy to change habits (particularly in younger athletes).

When these drinks are consumed closer to game action, however, the impacts are far different. In the previous chapter, you learned how carbohydrate-electrolyte drinks during exercise (particularly high-intensity work) have a definite impact on exercise capacity. This is the cornerstone of sport nutrition, and countless studies have confirmed its benefit, which is generally attributed to maintaining blood glucose levels and sparing glycogen. Carb drinks can also improve cognitive performance after prolonged, steady-state running (despite athletes still being in a normal glycemic state). It's also well-documented that player skills like shooting and passing decline during the second half, and carb availability is associated with faster visual discrimination, faster fine-motor speed, and faster psychomotor speed.[20] Halftime nutrition is a major potential advantage late in games when skill and decision-making decide the outcome.

When athletes consume too many simple sugars too far away from training or competition, the high-glycemic carbs spike blood glucose and insulin levels, leading to inhibition of pancreatic beta-cell function along with the surge of catecholamines that fuel performance. This scenario creates a big potential problem when athletes stop playing, such as during halftime, when significant drops in blood sugar levels occur. This rebound hypoglycemia is more common than coaches and practitioners realize. If your team often looks sluggish at the start of the second half (or during games), this could be a primary reason. It's still a common practice for players to knock back large volumes of sports drinks (with 30–60 g of simple sugars) at halftime while they sit and listen to coach instructions. By the time the game resumes 20 minutes or more later, their blood glucose levels will have hit rock bottom. It might be why so many teams start slow in the second half. If athletes could keep blood glucose levels stable, it seems that a performance benefit would result.

New research by Professor Emma Stevenson, PhD, and her team at Newcastle University looked into this question. Rather than using typical simple-carb solutions, Stevenson investigated the application of a traditional solution in an attempt to maintain stable blood glucose. Blood glucose levels in athletes were examined at halftime. The natural carbohydrate compound *isomaltulose*, found in abundance in honey, was given to one group of soccer players and compared to another group given the standard maltodextrin typically consumed during the halftime period. The results were eye-opening. After 60 minutes, blood glucose levels had dropped only 4 percent in the honey group compared to a 19 percent drop in the maltodextrin group.[21] Most important, in the last 15 minutes of a soccer game — when the vast majority of goals are scored — isomaltulose was far superior at keeping blood glucose levels stable compared to the standard sports drinks (when players had a halftime dose). This means the *type* of fuel you consume, the *timing*, and the *total* amount are all crucial to athlete performance. This research reveals how important a halftime nutrition strategy can be to the final score.

Caffeine can also play a major role as a halftime nutrition strategy, helping to buffer declines in skill and concentration due to fatigue.[22] Caffeine levels peak in the bloodstream 45–60 minutes post-consumption, which is often too long of a time period if you're attempting to apply halftime strategies to influence the outcome of the game. Caffeinated chewing gum provides a cutting-edge solution to this problem. Caffeine is absorbed much more rapidly via the oral mucosa, giving you a quick hit for the second half. A recent study in cyclists found 300 mg given 5 minutes before exercise improved cycling performance (yet no benefits were seen when given 1 hour before).[23] This is potentially a great solution for bench players and substitutes who never know when their number will be called, as these players often bring more energy into the game. Even for starters logging longer minutes, a second dose of caffeine might be helpful in important games that require increased work output compared to the norm. (Be sure to practice these strategies in training or simulated matches to assess individual player responses.)

What about sports like baseball, where play is highly intermittent and players have numerous occasions to fuel (or fuel inappropriately) during games? A baseball game is about three and a half hours long, and each inning players return to the dugout where snacking options are always available. In this case, constantly sipping on high-glycemic sports drinks can be a major problem. In a sport with a lot of sitting, standing, and waiting for play for unknown amounts of time, constant sipping can easily lead to rebound hypoglycemia. When this happens, players quickly feel more physically and mentally sluggish, which can kill their ability to perform in key at-bats or relief appearances. Having a preplanned strategy for players to stick to, rather than ad libitum food opportunities throughout the game, would help dial in the right dose for each player. The strategy will vary depending on a player's position, and whether the player is a starter or is coming off the bench. A great example of when to use nutrient timing, such as caffeinated chewing gum or carbohydrate drink, is when a pinch hitter enters the game in the seventh inning (versus 2 hours before the start of the game).

## It's All about Body Temperature

It's not just halftime nutrition strategies that can make or break a game. The research is uncovering that a number of therapeutic strategies could help support performance and reduce injury over a long season. New research shows that maintaining body temperature is crucial to performance. For every 1°C (1.8°F) an athlete's body temperature drops, peak power output drops by 3 percent.[24] In professional rugby union players, repeated sprint performance was improved after halftime when athletes wore "survival" garments to help maintain body temperature during the break.[25] For players who don't like the idea of wearing added garments, increasing the temperature of the locker room has also been proposed as a reasonable and practical way to maintain athlete temperature during extended pauses in action. Regardless if it's heated clothing, survival garments, heating pads, or warm locker rooms, the research shows marginal gains can be made by keeping athletes at the right temperature.

Halftime nutrition is a growing area of research and interest. It appears to be a potential strategy that can help influence the final score. What happened to Liverpool in that 2005 Champions League final? They beat AC Milan in a penalty shootout to become European Champions. Was this comeback attributable to their halftime nutrition? Maybe, although the old mantra "fitness won't win you the League, but it could lose it for you" seems to apply here. (Perhaps asking AC Milan what they did at halftime is a better place to start.) Nevertheless, in the high-performance world of marginal gains, halftime nutrition represents a big opportunity to influence the outcome.

## Compressed Competition Schedules: A Focus on Playoffs

For 15 years, Jim Mora was a highly successful professional football coach in the NFL. However, he unfortunately holds the dubious NFL record for most career regular-season wins (125) without a playoff victory. In one of his final seasons with the Indianapolis Colts, Mora gave one of the more infamous postgame press conference rants: "Playoffs? You kidding me . . . playoffs? We're just trying to win a game!" (Again, check out the YouTube video!) His emotional statement after a difficult loss highlights how things get magnified as the season progresses toward the playoffs. If athletes aren't fueling effectively during the season, it can leave them exposed during periods of compressed scheduling — like the playoffs — when games are played more frequently than normal. This can also happen in tournament-style play with multiple games in 1 day, or during international competitions with more frequent games over multiple weeks. Four key recommendations to consider if you're heading into a compressed competition (or training) window include:

- Adjust carb intake
- Ensure protein intake
- Rehydrate aggressively
- Cool inflammation and muscle soreness[26]

---

Competing intensely every game, night after night, takes its toll and changes the fueling needs of players. The recommended carbohydrate intake for strength and team sport athletes is typically 4–7 g/kg/day during regular training or competition conditions, but when things ramp up, carb intake needs to ramp up as well. During compressed schedules, topping up glycogen within 24 hours is crucial to put players in the best position to win the next day. The latest evidence suggests 7–10 g/kg/day of carbohydrates is the ideal range.[27] That's a lot of carbs, more than most athletes realize. Shawn Arent, PhD, at Rutgers University emphasizes that getting carbs in immediately postgame via liquid nutrition will kick-start the process. Then increasing meal frequency with more snacks ensures athletes get the energy (and carbs) they need to recover with a short turnaround. In real-world scenarios, athletes will often underconsume, especially when they're tired and run-down. Research shows team sport athletes who eat less than 6 g/ kg of carbs per day during periods of heavy competition and compressed schedules might be exposing themselves to increased fatigue, injury risk, and illness (or might be compromising their training camp gains).[28]

Protein intake is crucial as well. Most strength and team sport athletes seem to be getting enough protein, but I often see many endurance, youth, and recreational athletes fall short. In compressed competition windows, if you're taking bricks out of the wall faster than you're replacing them, eventually you'll run into some problems. Aim for at least 1.6–2.2 g/kg/day. And if you think you might be in a caloric deficit, take the advice of experts like Dr. Eric Helms and increase your intake above 2.3 g/kg/day (up to 3.1 g/kg/day) to help ward off illness, infection, and injury.

Hydration is also key. For every molecule of glycogen you lose, you lose three molecules of water. This can lead to dramatic weight loss and a more pro-inflammatory and catabolic milieu in the body. To rapidly restore hydration in a compressed time frame, aim to replace every kilogram of weight loss (from pregame to postgame weigh-ins) with 1.5 L of fluids.[29] Remember, it's best to start the process immediately after training while in a compressed training schedule.

Finally, let's cover inflammation and antioxidant support. In high-level athletes, inadequate intake of polyunsaturated fat (PUFA) has also been shown to be a limiting factor for athlete performance and recovery.[30] If you think about training adaptation, omega-3 fats play a key role in reducing pro-inflammatory eicosanoids (prostaglandins, leukotrienes, and thromboxanes), cytokines, and reactive oxygen species (ROS).[31] Athletes who eat diets higher in processed foods, vegetable oils (most often the oil of choice in restaurants and hotels), or animal proteins like chicken rather than omega-3 rich foods like fish or grass-fed beef, can skew their balance of omega-6

**TABLE 6.2.** Compressed Competition Fueling Strategies

| | TIMING | STRATEGY |
|---|---|---|
| 1 | Shake (liquid): immediately post | 40 g whey + 60 g high-GI carbs |
| 2 | Snack #1: 30–60 minutes post | 60 g of carbs |
| 3 | Meal: 2–3 hours post | 30 g protein + 80 g carbs + 20 g fat |
| 4 | Snack #2: up to 6 hours post | 40 g slow casein + 30 g low-GI carbs |
| 5 | Bedtime | Tart cherry juice |

*Source:* Mayur Krachna Ranchordas, Joel T. Dawson, and Mark Russell, "Practical Nutritional Recovery Strategies for Elite Soccer Players When Limited Time Separates Repeated Matches," *Journal of the International Society of Sports Nutrition* 14, no. 1 (2017), https://doi.org/10.1186/s12970-017-0193-8.

to omega-3 intake, leading to a more pro-inflammatory state. Today, the general population consumes a ratio of 10:1–20:1 of omega 6:3, compared to pre-industrial societies who likely consumed them at a 3:1–1:1 ratio.[32]

When athletes have to compete on back-to-back nights, or in multiple games in a short time frame, there is an opportunity to influence the outcome of the game or competition by strategically applying periodized nutrition strategies to accelerate recovery and rapidly restore fuels to maximize athlete performance. This is when postgame nutrition, in preparation for the upcoming match the next day, becomes crucial to player success. Table 6.2 provides a few examples of how to transfer the evidence-based science into your practice.

## The Biggest Rocks: Energy Balance and Macronutrient Intake

Let's review. Nutrition strategies that have the greatest influence on performance for team sport athletes ensure adequate energy balance and optimize macronutrient intake. Overwhelmingly, these are the "biggest rocks" impacting athlete health and performance. Put these fundamentals firmly in place and you'll be 80 percent of the way home. (The next biggest rocks are micronutrients, targeted supplementation, and maintaining hydration.) Energy balance is fundamental to athletic performance, but sometimes lack of sufficient fueling can fly under the radar and lead to symptoms that look a lot like overtraining. *Relative energy deficiency syndrome* (REDS) occurs when athletes aren't taking enough fuel onboard. This can impair athletic performance via reduced muscle glycogen storage, increased fatigue, impaired technical skills, diminished concentration, increased perception of effort, and increased injury risk.[33] Female athletes commonly get the most attention when it comes to REDS; however, men are affected as well. It doesn't just affect performance, but it also compromises athlete health, which ultimately impacts the outcome on the field.

As you've learned in this chapter, the culprit is seldom a lack of *protein* intake by athletes but rather a lack of *total caloric intake* (often due to insufficient carb intake). Carbs are a key fuel for muscle contraction, central nervous system function, and muscle glycogen storage, which means they can directly limit athlete performance on the field or in the gym. Expert nutritionist Ben House, PhD, from the United States, and consultant to many elite athletes, confirms that one of the most common things he sees in high-level athletes is under-eating.[34] Dr. House emphasizes the importance of eating as many calories as possible while remaining weight-stable and focusing on *both* food quantity and quality.

Expert Dr. Susan Kleiner, PhD, RD, performance nutritionist for the WNBA's Seattle Storm also sees many elite athletes under-eating in her practice. In our recent interview she emphasized the importance of athletes "eating consistently throughout the day," and added that "ensuring adequate meal frequency is a great way to achieve your energy goals."[35] This is great advice that is often forgotten by athletes, particularly when traveling, because regular meals — breakfast, lunch, and dinner — are provided, but extra snacks are rarely given. Of course, purposeful and strategic targeting of low carbohydrate availability, as described by Dr. James Morton and his work with Team SKY, might be appropriate during specific training sessions, but the applications for team sports are still being fleshed out. Numerous professional teams now seem to be incorporating more carb periodization throughout the week. Once the "big rocks" of energy balance and macronutrient breakdown are accounted for, practitioners can shift the focus to ensuring adequate micronutrient status (see table 6.3).

### THE NEXT "BIGGEST ROCK": MICRONUTRIENTS

Common micronutrients depleted by intense exercise include vitamin D, iron, calcium, and antioxidants (among others), which are all crucial for immunity, metabolism, and muscular adaptation. Vitamin D has garnered a lot of attention over the past decade as it relates to sport and performance. Early research in professional team sport athletes by expert Graeme Close, PhD, and his team at Liverpool John Moores University led to an explosion of interest in vitamin D, as they found significant improvements in strength, speed, and power with supplementation. The research by Close and others in the field found many athletes were vitamin D deficient, largely due to sun-shy lifestyles and poor dietary sources of vitamin D, even in those living in sunny climates."[36] When the UVB light from the sun comes into contact with your skin, a prohormone in the skin called 7-dehydrocholesterol gets converted into cholecalciferol, which then travels to the liver and gets metabolized into 25-hydroxyvitamin D, or 25(OH)D. This is the form typically measured when you run a blood test. The final conversion takes place in the kidneys, where 25(OH)D gets converted into 1,25-hydroxyvitamin D, the usable form in the body. As you learned in this chapter, 100 percent of the Brazilian soccer pros were deficient in vitamin D despite living and playing in Brazil. This illustrates how a sun-shy lifestyle and the inflammatory stress of training might contribute to deficiencies.

However, Dr. Close points out that over the years he has failed to replicate the performance-boosting effects of vitamin D supplementation. He believes the reason for such a widespread effect among this initial group was due to the fact they were all moderately vitamin D deficient (less than 25 nmol/l). In Dr. Close's research, athletes with moderate vitamin D deficiency were at greater risk of detrimental effects to muscle function, and supplementation with vitamin D improved function and performance. Mild vitamin D deficiency is also associated with impaired muscle regeneration; however, supplementation at this level does not confer any added benefits.[37] Dr. Close suggests athletes aim for at least 75 nmol/L (30ng/mL) from regular sunshine exposure, or a supplementation dose of 2,000–4,000 IU per day. (The reality is that most athletes will probably need to supplement during the winter months.)

Close's recent work with Daniel Owens, PhD, in England found that athletes mega-dosing with vitamin D once per week (between 35,000–70,000 IU) demonstrated elevated levels of harmful metabolites and detrimental effects to the target tissues by blocking vitamin D receptors.[38] Close and Owens assert the evidence supports lower daily doses of vitamin D as the most potent beneficial strategy, while also limiting the probability of negative regulatory molecules. They suggest the best practice is a daily dose between 2,000–4,000 IU.

Of course, a common mistake practitioners make is when they look at vitamin D status in isolation. Chronic inflammation might also drive down vitamin D levels. Such inflammation might come from intense training, chronic injury or illness, or it might be experienced by overweight clients who struggle with prediabetes and poor metabolic health. In fact, vitamin D status has shown promise in the research as a novel "health biomarker".[39] Also, if vitamin A levels or phosphorus (from drinking too much soda) are too high or calcium levels are too low, the result can be reduced vitamin D status.

Vitamin D status is also intimately linked with calcium status. Calcium is typically known for its essential role in the growth, maintenance, and repair of bone tissue. It's also critical for regulating muscle contraction and nerve conduction, both crucial to an athlete's training, recovery, and performance. Athletes who fall into a low energy availability state are at much greater risk of stress fractures. Incredibly, two-thirds of the pro soccer players in the Brazil study were found to have insufficient calcium intakes (below the

**TABLE 6.3.** Team Sport Nutrition Summary

| MACRONUTRIENTS | RECOMMENDED DOSE |
| --- | --- |
| Protein | Team sports: 1.6–2.2 g/kg/day bodyweight<br>Recommended *minimal* dose: 1.6 g/kg/day |
| Carbs | 4–7 g/kg/day<br>Increased to 7–10 g/kg/day in *compressed* schedules |
| Fat | Approximately 30% of total calories +/-5–10%<br>Do not go below 20% of total caloric intake |
| Meal Frequency | 4–6 meals per day<br>Minimum 20 g protein per meal (or 0.3–0.5 g protein/kg)<br>10 g EAA or 3.0 g leucine per serving |
| **MICRONUTRIENT** | **RECOMMENDED DOSE** |
| Vitamin D | 2,000–4,000 IU daily from the sun (20–30 min.)<br>or supplementation |
| Iron | *At least* 8 mg/kg/day (men) from animal protein<br>*At least* 18 mg/kg/day (women) from animal protein |
| Calcium | 1,500 mg daily from dairy, clams, bones of small fish |

recommended 1,500 mg daily). If your diet is low in dairy products, leafy greens, or seafood, or you're not taking a multivitamin, you might be at risk of insufficiency or deficiency. Also, drinking too much soda pop creates excess phosphorus that inhibits calcium absorption and can drive down calcium levels as well. It's important to remember that only significant deficiencies of calcium will appear on a blood test; therefore, like vitamin D, calcium should be assessed in conjunction with other nutrients. Chronic inflammation is also part of the vitamin D and calcium story. If inflammation levels are persistently high from intense training or poor health, calcidiol is more rapidly converted to calcitriol, thus impacting vitamin D and calcium status.[40]

Iron is also an essential mineral for health and athletic performance. Iron deficiency, with or without anemia, can hamper muscle function and limit work capacity, thereby compromising adaptations to training. Suboptimal or poor iron status is often seen in athletes with low intake of heme iron found in animal proteins. Your iron status can be impacted by menses, training at altitude, footstrike hemolysis, rapid periods of growth, and injury.[41] Athletes at the greatest risk of low iron status are distance runners, vegetarians, and females. Symptoms of low iron status or anemia might include fatigue, increased heart rate during exercise, light-headedness, pale skin, shortness of breath, and dry and damaged hair and skin. (If you suspect iron deficiency anemia, contact your doctor.) Ferritin is a reliable indicator of long-term iron stores, but it's also an acute-phase protein that increases with elevated oxidative stress and inflammation.[42] Chronic inflammation can drive up ferritin levels, masking a potential deficiency. The best way to increase heme iron intake is to ramp up the consumption of organ meats, red meats, and seafood. For vegan or vegetarian athletes, bioavailable nonheme iron is found in nuts, beans, vegetables, and fortified grains. Due to the reduced bioavailability of iron in a vegetarian diet, the RDA for vegetarians is 1.8 times higher compared to meat eaters.[43] For such athletes, supplementation is often advantageous for achieving daily targets. Just remember, iron supplements should not be taken immediately after strenuous exercise due to absorption issues.[44]

### OTHER MICRONUTRIENTS TO CONSIDER

Intense training leads to increased oxidative stress and inflammatory responses in athletes. This results in fatigue and delayed onset muscle soreness that can decrease performance. Omega-3 polyunsaturated fats have been shown to reduce ROS and inflammatory cytokines, as well as to exert immune-modulatory effects, which could be highly beneficial over the course of a long competitive season. Omega-3 supplementation might also benefit endurance athletes via increasing nitric oxide, and benefit strength-based athletes via augmenting the rise in muscle protein. Foods richest in long-chain omega-3 fats DHA and EPA are fish — black cod, wild salmon, mackerel, anchovies, sardines, herring — as well as mollusks, such as oysters, mussels, and scallops. Moderate amounts are found in the eggs from pasture-raised chickens and grass-fed beef.

Another crucial fat that gets less attention is arachidonic acid (AA). In fact, it's often associated with a more pro-inflammatory state, yet it is essential for many functions in the body. Arachidonic acid conversion into compounds, called resolvins and lipoxins, helps lower inflammation by cleaning up the leftover debris from an inflammatory reaction, which is crucial for health and performance. The main problem for athletes is that chronic inflammation and oxidative stress drive AA levels down, as does the regular use of NSAIDs like ibuprofen. Egg yolks are the best way to maintain your AA levels; aim for 3–4 per week (which should be easy for an athlete). Vegetarians and vegans can produce AA via consuming vegetable oils, but keep an eye out as insufficient intake of zinc, biotin, and vitamin $B_6$ can hinder conversion. Common symptoms of arachidonic acid deficiency include eczema, infertility, depressed immunity, persistent inflammation, and an increased risk of autoimmunity.

In addition, Vitamin A supports the innate "first line of defense" immune system, and a deficiency can leave athletes susceptible to more colds and flu. Common symptoms of low vitamin A status include bumps on the skin (typically on the backs of the arms), along with dry eyes, low sex hormones, and allergies. If you eat a lot of processed and packaged foods, which are loaded with pro-inflammatory omega-6, your vitamin A levels might also be low. If you don't eat animal protein, dairy, or egg yolks, or if you fail to consume enough red, orange, or yellow vegetables, then you might also be at risk. Finally, bodybuilders or figure competitors following low-fat diets might be low in vitamin A, as is anyone megadosing vitamin D supplements. If vitamin A is found to be low, zinc status should be investigated as well.

Zinc is indirectly connected to vitamin D and A status, highlighting the complexity of the human body (and the limitations of a reductionist approach). Zinc plays a key role in vitamin A metabolism, and thus can impact vitamin D status via its effect on vitamin A. Common symptoms of low zinc status are frequent colds and flu, slow wound healing, low testosterone levels, and hair loss. Low zinc status can impair vitamin A and D levels, as well as thyroid hormone production. Athletes with a low consumption of animal protein or who have a diet high in breads, cereals, and grains rich in phytates (which impair zinc absorption) are at the greatest risk of deficiency or insufficiency (this is more common in vegan or vegetarian athletes). Increasing your intake of oysters, shellfish, and red meat is a great way to boost zinc status. If you're vegan, targeted supplementation can be a supportive option. Aim for 50 mg per day with an 8:1–15:1 ratio of zinc to copper. If a practitioner advises taking 100 mg of zinc via supplements, be sure it's for no longer than four weeks and is accompanied by a multimineral formula. Dr. House highlights how lab testing can be highly beneficial for monitoring athlete health, but when it comes to micronutrients, be cautious about how you interpret the results; don't overreact — serum levels don't tell the whole story.

Magnesium also plays a key role in energy production (via ATP) and muscular and nervous system support in athletes. Common symptoms of low magnesium levels include fatigue, weakness, muscle twitches and spasms, and low vitamin D, calcium, or potassium levels. Large insufficiencies can lead to migraines, osteoporosis, high blood pressure, kidney disease, and more. For athletes, high sweat rates and high caffeine intake also increase the need for magnesium. Lab testing for magnesium can be done inexpensively via serum, which provides a more chronic picture; it can also be done by a more costly method via red blood cell (RBC), which is more sensitive to acute changes. Unfortunately, both markers have limitations. Athletes consuming diets high in processed foods and low in plant foods and leafy greens, coupled with large amounts of caffeine or alcohol, tend to be at highest risk of magnesium insufficiency (frank deficiency is not common in athletes).

The B-vitamin family, in particular vitamins $B_1$ (thiamin), $B_2$ (riboflavin), $B_3$ (niacin), $B_5$ (pantothenic acid), $B_6$ (pyridoxine), and $B_7$ (biotin), are also essential for energy metabolism, a crucial piece of the puzzle for all athletes. Excessive sweating and urination (from drinking too much water, caffeine, or alcohol, or struggling with prediabetes) can lead to lower levels. Some athletes who have low $B_2$ and/or $B_6$ levels might experience dryness and cracks at the corners of the mouth (angular stomatitis), along with swelling of the tongue or tingling in the hands and feet. Other factors impacting $B_6$ levels in athletes include inflammation, the regular use of NSAIDs, and oral contraceptives. Biotin (vitamin $B_7$) is also crucial for energy metabolism, and symptoms of deficiency include hair loss, fatigue, and depression. Rich sources of biotin include egg yolks and organ meats. Bodybuilders and physique-focused athletes should pay close attention to their diet, as the high consumption of egg whites (containing avidin) without the yolk can lead to low biotin status. Athletes with diets high in processed foods will be at increased risk of B-vitamin insufficiency. A simple heuristic for correcting low levels of B-vitamins is to increase animal protein intake and to eat more raw, leafy greens. For vegans, think about supplementation during periods of intense training. If you're taking a B-complex supplement, look for "activated" forms of riboflavin (riboflavin-5-phosphate), pyridoxine (pyridoxal-5-phosphate), folic acid (L-5-MTHF) and $B_{12}$ (methylcobalamin).

———

When it comes to the advantages that can be gained from planned, purposeful, and strategic nutrition strategies, the legendary quote from Hall of Fame football coach Paul "Bear" Bryant sums it up best: "It's not the will to win that matters. It's the will to prepare to win that matters!" Are you

## Folate and Methylation: Eat Your Greens

Among your 20,000 genes, the MTHFR gene — methylene-tetrahydrofolate reductase — contains the instructions for making the enzyme MTHFR that converts the folate from your food into methylfolate, which is the active form in the body. The MTHFR gene also initiates the methylation cycle, which involves adding a methyl group — one carbon plus three hydrogen atoms — to something like a gene or enzyme in the body. Methylation controls your genetic expression, determining whether a specific gene will be turned on or off. If you have a SNiP (single nucleotide polymorphism) or slight variation in the MTHFR gene, your methylation cycle will be disrupted and subsequently impair antioxidant production, cellular repair, energy production, inflammation, immune response, and brain chemistry, just to name a few. Expert in epigenetics and author of *Dirty Genes*, Ben Lynch, ND, from the United States, says common symptoms of poor MTHFR function include anxiety, brain fog, depression, irritability, short temper, and chemical sensitivities. Lynch also notes how methylfolate and methylcobalamin are key players in the methylation cycle, and that their teamwork is crucial for optimal function. If your folate, $B_{12}$, and homocysteine levels are frequently high, if you don't tolerate alcohol well, if you don't eat leafy greens every day, if you have low white blood cell counts, and if you experience low thyroid symptoms, then you might have sluggish MTHFR function. A genetic test can confirm your MTHFR gene status; however, Lynch warns against overinterpreting genetic test results. Instead, focusing on getting an adequate folate intake by eating your greens is a great place to start.

willing to put the time in to prepare your fueling strategy to beat the competition? There are still far too many elite athletes not taking full advantage of this area of performance.

In Part Two: Fuel, we reviewed the evidence-based insights from world-leading experts on the fundamentals of nutrition for improving physique, making weight, maximizing endurance performance, and supporting team sport athletes. However, the athlete's journey doesn't end there. To play your best every day, you need to maximize your ability to rest, repair, and recover, which comes next in Part Three: Recovery.

# Recovery

*Don't quit. Suffer now and live the rest of your life as a champion.*

— MUHAMMAD ALI

## CHAPTER 7

# Periodized Recovery

S tress is essential for survival. It is also a catalyst for growth. Without stress, athletes couldn't get bigger, stronger, or faster. Indeed, stress is an essential part of the training process and an essential part of life. Athletes need to train often and train hard, so physical stress is a given. But any good strength coach or trainer will be the first to tell an athlete that they don't get stronger in the gym, they get stronger from the adaptations that take place during rest and recovery. But what is recovery? It seems like such an obvious thing, but it's not very well defined in the scientific research. Sport scientist and recovery expert Shona Halson, PhD, of the Australian Institute of Sport believes a good working definition of recovery is that "[it] allows athletes to train at their highest level possible and compete to the best of their ability." Many factors can influence how well (or not so well) you recover from training. If you're a high-level athlete or pushing yourself hard in preparation for a local competition, then stress can come from a variety of factors. Busy training schedules, increased competition loads, frequent travel, changing time zones, and altitude all play roles in adding "stress" to the system.[1] Add on top the massive metabolic demands of competition, mental and emotional strain, and the physical toll of game day (especially in contact sports). Each of these factors cause fatigue and challenge the recovery process. Shawn Arent, PhD, the director of the Human Health and Performance Lab at Rutgers University, is quick to point out that "game day efforts just can't be replicated in the lab!" This makes recovery a crucial piece of the performance puzzle.

What you do in the other 22 hours of the day — when you're not training or practicing your sport — really matters. In terms of your ability to recover (and ultimately perform), it is equal to or even more important than what you do in the gym and/or the playing field. A decade ago the best sports teams in the business made this realization. After tracking, monitoring, and quantifying everything athletes were doing on the field or in the gym, they still couldn't put their finger on the exact recipe for success. But it did make them realize just how important the other 22 hours were on an athlete's total stress load.

Stress comes in many forms; it's not just the training you need to recover from. All the other life stressors — work, school, friends, family, daily living, and more — can heavily influence your total stress load, and ultimately your capacity to recover. For example, last summer you had a terrific off-season training program and made significant gains; however, this year you're working two jobs, lacking adequate sleep, and not preparing your food as diligently. Do you think you'll adapt in the same way to the old program? Probably not. Athletes are dynamic, training is dynamic, life is dynamic . . . You must be nimble and be willing to recalibrate your plan.

Perhaps the best way to look at the "recovery" question is to analyze how successful athletes respond to exercise. When high-level athletes push themselves hard in a specific training block, it's normal for them to feel tired and sometimes see a small performance drop. But when athletes rest and recover effectively, they experience a positive adaptation and a gain in performance. This *super-compensation* is a fundamental tenet of the periodization concept. It's what you see in training camp settings when athletes are preparing for an upcoming season, performing two-a-day sessions, and pushing themselves hard. But how do you *really* know how hard to push an athlete? What's the right amount of stress? Are there clear signs, symptoms, and biomarkers to track? These are difficult questions to answer.

What about the other end of the spectrum? Dr. Halson highlights another important question: Can you *over-recover*? Player monitoring is now deeply embedded in sport, and it seems as if every poor athletic performance is quickly followed by the phrase, "They need more rest." Is this accurate? At what point does taking days off in your training plan start blunting training adaptations? Most athletes intuitively know you can under-recover, but over-recovering can blunt the inflammation and muscle damage signals required to trigger positive adaptations to exercise. In theory, it seems reasonable to suggest if you're less tired and less sore, it should make you less likely to get injured, but the reality is not so straightforward. Finding the right dose of recovery is a delicate balance that sport scientists are constantly trying to manage. This is the evolution of recovery science, and there is still so much more the best sport scientists in the world are still trying to figure out.

Coaches periodize training, and nutritionists periodize nutrition to match the training goals; however, periodizing recovery has only recently been getting more attention. As an athlete, could you periodize recovery to enhance your training adaptations during a specific phase, or (perhaps if not followed correctly) blunt some of your precious gains? This chapter is written to help practitioners discover how to support athletes in-season in an evidence-informed and systematic manner to ensure they're physically and mentally ready to train and perform on game day.

In the following pages I'll review how sport scientists define various states of athlete fatigue, discuss the new concept of periodized recovery, highlight common themes among the recovery philosophies of great coaches, and outline nutrition strategies to support recovery in athletes.

## How Far Can You Reach?
## Acute Fatigue, FOR, NFOR, and OTS

To make progress in the gym, or in any training environment, you need to push yourself. To be the best in the world, you *really* need to push yourself. Successful training must involve overload, which means consistently pushing the body beyond its capacity to elicit the super-compensation effect and allow an athlete to progress. At the Olympic level, the best athletes in the world have the highest training volumes compared to national-level athletes. So if you want to make it to the highest level — or go up a notch from local to regional, or regional to national — then you need to put in the work.[2] It seems straightforward enough: just add more volume to your training. But it's actually far more complex than it appears.

The more you train, the greater your likelihood of sleep disturbances. The more you train, the greater your potential risk of cold and flu. The more you train, the more closely you walk the tightrope between healthy and harmful overload, not to mention flirting with the health and performance abyss of overtraining. It's a slippery slope. How far into the red "danger" zone do you want to push the accelerator? How much volume (or intensity) do you stack on before it breaks you? This is a vital consideration in team sports, where there is no singular competition to peak for, but instead, repeated events that occur over and over again throughout the season.

That's why successful training not only includes overload, but avoids the combination of excessive overload and insufficient recovery.

The sport science term for the right dose of overload is called functional overreaching (FOR). This is when you experience a short-term drop in your performance toward the end of a training block, but do so without significant adverse effects on your mood, immunity, health, and the like. Athletes bounce back stronger and fitter after a short period of recovery from FOR. This is the ideal scenario, and the concept applies to strength, aerobic, or team sport. A preseason training camp setting is a great example of this phenomenon.

When athletes fail to respect the balance between training and recovery, things start to go downhill. The fatigue, weakness, and poor performance you naturally experience during an overload linger, and you don't bounce back after rest. Your energy levels are low, your muscles ache more than normal, and the bar feels heavier than usual in the gym. You're stuck in a rut. This is known as nonfunctional overreaching (NFOR), or the bad kind of overreaching. You've pushed yourself too much, or you haven't had a sufficient amount of recovery (or worse, both!). It can takes weeks to regain your performance if you've dipped into NFOR, which could spell disaster if it happens before a big game or competition.

This is often where many recreational athletes go wrong. They get caught up into constantly trying to "confuse" their muscles, changing things up so much they don't achieve an effective overload. At first, you make progress. It's easy to overload when you haven't been exercising and are deconditioned. The fitter you get, the more specific and calculated you need to be to achieve an effective overload. Without that discipline you simply burn out your nervous system with intense sessions. Going "all out" every time will eventually lead to stagnation and symptoms of NFOR.

If this performance rut extends from days and weeks to months, you've pushed yourself into the abyss of overtraining syndrome (OTS). Renowned sport scientist Romain Meeusen, PhD, from Vrije Universiteit in Brussels, defines overtraining as "a plateau or decrease in performance consequent to training too often, too long or too hard, and not resting enough between training bouts."[3] In practice, athletes might be doing all three: training too much, training too hard, *and* not resting enough. This is a recipe for disaster in the long run, and it's why a good coach is a crucial piece of every performance puzzle.

Overtraining syndrome is a prolonged period of maladaptation that typically involves biological, neurochemical, and hormonal mechanisms that are far worse than NFOR. OTS can last for many months (sometimes up to a year or more) and is accompanied by symptoms of constant fatigue, pronounced performance declines, frequent or prolonged colds and flu, low mood and libido, and poor general health. In a practical sense, the main difference between NFOR and OTS is the amount of time your body needs to recover and bounce back to baseline. In a perfect world, both are completely avoided, but at the highest level, the line between positive FOR and detrimental NFOR is very thin.

How prevalent are NFOR and OTS? It occurs in about 10 percent of endurance athletes, but can increase to 21 percent in certain populations. Collegiate athletes are at particularly high risk. At the elite collegiate level, the first year in training is actually a huge predictor of future success or struggles. A recent study found that 91 percent of athletes with OTS in their first year at college or university would go on to struggle with it repeatedly (in one or more of the next three years), compared to only 34 percent of athletes who made it through their freshman year unscathed.[4] This issue likely has transfer to recreational athletes as well: If you get things right from the start, then you're far more likely to avoid the pitfalls of burnout as you go. OTS is far more common in endurance athletes, compared to strength and team sports, due to the nature of their training and the higher volumes of training that are required to compete. Expert physiologist Daniel Plews, PhD, a research fellow at the Sports Performance Research Institute New Zealand (SPRINZ) at the Auckland University of Technology, helped the New Zealand rowing team at both the 2012 and 2016 Olympic Games to win five gold medals. As an elite Ironman competitor himself, he is quick to point out that "endurance athletes walk the razor's edge between training stress and recovery." The job of a good coach or practitioner is to avoid maladaptive response to training like NFOR (and definitely OTS), because if an athlete is too rundown to train, they'll never beat the competition. They will always be two steps behind.

This is where athlete monitoring can play a massive role in supporting effective recovery. The earliest sign of athlete stress is acute fatigue, characterized by tiredness and a desire to rest. Acute fatigue is both physical and mental. With rest, it dissipates and the athlete becomes stronger. All athletes experience acute fatigue, and it's important to note that acute fatigue sets in before an athlete experiences FOR. Interestingly, in the research there is a clear difference between an athlete experiencing acute fatigue and an athlete experiencing functional overreaching. The super-compensation effect is greater in athletes with training-induced fatigue versus those experiencing functional overreaching (FOR), which means your ability to assess, monitor, and support effective recovery is crucial to athletic success.[5] Not only that, athletes dipping their toes into the realm of "good" FOR actually increase their risk of progressing to "bad" NFOR training maladaptation.[6] What does all this mean for the trainer or coach who should be keeping tabs on this? Applying effective recovery strategies, identifying the early signs of athlete fatigue (and FOR), and monitoring athletes are crucial pieces of the performance puzzle. If you wait until more pronounced symptoms show up, it makes the job that much more difficult (and it might even be too late if it's too close to competition).

If you're a coach or trainer, how do you know if your athlete's recovery is being compromised? When does an athlete cross the line from "good" functional overreaching (FOR) — where symptoms dissipate and functions return to normal after a few days (at most a week) — into "bad", maladaptive, nonfunctional overreaching (NFOR)? The most obvious symptoms include an inability to sustain effort during intense exercise, and increased fatigue during exercise and at rest. NFOR also tends to present with more psychological symptoms like periods of low mood, sleep disturbances, changes in eating patterns (sugar cravings, for example), and more frequent colds and flu.[7] It usually lasts for weeks (sometimes months), so identifying the earliest warning signs with clients is crucial in order to prioritize recovery and adjust the training plan. You want to catch them before they fall over the edge into overtraining. If your athlete is truly overtraining, it can take months or even years for them to recover. This effect occurs all the time in recreational athletes who train hard while logging long hours at the office. For these individuals, the other 22 hours is typically where the recovery roadblock lies. The accumulation of all of life's other stressors become too much for the system to cope with.

## Understanding Biomarkers: A Piece of the Recovery Puzzle

The biggest hurdle for expert sport scientists and doctors is distinguishing between acute fatigue, FOR, and NFOR states, as the differences can be incredibly subtle. Currently, there is no single gold-standard marker, biomarker, or collection of biomarkers to determine when an athlete is exceeding their limits.[8] The real-life symptoms aren't specific, they vary from athlete to athlete, and they can be numerous. Blood tests can be valuable biomarkers, providing a snapshot of the athlete's state of health and how well they're coping with stress. This information, in conjunction with the athlete's performance metrics and subjective feelings, can help to inform and guide decision-making as it relates to recovery strategies. Athletes at the professional level might get tested quarterly, whereas some collegiate athletes — such as Dr. Shawn Arent's teams at Rutgers University — might have the opportunity to get tested every month. The questions coaches and practitioners typically have  concern balance. Can biomarkers help flag overreaching and overtraining athletes? Can they distinguish between helpful (FOR) and harmful (NFOR) overreaching? Can the biomarkers tell you if athletes are pushing themselves too far over the line, or not hard enough? These are great questions, and the best experts in the world are still grappling with the answers. At the moment, there is no single biomarker, nor collection of biomarkers, that can specifically identify FOR, NFOR, and OTS. That said, gaining insights into specific key biomarkers can help athletes determine how they're responding to training and can also help them flag potential problems before they become major roadblocks. The following is a short list of commonly used markers.

## MUSCLE BREAKDOWN

The two most common biomarkers used for muscle breakdown are creatine kinase (CK) and lactate dehydrogenase (LDH). Creatine kinase is a very specific marker for muscle damage, and it is expected to be high when an athlete is training hard. Unfortunately, it's also highly variable in elite-level athletes, so you can't use the data alone to flag NFOR or OTS. Lactate dehydrogenase (LDH) can help shed more light on the picture. It's an enzyme found in almost all of the body's cells and is released into the blood when cells are damaged or destroyed. High levels are often, but not always, seen with high training loads. Again, this doesn't necessarily mean the athlete is struggling to recover effectively and adapt to training; it just means their muscles are working hard and tissue damage is taking place.

## INFLAMMATION

C-reactive protein (CRP-hs) is a biomarker for systemic inflammation, and intense exercise will cause a lot of inflammation. You would think it's a no-brainer to use CRP-hs to flag overtraining athletes. Unfortunately, it's not so straightforward. CRP-hs is also an acute-phase reactant, which means it responds to a lot of different factors in the body, and thus is not a very reliable biomarker during periods of heavy training when there's a lot of external noise. Interestingly, it might be a better bet when measuring athletes during periods of rest. Why? This is a time when you would expect their readings to return to baseline; thus, if you see an athlete with high CRP-hs during a rest period, it could be an early indicator of a potential problem.[9] Remember, these biomarkers are just a snapshot in time.

## Blood Glucose

Blood glucose levels can also provide you with insights about an athlete's health and recovery. Hemoglobin A1c (HbA1c) is a three-month estimate of blood glucose levels, and it gives you a glimpse into an athlete's nutrition regimen. More directly related to recovery, monitoring an athlete's morning fasting glucose can shed some light on the inflammatory load (and thus stress level) of the athlete. It's a cost-effective tool performed via a finger prick first thing in the morning. Daniel Plews, PhD, uses this test as a general assessment of overall stress load in endurance athletes. He raises a red flag when an athlete's level gets above 5.0 mmol/L (90 mg/dL). The use of continuous glucose monitors (CGM) is also gaining momentum, because it addresses the highly variable individual responses to food. CGM testing also provides a glimpse into how the "other 22 hours" are impacting an athlete's glucose control.

## Hormones

Hormones are often touted as key biomarkers that can be used to accurately predict how well an athlete is coping with stress, training, and competition. The classic hormone biomarkers for athletes are cortisol and testosterone, measured via urine, saliva, or blood. Low levels of cortisol, particularly seen during a stimulation test, are probably the most sensitive test for overtraining.[10] Unfortunately, for free and total testosterone there is only 26 percent diagnostic sensitivity for NFOR, and it's even worse yet in saliva and urine.[11] The use of a testosterone-to-cortisol ratio has also been implemented as a marker of overtraining. Typically this ratio decreases with training intensity and excess training volume. While a testosterone-to-cortisol ratio is useful acutely post-exercise, it doesn't pan out in the long term and can't differentiate between overreaching and overtraining.[12] That said, new research by Dr. Arent is finding that free cortisol, free testosterone, and free T3 thyroid hormone (in particular) are helpful in identifying athletes who are pushing the red line toward overtraining. Rather than focusing on absolute measures, Dr. Arent suggests keeping an eye on *relative* changes in individual athletes. To make informed decisions from biomarkers, it's important to run regular tests, rather than to perform one-off testing. This is because biomarkers are a snapshot in time, a piece of the puzzle that can help get a clearer picture of how the athlete is adapting and recovering.

Another biomarker used to assess an athlete's ability to tolerate training load is the adrenocorticotropic hormone (ACTH) to cortisol (C) ratio. Increases are seen in ACTH:C during recovery periods after exercise (due to a decrease in pituitary sensitivity to cortisol and tissue-sensitive changes in stress hormones) when an athlete is positively adapting to training.[13] Once again, the gray area is interpretation. Take for example endurance-trained men: on rest days their 24-hour cortisol output is normal and is exactly the same as age-matched *sedentary* men.[14] Also, cortisol output changes depending on the time of year. You can't compare tests done in the summer with another performed in fall or winter. Cortisol tests done in summer tend to provide lower readings, and in winter the readings tend to be higher. You can't compare the two due to this seasonal rhythmicity, because it's apples and oranges. Unless you can collect this data monthly, and have someone committed to analyzing the data, most sport scientists believe rest-day cortisol testing to be almost completely useless.

## CATECHOLAMINES

How about measuring catecholamine levels — such as epinephrine (adrenaline), norepinephrine (noradrenaline), or dopamine — over a 24-hour period? Surely the output of adrenaline, noradrenaline, and dopamine could help predict overtraining and help steer training advice? Unfortunately, it's another "maybe." The relationship between 24-hour urine output and performance or training monitoring is inconclusive and deemed "inappropriate . . . as a tool to monitor training status."[15] You can still measure it and add it to an athlete's profile, just don't hang your hat on it.

## HEMOGLOBIN

Blood serum markers like hemoglobin levels are also commonly used to assess and monitor athlete load. Declining levels of serum hemoglobin — the protein molecule in red blood cells (RBCs) that carries oxygen from your lungs to your tissues — is sometimes seen in trainees pushing the limits or struggling with OTS. The problem is hemoglobin is only 33 percent specific (I know, I know . . . I sound like a broken record!).[16]

Blood biomarkers provide a rough snapshot of what's going on. While specific, they aren't sensitive enough to tell with certainty if an athlete is struggling or adapting well to training. For example, let's look at common themes among athletes struggling with overtraining syndrome (OTS). During OTS, a small rise in pituitary hormones — ACTH, growth hormone, luteinizing hormone, and FSH — is seen in response to a stressful training stimulus.[17] This change in pituitary hormones can potentially be useful. The problem again is that while it's specific (meaning it tells you about overtraining), it's not very sensitive. Some athletes with low levels might struggle while others will perform and recover with no problem. How can you differentiate between the two in a real-world scenario? Training-induced catabolism can also spur reductions in IL-6, IGF-1, and insulin, but you must remember that these markers also decline when an athlete is in a chronic energy deficit. A failure to consume enough calories to support training and life demands — known as low energy availability — is often seen in endurance athletes, athletes in aesthetic sports during a weight cut, or sometimes in team sport athletes during the latter half of a long competitive season. If an athlete is chronically energy deficient, it will amplify stress hormone response and inflammatory cytokine response to exercise (mainly from depleted glycogen). This might be a trigger for NFOR or OTS in some athletes but not others. In short, similar patterns might be seen in athletes recovering well and those who are struggling to keep up.

At a certain point, it might seem daunting to make sense of all this complexity. While blood test biomarkers add important pieces to the puzzle, alone they cannot complete the picture. This is the danger of relying too heavily on data — an athlete's coach, nutritionist, or doctor shouldn't be steering the protocol based *solely* on these blood test results. This highlights the complexity of the problem and the importance of a good coach and performance team. You need to use this data in conjunction with physical performance metrics and the athlete's subjective experience (and symptoms) to fill in the gaps. More often than not, it comes back to the "coach's eye." Upgrading your skills as an expert-generalist can improve your ability to help athletes tread the fine line between positive adaptation to training stress and the pitfalls of maladaptation. This is what separates good coaches from great coaches.

## The Recovery Pyramid

A lot of people think of recovery as the isolated period directly after a training session. But recovery is also a preparation method for the *next* training session the following day, over the course of a week, or during a training block. Today, new technology allows sport scientists to more accurately assess internal and external training loads in athletes, and in theory create a better training and recovery plan. What is the ideal strategy to get athletes ready for their next sprint or Olympic heavy-lifting session? When athletes think recovery, they usually think of ice baths, hot tubs, massage, or compression garments. While these are all definitely tools and strategies for recovery, they're not the foundation. You're putting the cart before the horse if your recovery emphasis is focused on strategies. Expert sport scientist Lachlan Penfold, former director of performance for the Golden State Warriors and currently with the Melbourne Storm of the National Rugby League (NRL) in Australia, hammers home the importance of recovery to his players (and staff) by emphasizing a Recovery Pyramid (see figure 7.1). The base of the pyramid is the foundation for successful recovery—nutrition, sleep, and stress management (mental-emotional health). Penfold emphasizes to his staff, "If you're not sleeping or you're stressed out at home, you can take all the ice baths in the world, you won't recover effectively." This highlights the massive importance of the fundamentals, and this emphasis ensures that those fundamentals are applied in practice. Next up on the pyramid hierarchy is the training plan. Above that on Penfold's list comes athlete monitoring to help guide (not control) the decision-making process. This is followed by therapeutic treatments. The very top of the pyramid are recovery modalities, which are things like ice baths, cryotherapy, compression garments, neuromuscular stimulation, and the like. These recovery strategies alone won't make or break progress, but at the highest level they might provide the marginal gains needed to maximize recovery. Unfortunately, too many athletes—both recreational and elite—put their emphasis on the tip of the pyramid rather than the fundamentals at the base.

This philosophy is also shared by Shona Halson, PhD, at the Australian Institute of Sport. Referring to the sleep component at the base of the

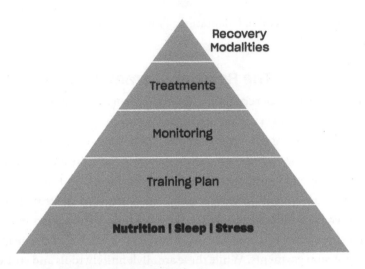

**FIGURE 7.1.** Penfold's Recovery Pyramid.

pyramid, she says, "If you're an athlete, sleep is the first place to start for re-covery. Especially for recreational athletes." Sleep isn't just crucial for athlete health, it's also a huge pillar for recovery. She warns that pushing the limits in training and at work at the expense of sleep will ultimately compromise performance. Recreational athletes keen on improving performance often get caught up in "trendy" recovery strategies, such as cold-water immersions and compression garments. But if those athletes are only sleeping 5.5 hours a night, those strategies mean very little. As we know, sleep is essential to overall health, so it makes sense that it's also essential for recovery. Not surprisingly, all the experts in the field of athletic recovery put a heavy emphasis on sleep. Dr. Halson emphasizes making adjustments in small, incremental steps with athletes. Adding extra sleep in 30-minute increments per night can lead to big gains down the line (a theme shared by sleep experts like Cheri Mah, MD, and Amy Bender, PhD, noted in chapter 1). But what happens if you have a bad night's sleep before a key training session or event? Dr. Halson says don't sweat the small stuff — you'll bounce back and perform fine. If it continues for a week or more, then it's time to reexamine sleep quality.

Another component of the foundation of Penfold's Recovery Pyramid is mental and emotional stability (that is, stress management). If you're stressed out from work or school, and if you're struggling within a relation-ship or family, do you think you'll adapt as well as you could to your train-ing plan? Likely not. All the stress you encounter in the "other 22 hours" when you're not training play a massive role in your capacity to recover. An athlete's mental and emotional stress is challenging for coaches and practitioners to assess because it's so subjective and highly individual. Nevertheless, the more mental resiliency athletes can build, the greater their capacity to recover. (In Part Four: Supercharge, I'll discuss how to support an athlete's brain and emotional health.)

Nutrition is the final component at the base of the Recovery Pyramid. The faster athletes can recover, the more training stress they can apply, the greater the adaptations. But if athletes fail to fuel themselves effectively, they will be more prone to harmful overreaching, and eventually overtraining. Let's now take a closer look at the latest evidence-based research when it comes to recovery nutrition.

## Recovery Nutrition Part 1: "The Big 3"

We've come a long way in the last decade in terms of nutrition and recovery. Most athletes and coaches know nutrition is a key component of optimal recovery, yet it's often still difficult to implement with maximal compliance. Nutrition can enhance recovery by promoting muscle repair, restoring glycogen status, reducing fatigue, cooling excessive inflammation, supporting immunity and digestive health, and improving overall health.[18] Another key principle of the new concept of periodized recovery is that athletes are not just recovering from the last training session but are also getting themselves ready for the upcoming session tomorrow, the rest of the week, and the remainder of the training block. Is tomorrow morning's training session an easy recovery run? Will it consist of hitting it hard with a heavy lifting session in the morning? The answers might influence nutrition choices the night before.

Nutrition is still an often-overlooked area when it comes to recovery, but it should be a fundamental focus. What coaches and practitioners want to know is how best to apply it in practice. What can move the needle for your athlete and give them an edge over the competition? What does the evidence-based research say, and how can it effectively inform your practice? Let's take a closer look at the Big 3: energy balance, protein intake, and carbohydrate intake.

### 1. ENERGY BALANCE

Energy balance plays the biggest role in the recovery process. In Part Two: Fuel, I highlighted how the biggest lever putting the brakes on the catabolic process is calories. When you ramp up training intensity or training volume (or both!), you need a lot more energy from the food you're eating to meet those demands. Your total energy intake is the biggest signal to your body to say "build." If you start ramping up intense training but forget to also ramp up your energy intake, you're setting yourself up for failure.

When you're in an energy deficit, the deficit itself is *the* major trigger for catabolism. Caloric restriction decreases muscle protein synthesis and key cellular signaling pathways for survival, and activates AMPK and sirtuins, which blunt muscle-building mTOR activity and ramp up protein turn-over.[19] In fact, even eucaloric conditions (when your calories in effectively match your calories out) are sub-optimal because the catabolism of proteins that occurs to fuel your vital organs are derived predominantly from your muscle tissue. In short, an energy deficit is a major problem for optimal recovery. Positive energy balance alone is a major stimulator of anabolism.[20] How much energy do you need to recover? It's a difficult question to answer. The International Society of Sports Nutrition recommends 50–80 kcal/kg/day for strength and team sport athletes. The recommendation for women athletes is a minimum of 40–45 kcal/kg/day.[21]

New research is investigating how your body attempts to offset the increase in energy you need to support intense training by slowing down your resting metabolic rate (RMR). If you don't eat enough, your RMR slows down. If you don't sleep enough, your RMR goes down. If you train too much, your RMR goes down. The work of Dr. Halson and her team has uncovered how RMR decreases with greater training loads, especially in endurance athletes.[22] This state of low energy availability (LEA) means there is less energy to support immunity, digestive and cardiovascular health, energy and red blood cell production, and bone health, growth, and repair. Traditionally, LEA is found more often in female and endurance athletes, but men and team sport athletes are not immune to it. Major red flags include amenorrhea (defined as loss of menses for three months or longer) and stress fractures, while secondary flags are more subtle — altered fasting glucose levels, lower insulin and free T3 thyroid hormone levels, and elevated cholesterol levels.[23] Performance dietitian Jen Sygo, formerly with the NHL's Toronto Maple Leafs and currently with NBA's Toronto Raptors, conducted a study in elite female sprinters. Sygo found that over 50 percent suffered from LEA by the end of a five-month indoor season.[24] This was eye-opening because most experts still believe low energy availability doesn't impact strength and power sport athletes. Perhaps even more concerning, 4 out of the 13 athletes presented to preseason training camp with LEA, which effectively means they were coming out of the gates into a new season at a disadvantage. For high-level athletes training intensely, or for recreational ones balancing work and sport, Sygo says it can actually be difficult to get in all the fuel you need to meet your demands. This constellation of symptoms, defined in the research as Relative Energy Deficiency in Sport (RED-S), reflects an athlete in sub-optimal health and highlights how insufficient energy intake compromises the Human First paradigm. If you consistently fall short on calories, Sygo highlights, you increase the risk of redlining or "circling the drain," the slang term performance nutritionists use to describe athletes who are headed toward the downward spiral of poor recovery and performance. If you can't recover, you won't be able to perform at a high level. It's that simple. Tailoring your total energy intake (and macronutrient balance of protein, carbs and fats) to suit your individual needs, your training block, and your ultimate goals is crucial.

## 2. Protein Intake

Protein is a building block for life. It promotes recovery in many ways, and chief among them are muscle repair and improved immune function. Athletes experience muscle damage from resistance training, and muscles need protein for repair. Team sport athletes run, cut, and move in multiple directions. Such activity is a massive contributor to training load, and it requires repeated eccentric muscle contractions that can lead to more muscle damage and soreness many days after competition (not to mention the physical contact that also damages body tissues).[25] Immunity also takes a big hit when training volume increases, making athletes more susceptible to colds and flu. Athletes whose bodies can't repair fast enough, or those who are always sick, won't be able to train intensely enough to pass the competition. This makes protein intake crucial for athletic recovery. Most athletes have heard the "eat more protein" mantra before from coaches and practitioners; however, many still struggle to achieve the *minimum* effective protein dose recommended for athletes of 1.6 g/kg/day, which is a figure based on the work of protein expert Stuart Phillips, PhD, and his team at McMaster University.[26]

Another key take-home for the expert-generalist regarding Recovery Nutrition is to pay close attention in the latter half of the season. This is when athletes get more run-down, lose lean muscle mass, and experience more bouts of cold and flu. When athletes are tired and run-down, they often eat less as well (which often goes unnoticed). Not only does this cause potential health issues due to energy deficit, it also tends to lead to a lower protein intake. Insufficient energy intake combined with inadequate protein intake is a recovery disaster waiting to happen. A recent study of collegiate weightlifters participating in off-season training found that all athletes failed to meet the International Society Sports Nutrition's recommendations for calories, protein, and carbohydrates.[27] This study highlights how easy it is for athletes to under-eat, which can easily compromise their ability to recover effectively.

If you're a figure competitor, bodybuilder, or physique-focused athlete and recovering in a caloric deficit, it becomes even more important to ramp up protein consumption. Recall the research on hypertrophy from Eric Helms, PhD, that suggests protein intakes between 2.3–3.1 g/kg/day (of fat-free mass) can help protect against lean mass losses. Higher protein intakes during periods of calorie deficit can also help to support athlete immunity and help injured players get back to health so that they can return to play. It's easy for athletes to fall into the trap of thinking, "Because I'm not training hard, I don't need to eat as much protein." Big mistake.

What about the "magic window" for protein intake post-training? Renowned expert Brad Schoenfeld, PhD, the director of performance at Lehman College in New York, has recently debunked this myth in his research. Recovery is a 24-hour process — it's nutrition over the course of the entire day that really counts. But if you're training in a fasted state or performing multiple sessions in 1 day separated by less than 4 hours, then you can consider nutrient timing strategies.[28] Schoenfeld suggests a good rule of thumb is for athletes to get at least four to six meals in daily, with a protein dose of approximately 0.25–0.4 g/kg (20–50 g) per meal, spread evenly throughout the day.

### 3. CARBOHYDRATE INTAKE

Carbs are a crucial fuel for recovery from intense training and in preparation for future performance. Low-carb and keto diets tend to dominate social media these days, and it's easy for athletes to get swept up in the deluge of anecdotal evidence they find online. Although both diets can be effective strategies for obese, diabetic, and metabolically challenged clients,

## Alcohol and Recovery

Depending on your age and your sport, drinking might be much more a reality in an athlete's life than a trainer or coach would like to admit. Collegiate athletes tend to binge drink, and sports such as rugby are renowned for their drinking culture when on competitive tours. Binge drinking is not only bad for your health, it's also bad for your muscles, because it impairs the body's ability to rebuild muscle post-exercise by inhibiting mTOR activation.[29] In short, if you know you're going to have a big drinking night, stay away from a heavy lifting session beforehand.

for athletes it's a different story. Athletes might, for example, start cutting carbs short (or out completely) at inappropriate times of the day or season. Unfortunately, if your fueling strategy doesn't match your goals (are you adapting or optimizing?), low-carb diets can easily lead to insufficient energy for recovery and performance. Many athletes don't fully understand just how important carbs are for the recovery process. For team sport athletes fighting through the rigors of a season, you might recall from the previous chapter that an evidence-based target is 4–7 g/kg/day of carbs to meet recovery demands.[30] Compare this to a bodybuilder or physique-focused athlete who might have periods where they drop carb intake to as low as 1–3 g/kg, or to an elite endurance athlete who might burn 6,000 calories a day and might need up to 10–12 g/kg/day of carbs to fuel all those long efforts. That's how far the pendulum can swing from one sport to another!

Athletes need carbs to fuel high-intensity training, to prevent fatigue, to fight off colds and flus (carbs are a big factor in immunity), to prevent the catabolic cascade of events that occur via energy deficit, and to overtraining or potential injuries.[31] If your glycogen stores aren't fully topped up, performance is going to suffer when pushing into your top gear during competition.[32] (However, planned and purposeful *training* with low-carb availability is an effective training tool, as discussed in Part Two: Fuel.)

If you're in a training camp–type setting, performing two-a-day sessions, or at a tournament with multiple games in a single day, then you need to be more proactive with refueling. Aim for 1.0 g/kg within the first hour post-training, and every hour thereafter up to 4 hours post-exercise to maximally top up glycogen stores.[33] This scenario is where higher-GI and rapidly absorbed carbs are preferred because they top up liver and muscle glycogen quickly. Of course, if your exercise intensity is moderate to low, if the duration is less than 90 minutes, or if you have at least 8 hours before the next session, then there is no need to take these aggressive proactive measures. If you're a recreational athlete training three to four times a week for 45–60 minutes, you don't need to worry about glycogen levels or rapid repletion. Remember, communication is key to help athletes make the right nutrition choices for recovery.

## Recovery Nutrition Part 2: Managing Micronutrients

Once you've established the fundamentals of Recovery Nutrition — energy balance, protein intake, and carb intake — it's time to dig a little deeper and mine for the smaller gains that might push you over the top. This is where a focus on micronutrients plays an important role in supporting health and recovery. If you're struggling with a health condition, lowered immunity, excessive inflammation, traveling frequently on the road, or really pushing the limits of your training capacity, then addressing micronutrient insufficiencies (or deficiencies) can be highly impactful.[34] Let's review the evidence-based micronutrients for recovery.

### INFLAMMATION, MUSCLE SORENESS, AND IMMUNE MODULATION

Recovery is essential to your ability to compete in the *next* game. The constant pounding, relentless intensity, and grueling demands of the season make it important to seek out all possible advantages. For athletes, omega-3 fats are capable of promoting muscle remodeling and repair via direct incorporation into the cell membrane of the muscle. This remodeling of the muscle cell wall triggers an activation of signaling proteins (within the cell membrane), such as the mTOR protein complex that triggers muscle protein synthesis.[35] Interestingly, the long chain EPA (eicosapentaenoic acid) is responsible for eliciting these effects, not DHA (docosahexaenoic acid). Omega-3 also plays an important role as an anti-inflammatory modulator. Intense exercise causes mechanical stress, metabolic stress, and tissue microtrauma, which trigger the beneficial adaptations to training.

Omega-3 supplementation has been found to improve feelings of muscle soreness and oxidative stress — especially after eccentric-based training — up to 2 days after training.[36] The supplement can make a big impact during heavy training blocks or late stages of a long competitive season. Omega-3 also plays a role in modulating your immune system via compounds called resolvins, which is important for high-level athletes exposed to the high training volumes that can crush the immune system. Unfortunately, vegetable-based omega-3 fats such as flax oil convert poorly to EPA/DHA, at a paltry 10 percent (up to 20 percent in women). Sea algae DHA supplements can do the trick; however, you need to consume a lot of capsules to achieve a therapeutic dose. Aim for 1,600 mg of combined EPA and DHA daily for men and 1,100 mg for women (regardless of bodyweight).

### VITAMIN D, SATELLITE CELLS, AND ACCELERATED RECOVERY

After intense exercise, a key component of recovery is repairing damaged muscle tissue, which occurs when satellite cells become activated by training-induced damage. There are many factors that support this recovery process, but researchers have recently found that vitamin D plays a role. There even appears to be a difference between upper- and lower-body recoveries. Research on upper-body recovery — as measured by an individual's ability to exert a maximal isometric force — found no recovery benefits with supplemental vitamin D.[37] On the other hand, lower-body muscle damage did show a significant improvement with added vitamin D.[38] A follow-up study in active men found that 6 weeks of vitamin D supplementation at 4,000 IU daily improved muscle recovery 48 hours after training and lasted up to 7 days; however, no benefit was shown for muscle soreness. Of course, the limitation with a lot of this research is that the subjects are not elite athletes (heck, many aren't even athletes at all!), making interpreting the data difficult.

Expert Graeme Close, PhD, from Liverpool John Moores University recommends athletes achieve a minimum level of 75 nmol/L (30 ng/mL), as this appears to be a threshold for the impact of vitamin D on satellite cell activity and recovery. If an athlete is deficient in vitamin D (below 50 nmol/L or 20 ng/mL), it can impair muscle regeneration and performance.[39] Exposure to the sun is the best place to get your vitamin D; when you get vitamin D from the sun, it doesn't spill over into systemic circulation (as it can with over-supplementation) and you lessen the risk of soft tissue calcification that can occur with excessive supplementation. On a sunny day, 30 minutes of exposure to your limbs or face nets about 10,000–20,000 IU of vitamin D₃; aim for midmorning and midafternoon to avoid peak sun intensity. Lastly, an underappreciated root cause of low vitamin D status in the general population is the widespread use of statins, high blood pressure drugs (thiazide diuretics), corticosteroids, and antibiotics. Antibiotics can reduce vitamin K levels by 75 percent, impacting the body's ability to utilize vitamin D effectively (another reason to add a probiotic if you need to go on antibiotics). As for supplementation, recall from Part Two: Fuel that the recommendation is 2,000–4,000 IU daily. Remember that it takes 4–6 weeks to ramp up your vitamin D status, so don't leave it until the last minute.

## POLYPHENOL POWER AND THE ANTIOXIDANT DEFENSE SYSTEM

For most Americans, coffee and tea provide over 50 percent of their daily polyphenol antioxidant intake. Next on the list are dark-skinned fruit, leafy greens, and cruciferous veggies. Athletes who eat a highly processed diet — like many high school, collegiate, and even pro athletes do — might have a low antioxidant status. Exercise is a major source of oxidative stress, kicking up free radical damage in the body. Of course, your body is hardwired with its own antioxidant defense system to help you repair and rebuild, but if you don't drink coffee (or tea) or if you struggle to eat your vegetables, you might be compromising your antioxidant defense system. Key players in this robust defense system include enzymes such as superoxide dismutase and glutathione peroxidase, whose role it is to scan the body for reactive oxygen species (ROS) and extinguish the pro-inflammatory sparks they create.[40]

The more you train, the more your body adapts by ramping up its own internal antioxidant production, increasing the workload on antioxidant enzymes and repairing the damage caused by exercise. When you stress your body, signals are generated telling your brain it's time to repair, and the internal cellular machinery is kicked into a higher gear to do the job. Humans are designed to adapt; it's what we do best. If you're still stuck in the "free radicals bad, antioxidants good" mindset, consider the following: ROS are key signaling molecules that trigger your muscles to grow, and even low levels of ROS are essential for supporting muscular force production.[41] If you want your athletes to be strong, healthy, and powerful, don't fear free-radical damage.

Now let's talk nuance. Food and drink aren't the only sources of antioxidants — you can also get them exogenously from antioxidant supplements.

The most common antioxidants studied with respect to athletes include vitamins C and E, as well as catechins (found in tea), quercetin (found in apples and raw onions), and anthocyanidins (found in blueberries, blackberries, and grapes). However, using high-dose antioxidant supplements post-training has been clearly shown to blunt some of the beneficial, adaptive training responses and dampen gains, an effect that is consistent in both strength and endurance athletes.[42] For example, even a 1,000 mg dose of vitamin C supplement after exercise might negatively impact training adaptations; however, dietary vitamin C from fruit and veggies does not exert this effect.[43] This is a great example of how nutrient timing can sometimes *negatively* impact training.

Actually, there are a lot of factors to consider when it comes to antioxidants, such as the athlete's baseline antioxidant status, uptake of antioxidants, timing and dose, and the athlete's training protocol. Long-term supplementation, in fact, seems to pose more risks than benefits, and if the best experts in the world aren't sure, the expert-generalist should take a conservative approach. Bottom line: Aim to get antioxidants from food.

### Functional Foods: Vegetable and Fruit Juice
Functional foods — concentrated fruit and vegetable drinks — have recently become the recommended source to support or accelerate recovery. In Part Two: Fuel we discussed the power of beet juice as an ergogenic aid. But it also has many recovery benefits, including offsetting losses in muscle function from training (a key recovery factor) as well as reducing muscle soreness after specific types of training.[44] Tart Montmorency cherry juice might also accelerate recovery, as it's been shown to reduce markers of inflammation and the perception of muscle soreness, and to improve antioxidant status after exercise.[45] The polyphenol quercetin, naturally found in cherries, kicks off a cascade of reactions that help to reduce upper respiratory symptoms (URS), and emerging evidence finds that cherry juice might also be a superior sleep aid via its phenolic compounds, which contain high concentrations of melatonin. Pomegranate juice also shows promise for reducing muscle soreness after eccentric exercise, as well as lowering CK and LDH biomarkers for tissue damage up to 48 hours after Olympic weightlifting.[46] Additionally, there is some evidence that black currant juice has an ability to reduce post-exercise muscular inflammation, although for only 24 hours post-training.[47]

The uses of natural vegetable and fruit juices is a rapidly growing area in sports nutrition research. But before you jump in with both feet and start adding exotic juices to your arsenal, think about what you're trying to accomplish. Are you in an *adaptation* period, like training camp? If so, then you don't really want to dampen the inflammatory signal that is essential for adaptation. On the other hand, if you're trying to *optimize* performance — peaking before a major event or playoff race — then your primary goal should be to maintain athletic qualities, which would therefore make this an appropriate time for more antioxidant support. I've said it before and I'll say it again: context is everything.

## Recovery Nutrition Part 3: Supplements

In terms of supplementation, certain recovery-specific supplements can accelerate an athlete's capacity to get back in the gym to train or be ready for another competitive game on back-to-back nights.

### CREATINE: THE FORGOTTEN RECOVERY ACCELERATOR

As noted in Part Two: Fuel, creatine ticked all the evidence-based boxes for supplements that can support strength, hypertrophy, and performance for athletes. What often gets overlooked is the ability of creatine to support recovery. If you're looking for a nutritional strategy that will enhance fuel replacement, increase post-training muscle protein synthesis, stimulate genetic growth factors, and reduce exercise-induced muscle damage and inflammation, then once again, creatine ticks all the boxes.[48] Research in lower-body-based eccentric exercise found that creatine reduced creatine kinase (CK) and lactate dehydrogenase (LDH) levels, which are reliable markers of muscle damage.[49] Creatine also improves delayed onset muscle soreness (DOMS), prevents reductions in range of motion from heavy training, and accelerates creatine resynthesis in muscles — all big wins if you're doing multiple sessions in 1 day.[50] Endurance athletes often overlook the benefits of creatine, thinking it's solely for power-based athletes. But multiple studies have found creatine loading in endurance athletes (20 g per day for 5 days) buffered spikes in muscle damage and inflammation after a 30-km run and half-Ironman.[51] Athletes saw reductions in both CK and LDH, as well as pro-inflammatory markers prostaglandin E2, interleukin-1 beta, and tumor necrosis factor alpha. If you're working with endurance-based athletes and their recovery time is a limiting factor in their ability to train or perform, creatine supplementation might provide a recovery advantage that will allow them to train more often or more intensely.

## CURCUMIN: THE SECRET FOR STRENGTH-BASED ATHLETIC RECOVERY

Curcumin is the active ingredient in the traditional Indian spice turmeric, and it exerts significant anti-inflammatory effects via COX-2 and TNF-alpha inhibition (among other pathways).[52] If curcumin supplementation can reliably reduce muscle soreness and inflammation in athletes, it might have a role as a potential recovery aid. For strength-based athletes doing eccentric resistance training, the results look promising. High-quality curcumin supplements at 400 mg daily reduced pro-inflammatory markers of muscle damage by 48 percent when taken 2 days prior and 4 days after the high-intensity training bout.[53] Another study found curcumin supplementation significantly reduced delayed-onset muscle soreness (DOMS) 24 hours and 48 hours after intense muscle-damaging training.[54] Interestingly, for endurance athletes the evidence isn't so clear. A 500 mg curcumin dose given 3 days before and immediately prior to training demonstrated no difference in muscle damage or inflammatory markers.[55]

## GELATIN AND COLLAGEN: BULLETPROOF YOUR JOINTS

Gelatin is the new kid on the block when it comes to sports supplementation and recovery. The work of muscle physiology researcher Keith Baar, PhD, from the University of California, Davis, has uncovered some incredible findings on the use of supplemental gelatin for joint health and recovery. Just like you can't build a strong wall without bricks, you can't build strong joints without collagen. Gelatin is found in the skin, bones, and connective tissues of animals (if you make bone broth at home, it's the stuff that floats to the top). At hot temperatures, gelatin presents in liquid form, and when it cools down it turns into a jellylike consistency. The process of hydrolyzation turns gelatin into supplemental collagen, which is soluble in both hot and cold water, making it a lot easier to use. Performance nutritionists often use gelatin in combination with cherry or pomegranate juice to make gelatin gummies for a preworkout snack.

Collagen is the main building block and structural protein in bone, tendon, and cartilage. A recent study found that when gelatin supplements (or the hydrolyzed form of collagen) are combined with vitamin C, collagen production increased threefold.[56] When timed 1 hour before training or rehab (mechanical loading) and combined with 40–50 mg of vitamin C, Dr. Barr and his team found that it doubled the amount of type-I collagen.[57] A 10 g daily dose has also been shown to improve cartilage thickness in the knee, as well as to significantly reduce knee pain in athletes.[58] This is a potential game-changer for athletes or anyone rehabbing from injury. If you have clients who suffer from osteoarthritis, then supplementation can improve joint function as well.[59] Interestingly, your joints prefer the gelatin or collagen peptides over supplements such as glycine or proline that contain only single amino acids. For athletes and coaches, some questions still need to be answered when it comes to collagen and gelatin supplementation. Does it accelerate a return to play post-injury? Can it improve performance via connective tissue-mediated adaptation to resistance training? The evolution of gelatin research will likely soon yield some exciting insights into these questions.

––––––––

In summary, recovery isn't just what happens after your workout. The best coaches and sport scientists in the world have a much broader view of what recovery means — it's how you plan your day, your week, and your training block to allow for optimal recovery from the last session, as well as to prepare for the upcoming session. In the next chapter, I'll discuss the fundamental role of athlete immunity and how it relates to recovery.

## CHAPTER 8

# Athlete Immunity

When Isaac Makwala of Botswana walked up to the gates of London Stadium for the IAAF World Championships in Athletics in 2017, he was ready to be a world champion. There was electricity in the air in anticipation of the main event of the evening: the 400-meter sprint final against South African rival and star Wayde van Niekerk. Makwala had been in incredible form in the lead-up to the World Championships. He was the first man to run a sub-20-second time in the 200 m and a sub-44-second time in the 400 m on the same day at an event earlier that year in Madrid. As Makwala approached the security gates of London Stadium, his night took a dramatic turn for the worse: He was banned from entering the building. In total disbelief and assuming there was some sort of misunderstanding, he waited for stadium security staff to clarify the situation. Unfortunately, they informed Makwala that he had been barred from entering by the sport's governing body due to illness: He was suspected of having contracted gastroenteritis. Makwala was banned due to risk of exposure to other athletes, and he never got to race in the final. This bizarre scenario triggered an uproar in the media and around track-and-field circles. The decision stemmed from the fact that 30 athletes and support staff had fallen ill with norovirus (a common gastrointestinal bug transmitted by close contact or touching contaminated surfaces) in the same hotel Makwala was staying, according to Public Health England. Makwala had been ill in the days leading up to the final, and based on this information, the International Association of Athletics Federations (IAAF) requested he be quarantined for 48 hours. The quarantine ended a day after the 400 m final, and so Makwala missed a golden opportunity to be a world champion.

Athletes often take their immunity for granted — that is, until they get sick. If you don't get the foundational pillars of recovery right — nutrition, sleep, mental-emotional stress — things can quickly derail and compromise your immune system. Your body will *always* prioritize survival over performance, and if you can't train because you're frequently sick, you'll never beat the competition.

In this chapter, I'll explore the following key questions. Are high-level athletes more prone to colds and flu? If you're frequently sick can you still be an elite athlete? Are symptoms alone sufficient to negatively impact performance? How do the "other 22 hours" impact an athlete's immunity? And, perhaps most important, what can you do to increase your odds of avoiding illness, or to reduce the severity and duration of colds and flu if you do succumb to an infection?

## The Modern Athlete: Stress, Load, and Travel

The International Society of Exercise and Immunology (ISEI) has confirmed in over three decades of research what most of us have come to find out the hard way: Training hard and pushing yourself to the limits takes its toll on the immune system. Expert exercise immunologist Michael Gleeson, PhD, of Loughborough University recently made this compelling statement: "There is now convincing evidence that an increased training load, competition load, and psychological stress together with international travel might all be risk factors for illness in the elite modern-day professional athlete."[1] But you don't have to be a professional or high-level athlete for this to impact you. If you work hard and train hard, this applies to you too. Regardless if you're gearing up for a marathon or are balancing work and family, training stress and general life stress all accumulate and impact immune function — sometimes for the better, but unfortunately, sometimes for the worse.

The modern-day athlete is exposed to higher training loads and an increasingly saturated competition calendar, whether they're a high school, collegiate, recreational, or high-level athlete. Emerging evidence indicates that inappropriate load management and/or prolonged bouts of strenuous exercise can significantly increase an athlete's risk of acute illness and temporarily depress immune function.[2] The emphasis on *prolonged* means that endurance athletes need to be even more vigilant about their training. These findings have led expert exercise immunologists to propose the "open window" theory, which suggests that after an intense (or prolonged) training session your immunity dips over the next 4 hours or so, increasing your risk of developing an infection.[3] Much of the research on the "open window" theory was performed on endurance athletes, and as most coaches or trainers will tell you, they do seem to suffer more colds than team- and strength-based athletes. Studies of marathon runners after the LA Marathon found them to be at much greater risk of infection in the 7–14 days post-race compared to age-matched controls who didn't race.[4] In South Africa, 33 percent of marathon runners got sick post-race compared to only 15 percent in the age-matched controls (non-racers).[5] Interestingly, researchers also found that the longer it took for participants to run the marathon, the greater their chances of getting sick. (It pays to be fitter in more ways than one!) Other factors like lack of sleep and inadequate nutrition can also depress immunity and lead to increased risk of infection.

This is the challenge for coaches, practitioners, and performance teams. As an athlete, your high training volumes need to be maximized, but this also increases your risk of harmful nonfunctional overreaching (NFOR), poorer sleep quality, and ultimately compromised immunity. You might be wondering if immunity really is *that* important for recovery and performance. Expert sport scientists in a recent study in the *Journal of Sports Science and Medicine* made a bold declaration, stating, "Elite athletic performance is incompatible with a high rate of infections."[6] This really hammers home an important point: If you're too sick or run-down, you *can't* show up every day to train and perform quality sessions. You'll be too far behind the pack and you'll never maximize your athletic potential. The key is having a strong immune system.

However, there is a curious outlier. The research clearly shows elite athletes competing at a national level get sick 40 percent *more* than athletes competing at the more elite international level.[7] Incredibly, this is despite international-level athletes having higher training loads. (Wait a minute, didn't I just say higher training loads equals more illness?) This is true across the board, except in the *most* elite athletes — they seem to be the outliers because they don't get sick at very high training volumes. How is this possible? Are they less sick because they're elite or are they elite because they get sick less often (and thus can train more)? Do nutrition or lifestyle strategies make a difference? At the highest level, the *British Journal of Sports Medicine* recently found "a negative correlation between infections and exercise training load among elite athletes is observed — the less sick you are the more you can train." In other words, the best athletes in the world have the highest training volumes (and don't get sick), while the rest of us struggle to ramp up training while staying free from colds and flu. Athletic success is predicated on a strong immune system. Put another way, if you're healthy, you can train — and if you can train more than the competition, you've got much better odds at beating them. But the question remains: How do the "best of the best" athletes train *more* and get sick *less* (even though increasing training loads is associated with more illness, *except* in this über-elite group)? Is it simply their genetics? Smarter training practices? Better load management and programming? This is a complex and challenging set of questions, but if you can figure out how to keep yourself from getting sick and feeling constantly run-down, then you can keep your training on track and give yourself the best chance of winning. Let's take a closer look at how exercise impacts immunity. From there, we can take a deeper dive into immunonutrition, a new term that describes specific nutrition strategies that support immunity (and ultimately recovery).

## The Impact of Exercise on Immunity

It doesn't matter if you're sedentary, recreationally active, or a high-level athlete — training impacts your immune system in different ways. Our understanding of these effects has evolved over the last few decades since the advent of the field of exercise immunology. In the early 1990s, renowned scientist and exercise immunologist David Nieman, PhD — cofounder of the the International Society of Exercise and Immunology — and his colleagues found that sedentary people were at an average risk of infection, compared to recreational exercisers who were at a lower risk of cold (and had improved their immunity with training), versus high-level athletes (who succumbed to more infections with their high training volumes and intensities).[8] This is known as the "J-shaped" immunity curve (see figure 8.1). It seemed like elite athletes were destined to catch more colds and flu.

Two decades later, science has progressed. The evolution in our understanding provides better clarity, and of course, a little more nuance. Expert exercise immunologist Neil Walsh, PhD, and his team at Bangor University in Wales discovered from their data the J-shaped curve might, in fact, actually be inverted. What does this mean for the athlete? Basically, the newbie exerciser is actually at the highest risk of infection (perhaps from the added and novel training stress), the recreational exerciser stills gets the bulk of the immune-boosting benefits of training, and the elite athlete is only at moderately higher

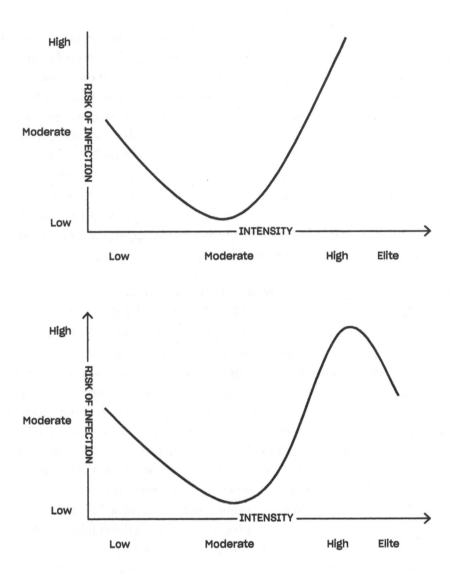

**FIGURE 8.1.** The original J-shaped curve (*top*) and proposed S-shaped immunity curve (*bottom*). From David C. Nieman, "Is Infection Risk Linked to Exercise Workload?" *Medicine & Science in Sports & Exercise* 32, no. 7 (2000), https://doi.org/10.1097/00005768-200007001-00005.

risk. Of course, if you're training at a high level this doesn't quite explain why national-level trainees experience more colds and flu compared to their more elite international-level colleagues. The answer might be in a third model of exercise and immunity: The S-shaped curve. The proposed S-shape curve suggests that increasing training volume into the high-level category does indeed increase infection risk (which most people who train hard would probably agree with), but once you hit a certain point at the highest volumes, you actually see a *reduced* risk of infection.[9] This is the "sweet spot," the area where very elite athletes are hitting their stride and not missing training or practice due to illness. While these competing theories are fleshed out by world-leading exercise immunologists, the take-home message for athletes looking to take their performance to the next level is that elite training is incompatible with frequent illness. Thus, the holy grail of recovery as it relates to immunity seems to be, "How do you get the highest training volumes without getting sick?" If you can figure that out, you've got a great chance of lapping the competition. Let's review the latest evidence-based research.

## The Power of Symptoms: "Don't Worry Coach, I'm Not Sick"

In high-level athletes, by far the two most common illnesses reported are upper respiratory tract infections (URTI) and general infections, at 30 percent and 32 percent respectively.[10] What makes the study of exercise immunology tricky is that not all infections are really "infections." Sounds confusing, doesn't it? Let me explain. Research at the IAAF World Championships in Athletics found 40 percent of the illnesses *reported* were URTI, yet when the athletes were actually *tested* for infection to confirm, only half of athletes had a diagnosed URTI. It raises the question, what did the other half suffer from if not an URTI? When you experience a scratchy throat, fatigue, or malaise, you often just assume it must be a cold or flu — but in fact, they're just symptoms. The other half of the athletes didn't have an infection, just the early warning signs that their bodies were struggling to keep up with the stressors of training (and maybe life!). These upper respiratory symptoms — known as URS in scientific speak — are very different from an infection. The athletes are not actually sick, but they don't feel well, either. It's really important to identify URS, because experiencing URS hampers the ability to train, recover, and perform! The other major causes of illness in athletes at the World Championships were exercise-induced dehydration, GI disturbances (12 percent and 10 percent, respectively), and most commonly norovirus, like Makwala experienced in 2017.

The common cold is one of the most frequent URTIs seen in athletes. It is usually acquired via airborne droplets or nasal secretion (the medical term for snot) from coronavirus, rhinovirus, or adenovirus, as well as the influenza and parainfluenza viruses. There are actually over 200 viruses that can cause a cold; of all these, the rhinovirus causes 40 percent of all URTI in athletes as well as adults in the general population.[11] What's the most likely way you'll get infected? Aerosol spray. This is the medical term for someone sneezing on you or near you. (Remember that last plane trip? If you're two seats away from someone sneezing due to a cold, there is an 80 percent chance you'll get sick.) Secondary infection routes come from touching infected surfaces and then touching your mouth or nose. I know, I know . . . it sounds like mundane stuff. This is low-hanging fruit – keeping yourself cold- and flu-free – but doing so could be the difference between winning and losing or missing out on a chance to compete in a world championship. So how can you protect yourself? Start by simply washing your hands, and often. It's hard to believe, but a recent study found frequent handwashing reduced URTI rates by a whopping 45 percent.[12] Athletes and the general public spend a lot of money on immune-boosting supplements and medications, but they neglect a fundamental pillar of immunity, which is regularly washing their hands with soap and water (it outperforms them all for prevention, and it's nearly free!). Finally, other common causes of illness are food poisoning (40 percent of cases occur in the home), contaminated drinking water, or competing in polluted waters.[13]

You might be wondering, "How does all this apply to me?" Consider this common scenario: You have a scratchy throat, mild congestion, and some dark circles forming under your eyes, but you're quick to tell your coach that you're not actually sick and can keep training. It seems reasonable – you haven't been diagnosed with an infection, you feel a little rough around the edges but nothing exceptional, so why not keep pushing forward? Here's the problem. Expert exercise immunologist Maree Gleeson, PhD, of the Australian Institute of Sport has shown that upper respiratory symptoms (URS) – without an active URTI – hinder exercise performance to the same degree as the infection itself.[14] Yep, you heard it right. It doesn't really matter if you have an infection or not, just having the *symptoms* is sufficient to cause poor recovery and subpar training. For some, it could be an early red flag that they're crossing into harmful nonfunctional overreaching (NFOR). These athletes should tell their coach and adjust their plans. In fact, simply having upper respiratory symptoms (URS) is predictive of poor performance, despite not having a full-blown cold (that is, URTI).[15] The bottom line for athletes and coaches is that symptoms matter. Professor Neil Walsh, PhD, echoes these statements, emphasizing upper respiratory symptoms (URS) are just as damaging to your performance as infections (URTI): "It doesn't matter if you have a cold or not, adverse symptoms negatively impact performance." Even though athletes and the general population get between two to four colds a year, athletes are at much greater risk of upper respiratory symptoms (URS), and symptoms are sufficient to derail progress if not monitored. England's Dr. Michael Gleeson notes that of the athletes who complain of illness at major competitions, 50 percent are related to symptoms (not actual illness). If symptoms arise when you're about to compete, it will be difficult for you to perform your best. Athletes can help offset this by applying nutrition strategies to support and bolster immunity.

If you're an endurance athlete, immunity should be a top priority when you think about recovery. Your immune system takes a major hit after prolonged exercise greater than 90 minutes. Regular intense endurance training at these longer distances triggers dramatic increases in free radicals, pro-inflammatory cytokines (IL-1ra, IL-6, IL-10), and stress hormones that lead to depressed immune system function.[16] Daniel Plews, PhD, describes elite endurance training as "walking the razor's edge" due to the tremendously high training volume required, which puts them at risk for increased illness (as they work their way to being elite athletes!). Interleukin-10 (IL-10) is a key player in keeping your immune system running on all cylinders. When IL-10 levels are too high from too much training stress and/or lack of recovery, it blocks key immune cells such as macrophages, natural killer (NK) cells, and T-cells. This leaves you more exposed to getting sick.

Paying careful attention to symptoms can be a game-changer for monitoring and supporting yourself or your athlete during training because these symptoms mimic the harmful overreaching state you're striving to avoid. Athletes who show up to train with upper respiratory symptoms (URS) are potentially treading a fine line between adequate recovery and NFOR. This is highlighted by the fact athletes in NFOR had far more upper respiratory symptoms along with much lower levels of secretory IgA (sIgA), a marker of their innate "first line of defense" immune system function.[17] This is a recovery double whammy and can turn the "open window" of infection post-training into a grand canyon of cold and flu risk. This doesn't mean you can't train *at all* if you feel a little rundown, but it's a sign you need to start monitoring yourself more closely and be more adaptable in your training plan, nutrition, and recovery support. Expert exercise immunologist Dr. Neil Walsh points out your exercise tolerance will be reduced during infection, and exercising with an infection can increase its duration or intensity. If your symptoms are "below the neck"—a chesty cough, achy joints, or shivering—then it's important to discontinue training completely.[18]

The last 40 years of research in exercise and immunology has birthed the term *immunonutrition* to describe how dietary (and supplemental) strategies might play a key role in keeping athletes healthy, ensuring they are cold- and flu-free, and most important, helping them be fit enough to continuously train and compete. New research suggests that applying targeted, individualized strategies might help buffer training-induced changes in immunity and reduce the frequency and severity of colds and flu. Immunonutrition represents the evolution of exercise immunology. But before we dive into the details, let's review how various forms of training impact immunity.

## Burning Matches, Long Rides, and "Two-a-Days"

Your body communicates via signals, and intense exercise is a pretty loud signal. So it's not surprising that hard training has significant impacts on your immunity. A single intense training bout "burning matches" with heavy glycolytic work elicits major changes in the number and concentration of your white blood cells (WBC), such as neutrophils, which are key soldiers in your immune system's innate first line of defense. These changes can last well into your recovery period. When you train hard, your WBCs ramp up because the stress hormone is released during exercise; WBCs can remain elevated for up to 6 hours after exercise (even longer if you trained for more than 2 hours).[19] In fact, your blood levels after prolonged exercise look just like those of a person who is struggling with a bacterial infection ($>7.0 \times 10^6$/ml), but with one key exception: The training-induced elevations will return back to normal after recovery.

Unlike neutrophils, lymphocyte soldiers from your adaptive "seek and destroy" immune system fall dramatically after intense or prolonged exercise—below the pre-exercise values within about 30 minutes post-training.[20] Again, if you were a patient seeing a doctor, this big drop could look like the result of a medical condition like an infectious disease, autoimmune conditions, or viral hepatitis. But, once again, this exercise-induced suppression of lymphocytes comes back to normal after 4–6 hours. The stress and inflammation from training is a necessary process that triggers these changes in immune markers, but recovery restores balance and homeostasis. That said, incomplete recovery elevates inflammation throughout the body, and this "noise" can drown out the key signals you're sending the body during training.

What happens when you kick things up a notch and train twice in a day (called "two-a-days")? Regardless if it's a 15-minute high-intensity workout or a regular team practice (2 hours at moderate intensity, for example), it takes an average of 3–4 hours to recover. But it's important to remember this doesn't take into account individual differences. If you read between the lines in the research, you'll see that the individual responses between athletes can vary between 45 minutes to up to 12 hours.[21] That is a massive difference! If it takes your teammate less than 2 hours after a morning session to recover, but it takes you 5–8 hours, then you can see how this could quickly lead to problems over the course of a training camp or season. The coach sets the training schedule, and athletes and practitioners need to figure out ways to survive it!

Amazingly, this variance in individual response is consistent across recreational, highly trained, and elite athletes. You'll almost certainly have athletes who take a lot longer to recover from training, and this in turn will expose them to catching more colds and flu. This is where the coach, trainer, nutritionist, or practitioner can make a difference. For example, natural killer (NK) cells make up 80 percent of the drop in lymphocytes; after 2 hours of prolonged exercise, they can drop by 40 percent below baseline for up to 7 days.[22] That's a massive open window for infection. The reality of high-level sports is that you have to play multiple back-to-back games throughout the year. In fact, high school and collegiate athletes probably do this the most, competing in tournaments with multiple games over a weekend. When you compete multiple times a day, your immune system is more heavily taxed after each subsequent session.[23] Over time, these repeated bouts of intense training leave your immune system running on empty. Secretory IgA (sIgA) levels drop by 40 percent compared to baseline levels, thus leaving you more susceptible to infection.[24] Incredibly, 82 percent of all reported illnesses show a decline in sIgA in the lead-up to infection (URTI).[25] All of this sounds very compelling, but it still doesn't guarantee that you'll be able to pin down the moment when you or your athlete will get sick. Biomarkers are associated with illness, but they can't *predict* with certainty. When your innate, first-line-of-defense immune system gets penetrated, sIgA kicks into gear with widespread antimicrobial activity against a wide range of viral and bacterial pathogens. It does this by inhibiting the invaders' ability to adhere and penetrate your cells (and thus your body).

In athletes, training load is generally negatively associated with sIgA levels. Studies in collegiate American football players show a big spike in URTI in late fall (toward the end of the season) as well as in late spring during exam time.[26] Athletes more prone to catching colds and flu exhibit the following patterns: increased weekly training hours (acute:chronic ratio), reduced secretory IgA levels, and increased IL-4 and IL-10 levels. In tennis players preparing for Wimbledon, sIgA levels bottomed out just before the athletes were about to get a cold or flu.[27] Monitoring in Olympic swimmers also revealed that low levels of sIgA and symptoms of sore throat were followed by two weeks of missed training due to feeling unwell.[28] During these periods, athletes are more prone to infection, and one big reason for this is the massive spike in IL-10 production due to intense training. Interleukin-10 is a key cytokine that inhibits a number of immune cells, specifically the Pac-Man macrophages that gobble up foreign intruders to keep you healthy. Incorporating strategies to support immunity is crucial to recovery, and ultimately performance.

## The "Other 22 Hours" and Risk of Infection

You've learned how training impacts immunity, but what about the "other 22 hours"? How do those factors play a role? Are you more likely to catch a cold or flu if you don't get adequate sleep? How about if you're constantly stressed (at work, school, or home)? Is your immunity at risk if you travel by air regularly? What about if your energy intake is insufficient to meet your needs? Let's take a closer look at how these factors impact immunity.

### Poor Sleep

How bad is lack of sleep for your immune system? People who experience poor sleep quality are at 4–5 times greater risk of catching a cold, and if your total sleep time is less than 7 hours per night, you're at threefold increased risk.[29] In Part One: Foundation, you learned how sleep is a fundamental pillar for health, and how athletes are extremely poor at rating their sleep quality — and, at the same time, commonly fail to get enough sleep. Making matters worse, high training volumes (synonymous with elite sport) impair sleep quality, which then hammers the immune system. You can see how things can start to snowball from there.

It's important to differentiate between acute versus chronic sleep problems. Struggling to sleep over a few days during a training camp (when you're sleeping in a new environment) or in the lead-up to competition is normal and will subside. Chronic sleep problems (characterized by at least 12 nights of 50 percent sleep loss) are a different story and can significantly increase pro-inflammatory markers (CRP and IL-6), setting up a major roadblock to high performance.[30] A key mechanism underpinning how lack of sleep can derail immunity is the excessive activation of your hypothalamic-pituitary-adrenal (HPA)-axis and sympathetic nervous system, leading to chronically elevated output of cortisol, adrenaline, and noradrenaline.

Lack of sleep also throws off your circadian rhythms, sparking inflammation and disturbing the rhythmic nature of your immune system. Experts believe this is likely responsible for the increased risk of infection and cardiovascular disease in shift workers among the general population.[31] If you're about to get a vaccine for travel, then make sure your sleep is on point first. Lack of sleep can compromise the effectiveness of the vaccine. A recent study showed that if you get less than 7 hours of sleep per night for 7 consecutive days, it significantly reduces your response to the hepatitis B vaccination, and therefore your clinical protection (this sounds like most collegiate or high school athletes or new parents, right?).[32] Remember this important point when you get your competitive travel schedule for the year.

## How Mental Stress Makes You Sick

Stress is a massive piece of the immune puzzle. Some people are naturally more stressed than others, but does this mean they're more likely to get sick? A groundbreaking study by Sheldon Cohen, PhD, in the early 1990s, published in the *New England Journal of Medicine*, put this theory to the test. He investigated how the common cold affected "stressed" people versus those who were more emotionally balanced. In this study, Dr. Cohen actually gave participants an active virus and then simply waited to see which group succumbed most to the infection. Perhaps not surprisingly, the more laid-back personality types were far less likely to get sick from the virus compared to the more stressed-out individuals.[33] In short, your perception of stress has a massive influence on your immunity. The more you perceive stress, the greater the likelihood you'll get sick. This highlights just how important mindset is for health and performance. If you struggle with frequent colds and flu, or if you miss regular training sessions due to sickness, it's time to prioritize recovery and immunonutrition to increase your resiliency.

### Air Travel and Avoiding the Sneezer

Airplane travel is a reality of high-level and professional sports. It's also one of the surest bets for getting you sick. You're in an enclosed tube with recycled air, and if you're seated next to someone who is sneezing or coughing, the chances of you catching a bug are really high. Recall, if you're only two seats away from a person coughing, you've got an 80 percent chance of getting sick.[34] Making matters worse, plane travel and crossing multiple time zones can acutely worsen your blood sugar control, throwing off circadian rhythms and increasing your risk of dysbiosis.[35] Not the best recipe for success. Athletes who travel frequently need to be proactive and support their immunity and circadian rhythm to avoid frequent and nagging colds.

### Micronutrient Deficiencies

If your vitamin D status is insufficient or deficient, you're at 3–4 times greater risk of catching a common cold. In the dark and cold days of winter, you won't be able to get sufficient vitamin D from the sun (in locations with a true winter climate), making supplementation an important weapon in your immune arsenal (and thus recovery). Recent work by Dr. Michael Gleeson found that individuals with blood levels of vitamin D at 120 nmol/L (48 ng/dL) had the highest correlation to improved immunity.[36] In winter, it is virtually impossible to achieve this level without a supplement. You simply cannot get enough vitamin D from fatty cold-water fish, egg yolks, and mushrooms to achieve that target. Athletes commonly struggle with vitamin D insufficiency or deficiency, so if you struggle with immunity, get tested and aim for 2,000–4,000 IU from November to March, depending on your results, skin tone, and health status.

## Immunonutrition Solutions

If you're sick too often, you can't train. If you can't train, you can't keep up with the competition. Avoiding frequent or persistent colds and flu is a crucial piece of the recovery puzzle. Even if you don't get sick, the upper

## Are You a Mouth Breather?

Do you ever wake up with cotton mouth? This is the dry, sticky sensation that leaves you looking for a quick swig of water to start the day. Dry mouth can be a major problem in terms of immunity. If your mouth is chronically dry, your salivary sIgA flow rate will decline significantly, compromising your immunity. This can also be a major side effect of dehydration, plane travel, and dry winter months. If you wake up regularly with a cotton mouth, it's a clear sign of reduced salivary flow rate. You can also have a dry mouth from being a "mouth breather," which is something far more common than most people realize. If you have some low-grade congestion in your sinuses, you end up breathing through your mouth rather than your nose. This is not what nature intended, and it leaves you more exposed to dry mouth and reduced salivary sIgA flow. If you struggle with food sensitivities to gluten or FODMAPs, it might result in mouth breathing and decreased sIgA flow rate. This means less protection from infection and poorer sleep quality. Both are harmful to healthy immune function. Mouth taping, the application of a small piece of tape to keep the mouth closed, is a new technique that has been shown anecdotally to help restore normal, healthy nasal breathing. (Give it a try and see for yourself!)

respiratory symptoms (URS) associated with the common cold can worsen training outcomes and performance. Monitoring is important so that athletes can successfully tread the fine line between progression and plateaus. To understand how the expert-generalist can help athletes, it's important to revisit how people fall victim to infection. In the last chapter, I talked about the foundation of the Recovery Pyramid, with a particular emphasis on sleep, stress, and proper nutrition. Consistently falling short on sleep, struggling with mental or emotional stress, or having a poor diet compromise immunity. Expert exercise immunologist Lygeri Dimitriou, PhD, at the London Sports Institute at Middlesex University London notes, "There are two things that must happen to get sick; your immune system must be compromised and you must be exposed to a pathogen." Immunonutrition highlights how your food (and supplement) choices can potentially improve immunity, prevent illness, or minimize the severity and duration of colds and flu. The other factor for warding off illness is limiting your exposure to infectious bugs, which is not always easy to do in a team sport, high school, collegiate, or workplace atmosphere. Good personal and oral hygiene, handwashing, and avoiding sick people is paramount to your success. (If you're a parent with young kids . . . good luck!) As an athlete, exposure to gyms, your teammates, training staff, sick friends, and your hygiene plays a big role in reducing your risk of infection.

### The Fundamentals of Immunonutrition

Handwashing is often overlooked by most coaches, practitioners, and athletes; however, it's the biggest hammer for nailing the door shut on pathogen exposure, and it is far and away the most effective tool for preventing illness in athletes. You don't need a PhD in *handwashing*, but thankfully expert exercise immunologists have an evidence-based approach for the most effective way to apply soap and water, perfecting the "art of handwashing" down to the smallest detail. (Hint: most people miss the fingertips, the backs of the thumbs, and the creases in the palms!)

If you're in an environment where teammates or other athletes are sick, or athletes are living in training camp or dorm situations, washing your hands frequently throughout the day (every 3–4 hours) and avoiding touching your mouth or nose is critical for prevention. Finally, don't share water bottles, because doing so can increases your risk of mononucleosis infection eightfold. This practice of not sharing bottles is especially important for at-risk high school and collegiate athletes.[37]

Carbohydrates also play a massive role in supporting your immune system during training. "When your blood glucose drops," explains Dr. Michael Gleeson, "you experience a marked increase in secretion of anti-inflammatory hormones and cytokines, which have a major detrimental impact on immune function." If you can prevent blood glucose from falling too low during exercise, your inflammatory response is much, much less. Dr. Gleeson emphasizes, "When training at high-intensities, or intense training blocks, it's crucial to have more carbs in your diet." This is especially important for high-level athletes because their training intensity is so much greater than recreational exercisers. Moreover, Dr. Gleeson points out that this practice still allows for days when you adjust carb availability to elicit a specific training response (the Train Low and Sleep Low strategies discussed in Part Two: Fuel). However, he also makes the point that these strategies should not be done day after day (after day). This is more common in higher-level recreational athletes compared to elite athletes working with performance staff. And Dr. Gleeson warns if training with low carb availability is done chronically and if you train at high volumes (or intensity) "you're going to get sick, have mood changes or sleep disturbances, etc."

Consuming carbs during prolonged or intense exercise (think endurance and team sport) has a significant and dramatic effect on limiting the spike in pro-inflammatory cytokines that occurs with training. It also has effects on neutrophils, natural killer (NK) cells, and lymphocytes.[38] Maintaining stable blood glucose levels during training helps blunt stress hormone and catecholamine release (adrenaline, noradrenaline, and the like) during and after exercise. This is when timing is key. If you consume a sugary drink 60–75 minutes before exercise — a common occurrence in pro sports, where athletes knock back sports drinks while coming off the team bus or warming up before a game — it can easily lead to rebound hypoglycemia (blood sugar levels falling dramatically below resting levels), just as you're about to play.[39] This is a disaster for performance. If you consume the same drink 10–15 minutes before a training session or a game, then you will prevent this blood sugar roller coaster and use the glucose immediately for fuel. This timing is really important during intense training, two-a-day sessions, or late in the season when fatigue is accumulating and your glycogen levels are low, and is important to bear in mind if you're adopting a Train Low, Compete High strategy. A higher-carb intake consistently buffers drops in immune markers following exercise after multiple sessions.[40] Extreme and chronic carb restriction during intense training sessions is a common pitfall for some athletes who follow low-carb and keto diets.[41] Be sure to tailor your approach to match your goals.

Protein is an often-overlooked area of support for your immune system. When athletes talk protein, muscle mass gets all the attention. However, your immune system needs protein to run on all cylinders, especially when you're pushing your training to the limits. Ensuring that you achieve the recommended 1.6 g/kg/day of protein for athletes is a great place to start. Aiming higher with your protein intake can make a difference if you're struggling

## Training Tips for Sick Athletes[43]

A lot of athletes ask me, "If I'm sick, can I still train?" Here is what the latest research says:

- Training during an infection can increase the severity and duration of infection.
- If symptoms are below the neck (chesty cough, joint aches, shivering, and the like), don't train.
- If you do decide to train, reduce intensity and duration.
- Your tolerance to exercise will be reduced during infection.
- If you're sick, isolate yourself from infected teammates.

with a scratchy throat or feel more run-down during an intense training block. Consuming greater than 2.2 g/kg/day of protein might provide added immune support, especially while in a caloric deficit, if you're struggling to meet the demands of a heavier training schedule, more travel, stress at work (or school), and the like. This increased intake of protein helps to minimize exercise-induced changes in lymphocyte profile after intense training.[42] This is very important to know if you're a coach, because research shows that a lower-protein diet, matched for calories and carbs, failed to produce the beneficial effects on athlete immunity. Of course, increasing protein intake can also increase satiety, so pay special attention to calorie intake to ensure that the total doesn't decline as a result. This highlights the importance of protein to immunity. (Pro tip: Add an extra shake during the day and/or before bed.)

If you identify athletes who are missing too many practices, training sessions, or games due to illness, it's important to get more information about why this is happening. Athlete immunity screening questionnaires (such as the Jackson Questionnaire) can be great, cost-effective tools that can help you flag athletes before issues arise. More in-depth lab testing can then help identify the root cause of the problem. Table 8.1 breaks down common immune biomarkers found on a CBC + Differential panel to help differentiate between the general population, healthy athletes, and overtrained athletes.

**TABLE 8.1.** Immune Biomarkers of Overtraining

| BIOMARKER | GENERAL POPULATION | ATHLETES | OVERTRAINED |
|---|---|---|---|
| Total leukocytes | 6.62 (+/−0.86) | 4.36 (+/−1.15) | 3.72 (+/−1.04) |
| Neutrophils | 3.83 (+/−0.86) | 2.46 (+/−0.87) | 1.92 (+/−0.86) |
| Lymphocytes | 2.02 (+/−0.27) | 1.36 (+/−0.20) | 1.25 (+/−0.28) |
| sIgA | 118–641 | Possibly low | Low to very low |

Source: Thomas B. Tomasi et al., "Immune Parameters in Athletes Before and After Strenuous Exercise," *Journal of Clinical Immunology* 2, no. 3 (1982), https://doi.org/10.1007/bf00915219; Neil P. Walsh et al., "Salivary IgA Response to Prolonged Exercise in a Cold Environment in Trained Cyclists," *Medicine & Science in Sports & Exercise* 34, no. 10 (2002), https://doi.org/10.1097/00005768-200210000-00015; A. K. Blannin et al., "Effects of Submaximal Cycling and Long-Term Endurance Training on Neutrophil Phagocytic Activity in Middle Aged Men," *British Journal of Sports Medicine* 30, no. 2 (1996), https://doi.org/10.1136/bjsm.30.2.125.

While there are still no definitive characteristics among all the immune parameters — some athlete profiles will look bad but they won't get sick, or vice versa — it provides the practitioner with a baseline to work from. Of course, this should always be assessed in conjunction with other athlete markers such as training load, session RPE, daily wellness questionnaire, and others.

Field practitioners need practical, evidence-based solutions they can use in real time with their athletes and clients. This is where secretory IgA levels can be a useful tool. Levels will decline for several hours after intense or prolonged training — and baseline levels will be lower — in athletes who are pushing the limits or are heading into NFOR.[44] Salivary tests are easy to collect and turnaround time is quick, but just like all the immune and recovery biomarkers, in isolation it's not predictive of illness. Biomarkers can first help you get a clearer picture of the athlete's state of health and recovery. Knowing this, you can *then* select the appropriate strategies to keep training and progress on track. Let's look at a few evidence-based options.

The bulk of the research on the benefits of probiotics for recovery is with respect to immunity. Probiotic supplementation has been found in a recent systematic review of 20 placebo-controlled studies to reduce the number of sick days and shorten the length of illness.[45] Another Cochrane Review

## Supplemental Vitamin C: Prevention or Treatment?

Vitamin C seems to always be the go-to when it comes to immunity. Vitamin C helps stimulate the production of immune cells and how well they function, thus it seems obvious to include it in your regime. The real question for athletes is this: Does supplementation help reduce severity and duration of colds? A recent meta-analysis sheds some light: If you're already sick, it's not likely to help out. If you're training intensely and regularly, take the supplement and you might get a modest reduction in colds and flu and less severe symptoms (the athletes who did supplement had half the colds of those who didn't). As noted in the previous chapter, if vitamin C is taken immediately post-training, it can actually dampen adaptation. However, if it's winter and you're run-down, then it can be a nice preventative (just don't take it immediately after training).

found that probiotics reduced URTI by 47 percent and cut short the average duration of illness by 2 days.[46] These are impressive results, but there is an important caveat: The subjects were nonathletes (this is still good news for the general population, however).

How do things stack up in athletic populations? Expert exercise immunologists Nicholas West, PhD, and David Pyne, PhD, at the Australian Institute of Sport recently conducted a research review and found that almost two-thirds of studies on probiotic supplementation and athletes revealed reduced frequency of illness.[47] Probiotic supplementation also appears to help maintain sIgA levels during periods of intense training, which is when you're at greater risk of infection.[48] This highlights the intimate role the gut microbiota play in immunity and augmenting resiliency. Other potential benefits of probiotic supplementation include reduced GI upset (such as "runner's trots") during marathons or ultramarathons, reduced endotoxemia during exercise in the heat, and reduced gut infections when traveling abroad. Probiotics seems to exert these benefits via increasing natural killer cell (NK) activity, enhancing activity of white blood cells (which gobble up pathogens), as well as impacting cytokines and immunoglobulin function. Most important, these effects aren't just local, but extend to distal mucosal areas of the body (your nose and throat), which highlights the complexity, integration, and interconnectedness of the human body. These evidence-based potential benefits shouldn't be ignored by coaches and practitioners. The research supports multistrain formulas that contain $10^{10}$ live bacteria per capsule of *Lactobacillus* or Bifidobacterium strains; however, expert probiotic researchers will tell you that probiotics do not repopulate your gut, but rather trigger signals to the gut microbiota. Thus, probiotic strains and cell numbers can vary markedly. Ideally, start probiotic supplementation two weeks before you, your athlete, or team will be at increased risk of infection.

Vitamin D plays a key role in both innate and acquired immunity via its impact on gene expression. Incredibly, approximately 5 percent of your entire human genome is impacted by vitamin D.[49] If your levels of this vitamin are insufficient, the expression of these genes (and the proteins they code for) and the activation of your immune cells will be subpar. Low levels of vitamin D means greater risk of colds and flu, and in athletes, higher levels of vitamin D in winter and spring are associated with reduced frequency of infections.[50] Vitamin D deficiencies pose the biggest problems during the winter months in colder climates. Ironically, these deficiencies can also present in athletes who train in warmer winter climates — like endurance runners in Kenya — because (due to extreme heat) these athletes often train indoors or cover up exposed skin when outdoors. Athletes with low vitamin D status have more days with upper respiratory symptoms and have higher symptom-severity scores — which, as you'll remember Neil Walsh, PhD, found, was just as problematic for performance as actual infections. Vitamin D also appears to boost sIgA levels in winter, and a recent study found that athletes supplementing with 5,000 IU for three months significantly boosted protective sIgA levels.[51] Dr. Michael Gleeson has found that athletes continued to see improvements in immune status up to vitamin D levels of 120 nmol/L (48 ng/mL). Consider supplementing with 2,000–4,000 IU of vitamin D during the winter months to maintain levels above 100 nmol/L if immunity is a concern. It's important to remember that vitamin D status is also tightly tied to overall health. If levels are persistently low, then

## The Glutamine Myth

Glutamine is one of the most prevalent free-form amino acids in the body, as well as one of the most popular supplements for athletes, physique-focused trainees, and the general public. It's claimed to support recovery, immunity, and digestive function. But what does the research *actually* say? With respect to recovery and performance, the overwhelming majority of studies actually show no significant benefits.[54] The claims for glutamine are misleading in regard to immunity, too. If you're a burn victim or receiving glutamine parenterally (via IV infusion), then it can help to support your immunity; otherwise, there is little in the literature to support better outcomes in athletes. The digestive front, however, is where glutamine can make a difference. The bulk of glutamine supplements are taken up by your enterocytes (gut cells), making them helpful for athletes who are struggling with digestive concerns. If your digestion is on point already, adding a glutamine supplement for immunity and recovery isn't worth the cost.

potential underlying issues might be chronically elevated blood glucose, high inflammatory levels, increased visceral body fat, or gut dysfunction (often related to autoimmunity).

If you've just gotten sick, it's time to call in the reinforcements. Zinc lozenges can be a quick, convenient, and evidence-based solution for athletes, as they've been shown to reduce the duration of common colds when taken within 24 hours of symptoms.[52] It seems to provide an added advantage for those suffering from a URTI and who need to target the nasal epithelium to reduce inflammation. I find zinc acetate lozenges to be more effective in athletes, but a recent meta-analysis found no definitive advantage of these lozenges over the more commonly used zinc gluconate lozenges. Aim for 75 mg divided throughout the day.

Vitamin A plays a key role in immunity, but it's often misunderstood. The vitamin A from animal sources is called retinoids (or retinol) while plant-sourced vitamin A is carotenoids. Retinol from animal sources is much more bioavailable than that from plant-based sources, which has to be converted into retinol in the body to be used. This conversion isn't always easy or efficient. For example, in terms of vitamin A, you need to eat over 4 pounds of carrots to get the same benefit as from 3.5 ounces of organ meat. The conversion from carotene to retinol is also inefficient in people who have poor blood sugar control, are following low-fat diets, have digestive conditions, or experience thyroid dysfunction. The traditional solution was to use cod liver oil in the winter to obtain vitamin D, A, and omega-3 in combination. (However, if you're trying to increase vitamin D levels, do *not* ramp up cod liver oil intake, as you'll likely increase vitamin A levels too high and risk toxicity.)

Eating mushrooms (fungi) might also support immunity. Regular consumption has been shown to improve immune status. A four-week study in healthy men and women found that eating 5 g of mushrooms doubled natural killer (NK) cell activity and increased T lymphocytes by 60 percent.[53] Interestingly, secretory IgA levels in the gut also increased alongside reductions in inflammatory CRP. The tricky part in practice is getting athletes to eat mushrooms at the quantity necessary to support immunity. This is where supplementation could be helpful.

----

The experts are in agreement: Being frequently sick is incompatible with elite performance, and incorporating immunonutrition strategies can help reduce the frequency, duration, and likelihood of illness. The fundamentals of the new science around peak performance are rooted in nutrition, sleep, and stress management (which all impact immunity). But how can you really tell how "stressed" an athlete is? How hard are you really pushing yourself? Athlete monitoring might be the answer, and we'll explore that in the next chapter.

# CHAPTER 9

# Athlete Monitoring and Recovery Strategies

Thomas Hoving walked into the room and immediately knew the statue was a fake. Despite the fact that other leading scientists had performed a battery of tests to validate the authenticity of the potentially priceless antiquity, in the blink of an eye, the world-leading expert Hoving knew it wasn't real. Malcolm Gladwell opens his terrific book *Blink* with this compelling story: How an expert can, in a split second — after years of observation, experience, and practice — instantaneously and intuitively see something others cannot. After Hoving's declaration, the Getty Museum reanalyzed the two-thousand-year-old statue and found the purported historic archaeological discovery was indeed a fake. Hoving's split-second deduction was correct. The knowledge accumulated through decades of research, practice, and experience yields an innate ability to know whether the outcome is appropriate or not (in a general sense). Experienced coaches and practitioners have this ability, too, although it presents a huge juxtaposition to the current massive surge in Big Data and the attempt to quantify everything, all the way down to our genes. Gladwell argues in his book that decisions made very quickly can be every bit as good as decisions made cautiously and deliberately. These heuristics, or mental shortcuts, are used to speed up the process of finding a satisfactory solution when an optimal one is impossible or impractical. Classic examples of heuristics include "rule of thumb," "educated guess," and "intuitive judgment." They can be powerful weapons in complex environments.

Instinct versus analysis: It's an interesting dilemma, particularly in sport, where the quantification and analysis of every aspect of the game is bringing new insights. This chapter will explore if athlete monitoring is leading to better player performance and reduced injury, or if it's creating a whole new set of problems. Let's see how elite performance staff strike a balance between the Hoving instinct and objective data.

In previous chapters, I discussed the importance of appropriate training stress — finding the right balance between helpful functional overreaching (FOR) and harmful nonfunctional overreaching (NFOR) — for athletic success, and how the "other 22 hours" play a major role in an athlete's total stress load. NFOR and overtraining are created via an imbalance between training stress, life stress, and recovery.[1] When coaches and practitioners deliberately apply periods of functional overreaching to spark physiological adaptations in their athletes, it yields positive results once the athlete is allowed to recover. During this period of adaptation, the athlete's performance might dip, but with a few days of rest or active recovery they bounce right back with superior fitness.[2] But what happens if they don't bounce back? Your deliberate overreaching period, which looked good on paper, ended up causing your athlete to feel adverse symptoms, be it prolonged and/or excessive muscle soreness, persistent fatigue, increased perceived effort, performance decrements, overuse injury, or mental symptoms such as low mood and loss of sense of humor (which can often persist over a long period of time).[3] What then? You've potentially crossed the line into maladaptation and harmful overreaching. Is it time to make decisions off the cuff and go with your gut, like Hoving? Or is it time to rely on all the data you've accumulated? To answer this question, you must first resolve this dilemma: How do you know when your athlete is pushing it too far into the red zone? Are the collection of blood tests or biomarkers sufficient? What about the athlete's subjective symptoms? Performance metrics? Unfortunately, even after decades of research there is no gold-standard diagnosis of nonfunctional overreaching (NFOR) or overtraining syndrome (OTS).[4]

If you or your athlete are chronically in a state of nonfunctional overreaching, it will eventually lead to overtraining. Push too hard or rest too little (or both) for too long and problems will emerge. Unfortunately, it's hard to know when OTS sets in because there are few clear separating factors (although endurance athletes will be much more prone to OTS than team or strength sport athletes). The clear distinguishing factor of overtraining syndrome is that prolonged recovery phases do not correct the problem. Recovery is a spectrum — from complete recovery to acute fatigue

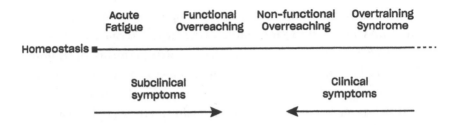

**FIGURE 9.1.** Recovery Continuum. Adapted from Rod W. Fry, Alan R. Morton, and David Keast, "Overtraining in Athletes: An Update," *Sports Medicine* 12, no. 1 (1991), https://doi.org/10.2165/00007256-199112010-00004.

to functional overreaching to nonfunctional overreaching to overtraining syndrome (see figure 9.1).

Here's the rub: You need to overload to elicit the training stress required to achieve the desired adaptive response. If you don't push yourself hard enough, you won't get fitter, faster, and stronger. On the flip side, if you push too hard or don't give yourself enough recovery, you'll also fail to get fitter and perform your best.[5] Prescribing the right training dose is paramount to supporting recovery. Lachlan Penfold, former head of physical performance and sports medicine with the Golden State Warriors and currently the performance director with the Melbourne Storm of the National Rugby League (NRL) in Australia, highlights the importance of getting your training process right to support recovery. Penfold states bluntly: "No amount of ice baths is going to help you recover from a poorly planned and poorly executed training session. . . . If you f*ck up the training session, it doesn't matter what you do in recovery. It's too late." Penfold emphasizes it's how you plan your day, your week, your training block that allows for optimal recovery. In order to do so effectively, you need to understand the athlete's training load and have evidence-based strategies to help you monitor the athlete's response to training and readiness.

## Understanding Workload: External versus Internal

The monitoring of training load has evolved massively in the past three decades. From cameras mounted on stadium rooftops to the use of cameras around the field to the addition of GPS monitoring devices, athlete monitoring is now a staple of every elite-level program. Sport scientists determine an athlete's total workload by assessing both *external* and *internal* training loads. Ramsey Nijem, DSc, head strength and conditioning coach for the NBA's Sacramento Kings, outlines the many external loads that can be put on athletes: It is the physical work the athlete performs, the training plan designed by the strength coach, the number of sets performed, the amount of weight lifted, the number of sprints run, the volume of miles cycled, and so on. As such, the external load is pretty straightforward to calculate. The internal load, says Nijem, is different. It is the effects that training has on an athlete's individual physiology (heart rate, for example) and perceived exertion (how hard they thought the training session was). What feels hard for one athlete might feel easier for another. Nijem notes that gauging internal load is much more difficult than gauging external load, but doing so can provide the insights you need to monitor a training plan effectively, and thus maximize recovery and performance.[6] Age, training history, fitness level, and injury history all play a role in these outcomes.

Why do experts like Nijem monitor the training loads of high-level athletes? They do this because it's an incredibly important tool for determining whether an athlete is adapting to the training program and for minimizing the risk of harmful nonfunctional overreaching, injury, and illness.[7] Of course, the common misconception is that monitoring is used to tell you to add more rest to an athlete's regime. While this is sometimes the case, not training hard enough can also cause some serious recovery and performance roadblocks.

The early research on training load by renowned experts such as Tim Gabbett, PhD, from Australia, suggested that the greater an athlete's training load, the greater their risk of injury.[8] It also suggested that the more high-speed running you do, the greater your risk of soft tissue injury.[9] However, something very unexpected began happening over the decade that followed: Athletes with higher training loads got injured less frequently.[10] They didn't need more rest, they needed more training. Not only that, athletes with low training workloads also saw more injuries. Hence, both over-recovery and under-recovery can increase injury risk and compromise performance.[11] Experts began to nail down a dose-response relationship between training volume and injury risk.

One of the first studies to reveal that high training loads can protect athletes from injury was in cricket bowlers — the ones bowling the most balls (quite like a baseball pitcher throwing fastballs) over a four-week period had the lowest risk of injury.[12] Subsequently, this trend was found to hold true in other sports as well.[13] It turns out your acute workload (how much work you do in a week) in relation to your chronic workload (how much you do in a month or training block) was the best predictor of injury. When the acute:chronic workload ratio was approximately 0.8–1.3, the odds of athletes getting injured was much lower. When it was above 1.5 (that is, you're doing much more in a week than you've done previously) injury risk ballooned upwards.

How is this possible? Experts believe the benefits of workload are two-fold: Exposing athletes to greater loads allows them to tolerate greater loads, and training develops the qualities athletes need to protect themselves from injury (that is, strength, high-intensity running, and aerobic fitness). In his terrific book *Game Changer*, Dr. Fergus Connolly makes the very astute observation: "There is no such thing as full recovery after training; there is simply adaptation to training. Your body is constantly attempting to adapt and learn so it can survive." A great example is high-speed running. It can definitely increase the risk of injury, but this effect is blunted when you expose the athlete to higher training loads.[14] Remember, be judicious when you apply increased loads into your training plan. Expert strength and sprint coaches such as consultant Derek Hansen agree that the start of a training session, or earlier in the training week when athletes are most recovered, is the best time for high-speed running. It's very taxing on the nervous system, and as Hansen describes, "Sprinting is perhaps the purest expression of the fight or flight response."

Does this mean the acute:chronic workload ratio is the magic bullet for athlete monitoring? Unfortunately not. Dr. Ramsey Nijem is quick to point out there is a lot of nuance in monitoring this ratio. The evidence-based research provides a foundation, but of course, it becomes much more complex in real-world practice. If you train too little or too much, then you can increase your likelihood of illness or injury. If you're sick, you can't train. If you're injured, you can't train. Ultimately if you can't train, you won't be able to adapt and grow stronger. Monitoring can be a tool to help flag athletes when they are at risk.

## Daily Wellness: How Do You Rate Yourself?

You've learned so far that there is no gold-standard diagnostic tool or bio-marker to flag harmful overreaching or overtraining, yet athletes do need to push themselves hard and walk the razor's edge to achieve the positive adaptations required to be the best. The human "machine" is incredibly complex, and as you'll learn in Part Four: Supercharge, your emotions trigger the quickest responses by your brain. Perhaps it's no surprise, then, that changes in mood and emotional state are well documented as some of the earliest signs of harmful overreaching (and overtraining) in athletes.[15] In fact, the most pragmatic and effective ways of identifying harmful non-functional overreaching (NFOR) or overtraining syndrome (OTS) seem to be psychological markers and/or performance decrements.[16] How you feel matters.

Coaches and athletes are often so focused on the training and competitive aspects of sport, they forget that the rest of the athlete's life imposes major demands on their ability to recover. Keeping up-to-date with your athletes on how they're feeling is a major piece of the recovery puzzle, as the research clearly shows a dose-response relationship between mood states and training load, making it a highly useful tool for coaches.[17] Using a daily wellness score, athletes are asked to rate their subjective feelings on a scale of 1–5 for the following five factors: fatigue, sleep quality, general muscle soreness, stress levels, and mood. This can help determine how well they're responding to training. A recent study in the *Journal of Strength and Conditioning Research* surveyed an Australian Football team for an entire season and found the subjective ratings of daily wellness accurately reflected changes in weekly training plans.[18] The players reported better sleep and less physical strain during the week (allowing for optimal recovery), while scores expectedly dropped after intense games on the weekend. During periods of deloading (reductions in training volume, intensity, or both), wellness scores also improved dramatically. Perhaps the greatest strength of using daily wellness scores in team sports is its ability to pick up on individual differences between competition and training for things such as muscle strain.[19] Daily wellness scores provide a simple, cheap, and validated method of seeing how hard (or not-so-hard) your athletes are working. And if you work with clients on a one-on-one basis, it's also a useful tool for better tracking and monitoring of your athlete (this is an especially good tool for online coaches).

A training plan is a road map from a starting point to a goal, but rarely does it progress linearly from start to finish. A coach's ability to be nimble and adapt the plan to suit the needs of an individual athlete is critical. How does your athlete look, feel, and perform in your mind? You can't just sit behind a computer and analyze the data; you need to engage with the athlete. A daily wellness score is where the art meets the science. However, in some high-performance environments, it can be difficult to apply this to a complex real-world scenario. Getting answers from athletes can be a chore (most hate extra homework); collecting the data, analyzing it, and interpreting the results takes time, and most practitioners don't have a lot of extra time. This can be a challenge even at cutting-edge performance facilities such as ALTIS in Arizona — home to some of the best strength coaches and sport scientists in the world, and a key training base for elite Olympic track and field athletes. Dr. Jas Randhawa, the director of sports medicine and performance therapy Lead at ALTIS, describes the tremendous value of coaches talking with each athlete before the session and knowing how to ask conversational (nonconfrontational) questions to tease out how athletes are adapting and progressing. Highly skilled professionals with years of experience asking the right questions can provide incredible insights. So much so that, despite having access to all the latest technology, ALTIS would rather invest in people (rather than technology) to best support their world-class athletes. Context matters — it's important to find the tool that best suits your individual or team needs.

## The RPE Scale: How Hard Did Your Workout Feel?

Sport scientists love objective measures. Today, data is everywhere, and coaches are making more and more decisions based on analytics. The results of those decisions are evident on the playing field: The dramatic rise in three-point shooting in basketball, defensive shifts in baseball, football teams going for more two-point conversions — the list goes on and on. But subjective ratings of perceived exertion provide a valuable and reliable snapshot into both acute and chronic training loads. In fact, they might even be *more* sensitive and consistent compared to tech-driven objective measures. When acute training loads go up, subjective well-being goes down. If training load is decreased, subjective well-being improves. The same story applies to chronic training loads. It seems obvious, but despite a wide array of advanced testing and physiological, biochemical, and immunological biomarkers, simply asking an athlete how they feel is arguably the most effective (and practical) method of detecting harmful overreaching.[20] (It's really cost-effective too!)

Rating of perceived exertion (RPE) is a subjective way of assessing an athlete's internal load. Athletes provide a number value for their effort level in a specific session. The RPE scale was originally developed in the 1970s by Gunnar Borg, who called it the Borg Rating of Perceived Exertion. The scale went from 6–20, which might seem odd, but it correlated to the athlete's heart rate when multiplied by a factor of 10 (see table 9.1). For example, a score of 9 reflects very light exercise like walking; 13 is somewhat hard, but you can continue to train; 17 is very hard and you're having to really push yourself to continue; and 19 is the most strenuous activity you've ever experienced (20 is basically running for your life!). It's a great way to monitor your internal training load, because it is specific to each individual.

More recently, the Borg scale has been modified using a 1–10 range (see table 9.1). Most coaches and athletes find this more straightforward to use, and color-coding the numbers helps athletes determine the right effort rating. If you take the athlete's RPE score and multiply it by the duration of the session in minutes, you end up with a score called arbitrary units. These are used in collegiate, elite, and pro sports to provide some insight into athlete internal training load.

You can change an athlete's training load by changing the training frequency, intensity, time, or type (this is the FITT principle). In real-world application, intensity is the key differentiator between practice and games, and it's also the easiest factor for trainer and coaches to manipulate. RPE helps you plan out your training week to provide varying activities to the athlete and allow for adequate periods of rest and recovery. The trends you start to see for individual athletes will help you flag players when an abnormal reading pops up. This doesn't mean the athlete can't train, it's just a cue to start a conversation between the athlete and coach (or performance staff) to determine what's going on — is this just a blip on the radar — or is it something to actually worry about? A recent study in combat sports found the rating of perceived exertion (RPE) can be used as an indirect marker to determine the level of effort and stress across bouts, successive matches, and training in athletes.[21] Researchers also used two separate heart-rate-based methods to confirm that session RPE was indeed reliable, highlighting that the correlation was greatest in adults and in the precompetition period. They concluded that session RPE is a low-cost, noninvasive, and valuable tool for coaches, sport scientists, and athletes for monitoring training loads in combat sports, particularly in sessions with a higher percentage of aerobic exercise.

It looks like RPE is an effective tool for team and combat sport athletes. But what about endurance sports? Renowned endurance expert Trent Stellingwerff, PhD, at the Canadian Sport Institute Pacific, enthusiastically supports the use of RPE (along with an external load metric) to monitor and track progress in elite endurance athletes. What about in recreational athletes?

**TABLE 9.1.** Rating of Perceived Exertion (RPE)

| BORG SCALE | | MODIFIED BORG SCALE | |
|---|---|---|---|
| 6 | | 0 | At rest |
| 7 | Very, very light | 1 | Very easy |
| 8 | | | |
| 9 | Very light | 2 | Somewhat easy |
| 10 | | | |
| 11 | Fairly light | 3 | Moderate |
| 12 | | 4 | Somewhat hard |
| 13 | Somewhat hard | 5 | Hard |
| 14 | | 6 | |
| 15 | Hard | | |
| 16 | | 7 | Very hard |
| 17 | Very hard | 8 | |
| 18 | | 9 | |
| 19 | Very, very hard | | |
| 20 | | 10 | Very, very hard |

*Source:* Gunnar A. V. Borg, "Psychophysical Bases of Perceived Exertion." *Medicine & Science in Sports & Exercise* 14, no. 5 (1982), https://doi.org/10.1249/00005768-198205000 -00012.

Can perceived exertion help guide their training protocol and plan? A recent study was the first to show that RPE in runners was effective, for both men and women, at gauging their time to complete the task.[22] Runners completed an in-lab assessment test, and then were asked to complete a competitive 7-mile run followed by a half-marathon in the following week. Of course, it seems obvious the rate of perceived exertion was higher in the shorter 7-mile race, as the athletes were running faster. But when RPE was plotted against the percentage of time to complete the race, the RPEs were very similar. This phenomenon occurred despite the runners being instructed to use different pacing strategies. The study's authors suggested that "your brain regulates perceived exertion and physical performance in an anticipatory manner" and that this awareness is based on fuel reserves and biomechanical performance.

This analysis supports classic research by Tim Noakes, emeritus professor in South Africa, and the central governor theory, whereby the brain acts as the principle governor of physical output. Your brain effectively knows before the race even starts how hard it's *willing* to let you push yourself, and this anticipatory ability sets the endpoint for how hard you can push. In short, RPE works well for endurance training, too.

However, like all measures, RPE has its shortcomings. One of the biggest hurdles in team sports is that the best players play a lot, and the substitutes play much less. So when it's time to practice the day after a game, problems can arise when the starter who logged heavy minutes in the previous day's game is asked to do the same amount of work as the substitute who didn't play. Not surprisingly, these starters can look sluggish in practices while the substitutes seem to have boundless energy. You have some athletes training too much and others training too little, which presents a major performance problem.[23] (In a real-life scenario, players often don't want to tell the coach they're too tired to practice.) Other elite athletes, often endurance types, simply refuse to admit they perceive *any* fatigue — they view it as a weakness and keep reporting a 7 when the exercise physiologist can obviously see they're about to blow a gasket! Another shortcoming is if you're working with a large group of athletes. It can be really difficult to collect all the RPEs for each player on top of your other duties as the lead therapist or strength coach. Yet another roadblock is when coaches decide to ramp up the intensity during a planned longer training day, transforming it from a planned RPE of 4 (less intense) into a 7 or 8. Players then kick it up into a higher gear and become run-down and exhausted heading into the rest of the week or upcoming games. All of that said, RPE is still an evidence-based tool for assessing training load. The best time to collect RPEs is typically either 10 minutes or 30 minutes post-training.[24]

## Athlete Performance Output: Potential Recovery Markers

An athlete's performance during training is another opportunity to flag overreaching and impaired recovery capacity. One of the most consistent findings in the sport science literature is that a diminished maximal lactate concentration appears during all-out effort — with both strength and endurance athletes — while values below max threshold remain about the same (sometimes lower, sometimes not).[25] Multiple exercise tests can also be used to assess recovery. If an athlete cannot perform a second bout of exercise after a standardized first bout, then that might be an indication of overtraining — and more important, can help the practitioner distinguish it from a normal training response. In reality, unless you're working in a collegiate, pro, or research environment, you're not going to have access to these tests. How can a field-based practitioner get a glimpse of an athlete's internal load? It's very subjective; what an intense training block does to one individual's recovery will probably do something very different to another, despite exactly the same training plan. Table 9.2 offers a quick list of signs of symptoms to watch out for in athletes who are approaching harmful nonfunctional overreaching.

Of course, don't be fooled into thinking just because your athlete doesn't experience any of these symptoms means that they're "good to go" for intense training. It's not that simple. Let's take a closer look at a more tech-driven assessment strategy, heart rate variability (HRV), which can help provide deeper evidence-based insights into athlete recovery and readiness to perform.

**TABLE 9.2.** Symptoms of Potential NFOR and Overtraining Syndrome in Athletes

| BIOMARKER | SYMPTOM (INCREASES) |
| --- | --- |
| Morning resting heart rate | Increased by 10 beats or more |
| Exercising heart rate | Increased by 10 beats or more |
| Blood pressure | Increased by 10+ mmHg |
| Subjective complaints | Session RPE increased |
| BIOMARKER | SYMPTOM (DECREASES) |
| $VO_2$ max | Decreases |
| Maximum heart rate | Decreases |
| Maximum lactate | Decreases |
| Maximum power | Decreases |
| Postural hypotension | Decreased by 10+ mmHg (after standing measure) |

*Source:* Romain Meeusen et al., "Prevention, Diagnosis, and Treatment of the Overtraining Syndrome: Joint Consensus Statement of the European College of Sport Science and the American College of Sports Medicine," *Medicine & Science in Sports & Exercise* 45, no. 1 (2013), https://doi.org/10.1249/mss.0b013e318279a10a.

## Heart Rate Variability and Athlete Monitoring

Training and recovery are incredibly complex processes that become even murkier when you try to apply a reductionist approach. For example, just because cortisol is low, it doesn't mean your athlete is in trouble. Similarly, just because free testosterone is in the normal range, it doesn't mean your athlete is all good. It all depends on context. Where are you in your training plan? Are you adapting or optimizing? Is the athlete responding effectively to training and progressing or stuck in a plateau? The answers to these questions are crucial to determining the right strategy. The challenge with blood, salivary, or urine biomarkers is they're just a snapshot in time. If you run them twice a year, will that really tell you anything about your athlete in the short term? It can help flag overt problems, but you might lack sufficient data to reveal more nuanced and dynamic dysfunctions that fly under the radar. To get a better idea of the full athlete picture, you would need to run these tests much more frequently (daily, weekly, monthly, and so forth), which can be incredibly costly. To add more insight into these biomarkers, elite teams and coaches use a variety of monitoring tools to assess athlete stress; one in particular is heart rate variability.

Heart rate variability (HRV) is the changes or variations that occur between each successive heartbeat. For example, if your resting heart rate is 60 bpm (beats per minute), you would have approximately one heartbeat per second; however, on closer inspection, there is considerable (or very little) variability between each one of those 60 heartbeats. This variability between heartbeats acts as a proxy for assessing an athlete's autonomic nervous system function, and in particular the balance between the sympathetic and parasympathetic systems. Your autonomic nervous system (ANS) is made up of two branches: the "fight or flight" sympathetic and the "rest and digest" parasympathetic. Like the gas pedal and the brake, these two systems react and respond to all the stimuli and stressors you're exposed to. They're not under your conscious control. HRV has become a very popular strategy for measuring stress (and thus recovery) in athletes and active people. Expert Marco Altini, PhD, from the Netherlands explains that your heart doesn't beat like a metronome. Rather, it has small variations between beats. These variations provide a window into your autonomic nervous system function, and more specifically your parasympathetic system. HRV is considered a highly reliable proxy for parasympathetic activity (and thus recovery).[26]

Let's dig deeper into the mechanisms of how HRV works. Your para-sympathetic nervous system communicates with the SA node of your heart (its pacemaker) via release of acetylcholine (ACh) neurotransmitters from nerve cells that bind to specific receptors on the heart. This communication occurs *very quickly* between acetylcholine and the muscarinic receptors on the heart. Your sympathetic nervous system also communicates with the SA node of your heart, but via the release of a different neurotransmitter called norepinephrine (NE). Norepinephrine has a little bit more *delayed* effect on the heart; this subtle difference in response time between your para-sympathetic (NE) and sympathetic systems (ACh) gives you a glimpse into how each system is affecting your body. By analyzing the micro-changes in heartbeats, research scientists are able to capture an idea of the physiological stress on your body. This measure is your HRV score.

In general, the fitter you are, the higher your HRV. This reflects greater variability between your heartbeats and thus a greater capacity to adapt to stress and novel challenges. This is typically a good sign (most of the time), but HRV can vary depending on training blocks. Typically, the higher your HRV, the more adaptive or resilient you're likely going to be. If you're over-weight, out of shape, or deconditioned, you'll tend to have a lower HRV score. This reduction in variability reveals a sympathetic nervous system dominance (you're stuck in "fight or flight") and a reduced capacity to adapt to stressors. Your heart starts to beat at a very constant rate — like a metronome — with very little variability between beats. Therefore, the lower your HRV, the less resilient or adaptive you are. (Remember, these are generalizations to help better understand the concept; there is a lot nuance within these themes.)

## The Recovery Pyramid and HRV

Your autonomic nervous system (ANS) plays a massive role in your re-sponse to exercise. Unfortunately, it's not under your conscious control. What's more, the ANS response to training is remarkably variable from one person to the next. Do you thrive with more high-intensity work inter-spersed with more rest? Do you need longer, slower sessions to achieve your goals? Your ANS response is heavily impacted by your genes, how much sleep you get, your nutrition, your chronological age as well as your train-ing age, and psychological factors. Until recently, when an athlete decided to back off training, it was primarily driven by the coach's eye, experience, and the athlete's best guess as to how they felt. While you'll always benefit from an experienced coach's feel for your progress, using a monitoring tool like HRV (along with other metrics) can help clarify the situation when the coach's eye isn't enough, such as when to back off training (and emphasize recovery) and when to push harder. Heart rate variability doesn't just measure your training stress; it also takes into account life stressors like alcohol, caffeine, travel, work stress, mental stress, emotional stress, and lack of sleep, which all play their role in your training load and thus your ability to recover effectively.

HRV can provide a wealth of valuable data — yet alone, it cannot tell you everything about an athlete. HRV is based on cardiac output and therefore tends to be more easily applied to endurance compared to strength and team sport. Also, it isn't able to capture your stress *during* training, the mechanical and muscular stress of a lifting session, or other aspects such as muscular pain and discomfort. In the short term, acute stressors have the biggest impact on HRV, whereas in the long term, factors such as circadian rhythm start to play a much greater role. Let's take a quick look at how sleep, blood glucose control, and mental and emotional stress can impact HRV.

### Sleep, Blood Glucose Control, and Stress

If you're training hard to prepare for a competition or to achieve a personal best, you're likely up early in the morning or out late at night to train. If you don't get enough sleep or constantly alter your sleeping and wake times, it can significantly increase your daytime resting heart rate and decrease HRV.[27] Sleep expert Cheri Mah, MD, hammers home the importance of sleep for recovery, stating bluntly, "It's a non-negotiable," while recovery expert Dr. Shona Halson from the Australian Institute of Sport says that sleep should be the first thing you emphasize for recovery. You can't sacrifice sleep and optimize recovery.

In pro sports, sugar consumption (even addiction) is legendary. Just ask Cate Shanahan, MD, author of *Deep Nutrition* and former medical lead for the LA Lakers who helped NBA All-Star center Dwight Howard curb his late-night habit of knocking back bags of Oreos after evening games. He's not alone in his sugar addiction; a few seasons ago, Toronto Raptors All-Star point guard Kyle Lowry dropped significant weight and dramatically improved body composition by simply shifting away from late-night snacks such as candy and cookies after games. It's not just in team sports; endurance athletes are perhaps the most prone to chronic sugar cravings.

In overweight individuals, the research is showing a clear trend that higher fasting glucose and glycated hemoglobin levels (HbA1c) are associated with a lowering of HRV scores.[28] Studies also show that insulin sensitivity — as measured by the homeostasis model assessment of insulin resistance (HOMA-IR) — is also negatively associated with HRV, with researchers finding "altered heart rate variability . . . during everyday life is linked to insulin resistance." It's important to remember these studies are not performed in athletes. However, they highlight the need to achieve the right energy balance to drive performance while not sabotaging health.

And as mentioned previously, athletes are not immune to depression. Recently, NBA All-Star DeMar DeRozan admitted he's struggled with bouts of depression in the past, and NBA All-Star Kevin Love revealed he's battled anxiety for some time. Many type-A personalities are stuck in a constant sympathetic drive, which can lead to exhaustion and low mood, as well as anxietylike symptoms. Exercise is a great mood-enhancing tool for most people, ramping up brain-derived neurotrophic factors (BDNF) in the brain; however, the intensity and volume at elite levels can push athletes into overtraining and increase risk of mood disturbances. As classically described in sport science literature, mood state disturbances increase in a dose-response manner as training stimuli increase. A recent meta-analysis also found that depression is associated with reduced HRV, and that it decreases with the increasing severity of the depression (in people without cardiovascular issues).[29] The use of antidepressant medications didn't alter this finding.

## HRV AND DEHYDRATION

Most people know hydration is crucial for athletic performance. A mere 2 percent drop in hydration might confer a 5–8 percent drop in performance for endurance athletes, while strength and team sport have a little more wiggle room at 3–5 percent.[30] Plasma is the liquid portion of your blood — made up of 92 percent water — and constitutes 55 percent of your total blood volume. So if you don't drink enough water, sweat excessively in training, or overconsume caffeine or alcohol, your plasma volume will drop below normal. Consequently, your sympathetic system kicks into gear, which instantaneously increases your heart rate to offset this loss of fluid and restore your blood pressure. This takes its toll on your nervous system, dropping your HRV. A recent study of collegiate athletes on the impacts of dehydration on

## Heart Rate Variability and Longevity

If you're looking to eat, train, and recover to promote your best health into your senior years, then HRV might be a pretty useful biomarker. Consistently high HRV levels are associated with reduced all-cause mortality, and is a reliably predictive marker of healthy aging and longevity.[32] Of course, as you get older your HRV tends to drop. The experts note the mechanism for this HRV drop could be caused by cardiovascular structural changes, decreased arterial flexibility, or other regulatory processes that occur during aging.[33] If you keep yourself fit, you can potentially slow the drop seen in the general population. If you're a coffee drinker, there is more good news. Coffee has also been shown to increase HRV, as well as lengthen telomeres, another reliable biomarker of healthy aging.[34]

HRV found the group failing to adequately rehydrate 4 hours after a training session experienced a significant drop in HRV.[31] When you rehydrate, your plasma volume increases, which increases the venous return to your heart, and thus boosts the amount of blood per heartbeat you can pump out. This is what happens when you're fit — more blood comes back to the heart, thus your resting heart rate lowers because you can pump out bigger volumes per heartbeat. This reinforces the importance of hydration to recovery.

## How Can Training Impact Recovery?

How does knowing your HRV impact your ability to adjust your training plan or support recovery? The work of Andrew Flatt, PhD, from Georgia Southern University, found that when training camp starts for collegiate female soccer players, all of the athletes have a large degree of fluctuations in their weekly HRV scores (this is called the coefficient of variation, or HRV CV).[35] By the third week, the athletes making the greatest progress had very small daily fluctuations, demonstrating they've adapted to the stress of training and become fitter. On the other hand, the players struggling to keep up and making the smallest gains — or even regressing in their performance — experienced high daily fluctuations in HRV. This doesn't imply they're "bad" players, or even unfit — it just means they're not responding to the training stimuli appropriately. The HRV monitoring tool can help identify and target athletes who might need individualized changes in their recovery strategies so that they can adapt more effectively to training.

There is a big aerobic component to HRV assessment; thus, endurance experts like Daniel Plews, PhD, and Professor Paul Laursen, PhD, typically see the highest value for using HRV with endurance athletes. Classically, in endurance training you can effectively follow a spreadsheet-like program and achieve performance gains; however, adding HRV into the mix allows for more personalization as it takes into account how the athlete is adapting to the program. These day-to-day changes are more meaningful for endurance trainees, and the training plan can be adjusted in real-time in response to the data collected. In short, for aerobic-based training, HRV is a very good measure of recovery. In team and strength-based sports, however, it's more difficult to filter through the noise. Andrew Flatt, PhD, notes that "reductions are more consistent, more linear after aerobic workouts. With strength-based sports it's not so straightforward." Dr. Flatt says he only sees dramatic changes in HRV after "very intense" sessions, and that this is typically only seen in really high-level, elite lifters and athletes. He's quick to note it's simply one tool, and not all decisions are based on HRV.

Other limitations exist, too, for using HRV, including the fact that you can't use it to estimate an athlete's $VO_2$ max. However, what you can do is look at the baseline mean HRV values — the 7-day rolling averages — and compare them to an athlete's normal values. Are they lower? Are they a lot lower? It might or might not be a problem; it all depends on the context. Maybe it's time to postpone intense training blocks and ramp up recovery time or recovery workouts. A recent study looked at just that. A group of overreaching endurance athletes were divided into two groups; one would postpone heavy training (based on HRV data) until adequate recovery, while the other would continue as usual. The group who rested outperformed the group who gritted their teeth and trained through the pain.[36] That's right . . . the group that did *less* got a better outcome. It's not always about training hard, but about training smart and individualizing the training stimulus and recovery program to maximize gains.

It's important to keep things in context. The role of HRV is to give you a snapshot of the stressors imposed on your body so that you can

## Pitfalls of Game-Day Assessments

Make sure to avoid the pitfall of reacting acutely to individual HRV measures. The research tends to show that most athletes have significantly lower scores on competition day, which is thought to be due to natural anxiety and increased likelihood of poor sleep before competition. Therefore, it's important to avoid overinterpreting the data and thus overreacting to it. The research shows HRV doesn't impact performance. For example, sprinters who performed the best over 100 m also had notably lower scores on race day. This might be reflective of increased sympathetic activity on race day (which is a very good thing!). This is why it's important for you to decide if and when it's appropriate to show your athlete HRV (or other) monitoring scores and how they're trending. It will be highly individual depending on the athlete and coach.

monitor training loads to maximize training response. The athlete's goal is definitely *not* to have the "best" HRV in the club or team. Monitoring can allow you to replicate your training plan in a methodical, systematic manner in order to make performances more consistent. Dr. Plews outlines three important questions HRV can help you answer when it comes to endurance training.

1. **Is the type of training right?** Is it time for a recovery session today? Are you pushing yourself hard enough to get the gains you want? HRV helps to guide (not control) the type of training you perform to ensure you're on track.
2. **Can you do it consistently?** Consistency is key in high-level endurance sport. HRV can help identify the right training intensities and volumes over the course of your training block so you can make it through your training mesocycle effectively. Are you too fatigued to continue? Are you redlining? Dr. Plews says he's amazed at how many endurance athletes still "train in the dark," and do not assess how their body is reacting to training.

3. **How are you tracking?** How far away are you from your goal? Are you progressing toward your target or are you lagging behind? Perhaps you're performing well but at a great energy cost, suggesting the need to back off and prioritize recovery. Dr. Plews highlights the value of collecting data by emphasizing, "If you're not sure, the data gives you greater clarity. . . . It reduces uncertainty." HRV is roughly telling you the internal cost of performing the training session. If your acute load is much greater than your chronic load, then you're likely doing something wrong. Reassess your training plan and make the necessary adjustments.

HRV validation apps like HRV4training or Elite HRV are simple and effective tools that both clients and athletes can use.[37] But the bottom line is that you can't just look at HRV in a vacuum and make recommendations, as a reductionist approach won't work in the long-term. In summary, here are some tips from the experts about implementing HRV:

- HRV shouldn't be the first thing you add to your monitoring tool box.
- Don't adjust your training solely based on HRV (use it as a secondary marker).
- Understand that "high" is not always good and "low" is not always bad.
- HRV is simply a tool; having a coach or practitioner to support you in the monitoring process is recommended.
- Don't track everything; start with one or two variables.

## Ice Baths, Cryotherapy, and Compression Garments

Now let's talk about the top of the recovery pyramid: recovery strategies. Performance director Lachlan Penfold's Recovery Pyramid (see figure 7.1) emphasizes the importance of the fundamentals: nutrition, sleep, and stress (mental-emotional health). The next most important part of recovery is getting your training process right. As Penfold says, "It's never perfect, but you get as close as you can." Once you've ensured every level of the pyramid has been addressed, then you can cap it off by chasing marginal gains by way of using ice baths, hot tubs, cryotherapy, and the like. It's important to point out Penfold gives his players options so that they can choose the strategy they prefer. This is a great way to increase athlete compliance and ensure each member of the team gets their daily dose. The following is a quick review of some popular evidence-based recovery strategies currently in use.

### COLD-WATER IMMERSION (CWI)

Ice baths seem like a rite of passage for every elite athlete. I'll never forget the first time I saw a picture of William "The Refrigerator" Perry, famous defense lineman for the Chicago Bears in the 1980s, climb into a keglike bucket full of ice just to cool down post-practice in training camp. (It looked excruciating!) Intense training can quickly lead to significant delayed-onset muscle soreness (DOMS), reduced muscular function, and even reductions in performance. The study of ice baths, defined as cold-water immersion (CWI) in scientific circles, has exploded over the past decade as researchers race to attempt to uncover how (and if) it supports recovery. A recent meta-analysis study on CWI investigated its effects on recovery after eccentric and high-intensity exercise. Athletes performed drop jumps, sprints on a bike, and simulated team sport games, followed by post-exercise cold-water immersion. What happened? The ice baths did reduce muscle soreness up to 96 hours (4 days), and athetes had a small reduction in their creatine kinase levels.[38] Interestingly, the athletes saw an improvement in muscular power within 24 hours following CWI, but not muscular strength. It appears cold water might provide a recovery advantage for faster-twitch, high-velocity, and type II muscle fibers.

How does cold-water immersion work? Most people think ice baths help to reduce the inflammatory response from intense training, thus aiding recovery. New research from Jonathan Peake, PhD, of the Australian Institute of Sport found that CWI after intense training didn't change the inflammatory response compared to active recovery.[39] If CWI doesn't blunt inflammation, then what? Experts are still trying to decipher the exact mechanisms, but they believe redistribution of blood flow, localized cooling, and its analgesic (painkilling) effects might be at the root.[40] Although experts are in general agreement that CWI can help reduce athlete muscle soreness, there is a lot more skepticism on whether it benefits muscle function and performance.[41] Some studies show minor benefit, while many others do not. It's still up for debate. The research does support CWI as superior to passive rest for improving muscle soreness post-training; the next questions are "how cold?" and "for how long?" The research varies in terms of temperature and length of time, so you've got room to personalize your approach. Studies have varied in length from 3–20 minutes, and immersion depth from waist to shoulder. The general consensus from recovery expert Dr. Shona Halson is 11–15 minutes in a tub at 11–15°C (59°F) is a good evidence-based option.[42]

### Hot-Water Immersion (HWI)

Hydrotherapy can also involve the application of hot-water immersions (HWI), typically performed at temperatures of 36°C (99°F) for 10–14 minutes. The effect of HWI on exercise performance has not yet yielded much evidence that it can assist performance (competition) recovery. One study found the daily application of a 14-minute HWI at 38°C (100°F) had no effect on cycling sprint or time trial performance.[43] That said, in another research study using the same protocol, the authors found daily HWI improved recovery from isometric squats for 72 hours post-training.[44] With only limited findings, experts agree that hot-water immersions cannot yet be recommended as recovery technique after quality training sessions or competition. How can you use hot-water immersions to support athlete gains? This is a great example of the application of periodized recovery. Dr. Shona Halson uses the table shown in figure 9.2 as a guide for when to incorporate hot- or cold-water immersions.[45]

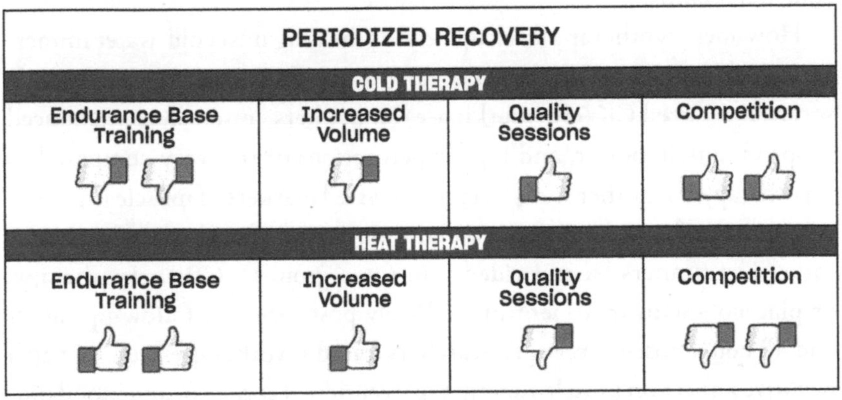

**FIGURE 9.2.** Periodized Recovery Strategies. From Shona Halson, "Controversies in Recovery," (presentation, University of Notre Dame and Australian Catholic University Human Performance Summit: The 24 Hour Athlete, South Bend, Indiana, USA, June 2018).

## CRYOTHERAPY

Cryotherapy has been the latest buzzword in recovery over the past few years. Whole-body cryotherapy (WBC) is like something out of Star Trek: You stand in a tank (up to your neck) that blasts freezing temperatures (-80 to -190°C; -176 to -374°F) over your body for 2–4 minutes. The proposed benefits of WBC include buffering post-training inflammation, edema, and muscle damage as well as reducing muscle soreness. What does the research say? The best results from cryotherapy come when it's used repeatedly over multiple days. Several studies have shown three and five sessions of cryotherapy encouraged faster recovery in peak muscle torque and reduced pain perceptions.[46] Immediate exposure to cryotherapy after drop jump training was also able to accelerate recovery of muscular strength (whereas no benefit was found if applied 24 hours after training).

There are some serious limitations when it comes to cryotherapy. A major selling point is the incredibly cold temperatures the body is exposed to, which make it seem like a better bet than ice baths. Interestingly, when you compare a cold bath at 8°C (46°F) versus a cryotherapy session at -110°C (-166°F), both elicit the same effect on muscle and core body temperature. How is this possible? Air has poor thermal conductivity compared to water, and thus prevents significant cooling of subcutaneous and core tissues. Cryotherapy definitely makes your skin a lot colder, but this effect dissipates after 60 minutes, which is a faster return to baseline than cold-water baths.[47]

How does cryotherapy stack up head-to-head against cold-water immersions? Athletes using CWI as a recovery strategy had lower levels of muscle soreness, reduced CK (creatine kinase) biomarkers, lesser exercise-induced drops in muscle power, and higher perceptions of recovery compared to cryotherapy.[48] Another study in runners tested markers of muscle function, perceptions of muscle soreness, and training stress after the London Marathon. The runners were divided into three groups — CWI, cryotherapy, or placebo — with treatment immediately post-race and follow-ups at 24 and 48 hours post-exercise. Researchers found cryotherapy actually had a negative impact on muscle function, perception of soreness, and blood biomarkers compared to cold-water immersions. In fact, cryotherapy was not better than placebo in this study.[49] It appears that cold-water immersions are superior to cryotherapy. But in practical terms, it's much easier to get an athlete to do a 3-minute cryotherapy session than to sit in a cold tub for

5–15 minutes. It's also worth noting that the performance staff of certain elite pro teams use cryotherapy regularly with their athletes.

### COMPRESSION GARMENTS

Turn on your favorite sporting event and you'll probably see an advertisement for compression gear. Popularized by the NBA's Allen Iverson many years ago with the "sleeve" (originally thought to be used to cover up tattoos, which are now accepted), the use of compression garments has blown up over the last decade. Compression garments are supposed to enhance blood flow and thus help remove the buildup of metabolites in muscle (that limit recovery) after intense training. Does the science back up the claims? Like all the recovery-specific strategies, the results are mixed. A recent meta-analysis found compression garments worn during, or during *and* after, strenuous exercise were able to moderately reduce muscle soreness, reduce levels of creatine kinase, and improve muscle strength and power recovery.[50] When it comes to endurance exercise, the benefits aren't so clear. Runners wearing lower-limb compression garments 72 hours after exercise saw no benefit to muscle damage or inflammation compared to placebo.[51] The biggest confounder when it comes to compression garments is the amount of pressure exerted. Experts believe it's the pressure that provides the recovery benefit. If the pressure isn't high enough, it won't elicit a recovery effect, but if it's too high it can actually exacerbate the damage and swelling.[52] You need to find the right dose for you.

## Athlete Monitoring Solutions: From Science to Practice

Before you race to apply a few of these strategies to your own recovery plan, there are a few important principles to understand. The first is context. You must apply a strategy that enhances your training plan. If you're in an adaptation phase, limiting inflammation might not be your best bet. Athletes using cold-water immersion during a lower-body strength training phase (twice weekly for 12 weeks) had significantly lowers gains in muscle mass, max strength, and rate of force development compared to controls.[53] In a follow-up study, the authors identified that CWI suppressed satellite cell activity and p70S6 (a regulator of mTOR) during recovery from strength training. Again: context matters. Just because you *can* use a recovery strategy doesn't mean you *should*. Understanding the context and the nuances of application is crucial for success. Therefore, its best use is likely around competition, and not during adaptive training phases.

On the other hand, if you're entering a competition phase and need to bounce back as quickly as possible, it might be ideal. Change the context and you might get a different result. In endurance athletes, Dr. Halson found elite cyclists using CWI four times weekly improved performance over a 5-week time frame.[54] It appears that cold-water immersion might help support mitochondrial biogenesis via activation of PGC-1alpha, which is well established in scientific research as the primary regulator of mitochondrial biogenesis in skeletal muscle.[55] In fact, just the application of cold-water immersion upregulated this pathway, although not to the same extent as exercise plus cold-water immersion.

---

In summary, recovery is a crucial aspect of an athlete's ability to recharge after a workout, as well as to prepare for the next training sessions. The use of biomarkers, Big Data, and old-school subjective markers all play a role in painting the picture of the athlete's state of health and readiness. Performance expert Doug Kechijian, DPT, from New York stresses the importance of using monitoring tools to alert you when it's time to have a conversation with your athlete, and he cautions against the over-inter-pretation of data. Engage with your athletes; talk to them. The language you use is also highly impactful, particularly as it relates to recovery. Dr. Shona Halson is always reminding coaches to "never say fatigue is bad . . . never say soreness is bad . . . never say tired is bad . . . it's not about reducing fatigue, it's about managing it." This is a hugely important point. Halson also suggests a simple rule when deciding what recovery modality (if any) to choose from, stating, "If an athlete feels better using a recovery strategy, that's likely going to help them in the long run because how an athlete feels is crucial to performance." If an athlete feels flat, it affects performance.

Muhammad Ali didn't have access to this recovery science when he said famously: "Don't quit. Suffer now and live the rest of your life as a champion." Prioritizing recovery will not only make the process a little more tolerable, the science shows it can amplify your gains.

# PART FOUR

# Supercharge

*Your biggest opponent isn't the other guy. It's human nature.*
— BOBBY KNIGHT

# CHAPTER 10

# Brain Health and Concussions

I t was 2017, and quarterback Tom Savage of the Houston Texans was on the ground, knocked unconscious after taking a big hit from San Francisco 49ers defensive end Elvis Dumervil. Savage's head hit the ground violently and he lost consciousness, his hands visibly trembling as if he was experiencing a seizure. It was a frightening scene, and when Savage regained consciousness, he was noticeably shaken and struggled to make it over to the sidelines. The seizure happened in a flash, and unbeknownst to the neurotrauma consultant on the sidelines about to evaluate Savage. While the assessment took place, the video replay was shown multiple times on the stadium big screen, and even hardcore football fans were left stunned by the gruesome scene of the trembling Savage laying unconscious on the field. Five minutes later, after taking the enormous hit, Savage was cleared by the medical staff and sent back in the game. The medical staff, having not seen the replay, were then alerted about the video footage and Savage was pulled from the game. This was an astonishing example of the risk professional football players take every time they step on the field, and how difficult it can be for medical professionals to react effectively.

The incidence of concussion is on the rise in the NFL, and teams are attempting to support player health by providing independent neurotrauma consultants to perform on-field tests. It's an incredibly difficult environment to perform the necessary tests in a short time frame. While most players and coaches would agree it's a step in the right direction, medical experts like Chris Nowinski, PhD, CEO of the Concussion Legacy Foundation and co-director of Boston University's Chronic Traumatic Encephalopathy (CTE) Center, are not impressed. Nowinski's tweet in response to the incident highlights this contempt: "Disgusted the Houston Texans allowed Tom Savage to return to the game after 2 plays after showing these horrifying

#concussion signs (is that a seizure?) after a head impact. I would not let my worst enemy go through the 2017 #NFL sideline concussion protocol . . ." It's a clear sign the situation is reaching a tipping point.

But it's not just obvious headshots and acute head trauma that affect an athlete's cognitive health. The cumulative effect of taking hits over a career can cause myriad problems. This was easily apparent in a recent interview with two-time NFL All-Pro quarterback Mark Rypien of the Washington Redskins, considered one of the best deep-ball passers of his generation, who was fighting back tears. No, these were not tears of glee, as they might have been in 1992, when Rypien won Super Bowl XXVI with Washington by beating the Buffalo Bills 37–24 and winning MVP honors. It was 2018, and Rypien was 55 years old. In the interview, he described how he attempted suicide by taking 150 pills and a bottle of alcohol. Since retiring from pro football in 1998, Rypien has struggled massively with mental health issues, and he shares how over two decades of football led to "mental health conditions, dark places, depression, anxiety, poor choices and poor decisions brought about from dozens of concussions and thousands of subconcussive injuries from playing [football]." Rypien's situation is not an isolated incident in the NFL, and sadly his story has become increasingly common in other professional contact sports — something pro hockey players, for example, know all too well.[1]

Nick Boynton played 11 seasons in the NHL as an enforcer, going out every night on the ice to impose himself physically on the other team. In a recent interview for the *Players' Tribune*, Boynton admitted: "I've struggled a ton since I retired from hockey in 2011. . . . I've faced a lot of different personal demons." He was talking about his state of mental health and the fate of fellow NHLers and friends Steve Montador, Wade Belak, Derek Boogaard, and Rick Rypien, who all died after struggles with anxiety, depression, and substance abuse.[2] While he's the first to admit he's made many poor decisions throughout his life, Boynton says death often seems to him a form of release, an escape from the suffering. Suffering is a common theme among pro athletes struggling with the effects of repeated head trauma.

Until relatively recently, the awareness of the impact of physical contact on brain health was largely unknown. This all changed in the late 1990s, when expert pathologist Bennet Omalu, MD, discovered something out of the ordinary when performing autopsies on deceased former NFL football players. Dr. Omalu found a disturbing pattern of brown stains on the thin slices of the player's brain tissue. He recognized them immediately as tau proteins, the well-established hallmark of Alzheimer's disease, a chronic neurodegenerative disease that progressively and irreversibly destroys brain cells, leading to memory loss and cognitive decline.[3] Alarmingly, the magnitude of the staining was reminiscent of what Dr. Omalu might see in advanced Alzheimer's patients in their late 80s, not in an otherwise healthy ex-professional football player in his mid-40s. Dr. Omalu's findings led to the discovery of chronic traumatic encephalitis, or CTE — made famous from his portrayal by actor Will Smith in the movie *Concussion* — and his published results have changed player safety in the NFL. That said, the initial reaction from the NFL was denial. They refused to admit any connection between brain trauma and the game of football. But as the cases mounted, the league acknowledged it was time for action (although the league still continues to deny causality). In 2017, a research team at the Boston brain bank examined the brains of 202 deceased football players and found almost 90 percent had some degree of CTE. Among the deceased NFL players examined, shockingly, 110 out of 111 were found to have traces of CTE.[4] The NFL and NHL still deny the claim of causation and are holding strong it's only one of association. Today concussion protocols have been implemented in both leagues; however, as you can see from the case of Tom Savage and many others, it's difficult to execute successfully from the sidelines. What's more, a big hit can lead to brain trauma even if the player doesn't lose consciousness and undergo the concussion protocol. Of course, head trauma isn't just a problem for pro athletes.

## Traumatic Brain Injuries: Looking Deeper

The medical term for a concussion is mild traumatic brain injury (mTBI), and it affects an estimated 1.7 million people across America, contributing to one-third of all injury-related deaths every year. Three to four million people are diagnosed with head injuries in America every year, and among the 45 million kids playing youth sports, nearly two million children aged 19 or younger are treated in emergency rooms for sports and recreational-related concussions. The list of activities and sports with increased risk of head trauma include soccer, hockey, football, horseback riding, lacrosse, wrestling, skateboarding, cycling, playing on playgrounds, and falling. In fact, it's not even male football players who have the highest rate of concussion, but actually female ice hockey players. Interestingly, high school and collegiate girls and young women suffer concussions at higher rates than boys and young men. For example, female soccer and softball players experience concussions at twice the rate of male players. Experts aren't sure why, but speculate it might be related to female hormone levels or weaker neck musculature that contribute to the increased susceptibility.

Statistics from the Centers for Disease Control and Prevention (CDC) show that of all reported brain injuries, 75 percent are due to mild concussions (mTBI), although the number of unreported concussions and patients not seeking medical help is likely high as well. What happens to the brain during a concussion? How did all those hits that Mark Rypien took over the years from defensive linemen, or all the punches to the face Derek Boogaard endured against other enforcers, impact brain physiology and health? It's a complex phenomenon, but here's what researchers know to date.

Your brain sits bathed in fluid to prevent shocks, perturbations, and trauma, as it doesn't like to be bounced around inside your skull. Neurons are brain cells that perform the majority of the information processing in the brain, while other supportive cells are crucial for keeping your neurons happy and running on all cylinders (you can think of them as "role players"). In particular, astrocytes and microglia are key role players responsible for protecting your precious neurons from threats, helping them heal after injury, and providing them energy.[5] In a healthy brain, the tiny astrocytes monitor the health and activity of surrounding cells by creating a network of thin filaments, effectively establishing a surveillance system to ensure the brain avoids threat. If your brain is injured, explains expert neuroscientist and author of *The Hungry Brain* Stephan Guyenet, PhD, "these cells go into overdrive, increasing in size and number to counter the threat and accelerate healing." Astrocytes and microglia enlarge, proliferate, and entangle themselves, something not seen in a healthy brain. In fact, Dr. Guyenet states that "the activation of microglia and astrocytes is a universal marker of brain injury."[6] This overlapping of filaments can easily occur from the trauma in contact sports: a hit from an opposing lineman, a bodycheck in hockey, a collision between two players in soccer, or simply an accident or fall.

It's not simply the initial trauma of the hit or fall that causes the problem, but the activation of a cascade of secondary reactions that kick off many of the adverse symptoms experienced during and after the concussion. These secondary effects of concussion can occur after taking a big hit (despite not losing consciousness) and include the following:

- Ionic flux
- Disruption of cellular function
- Free-radical damage
- Activation of microglia

- Chronic inflammation
- Derangement of blood flow
- SNS and ANS dysfunction
- Leaky blood-brain barrier

These secondary effects are largely responsible for the myriad symptoms people experience post-concussion, such as headache, dizziness, fatigue, irritability, anxiety, insomnia, loss of concentration and memory, and ringing in the ears.[7] These symptoms can drive players to look for medications to temper the persistent pain and suffering. How long does it take to recover from a mild concussion? The evidence shows that 70–90 percent of concussions resolve within 10–14 days.[8] Of course, the timing of subsequent head traumas also plays a large role in how well you can recover. If you suffer another trauma to the head within a week of your previous concussion, the symptoms will worsen. That's why experts put so much emphasis on the first few weeks post-concussion, because if another concussion occurs more than 15 days after the initial trauma, there is no difference in response compared to the initial injury. If you don't allow your brain enough time to recover, subsequent head traumas exert more harmful effects, such as altering the metabolic and inflammatory terrain, worsening symptoms, and reducing the ability to get back to normal functions.

Making things even more challenging today is that there is currently no reliable biomarker or imaging test to diagnose concussion or confirm the athlete is ready to return to play. So when players suffer a blow to the head and symptoms subside, athletes are simply cleared to return to play. The problem with this approach is that *clinical* recovery — which means complete cessation of symptoms — does not equal *physiological* recovery.[9] This means even if athletes have no symptoms, the harmful cascade of secondary effects is still present, compromising the athlete's brain health. Unfortunately, despite improved concussion protocols in recent years, the typical return-to-play decisions are still too often made before full physiological recovery. Let's be honest: elite players also have a lot of pressure from coaches and management to get back on the field as quickly as possible.

Approximately 30 percent of concussion sufferers will experience post-concussion syndrome (PCS) when symptoms persist past 30 days; symptoms include headaches, fatigue, dizziness, irritability, reduced tolerance to stress, and cognitive impairment.[10] Although experts can't exactly pinpoint the mechanism contributing to these symptoms, they do believe it's some combination of blood flow or metabolic dysfunction, biopsychosocial factors, reduced cognitive reserve compared to pre-injury, and persistent inflammation. In fact, elevated CRP (C-reactive protein) levels — a biomarker for systemic inflammation — after three months are linked to greater risk of depression, fatigue, and cognitive impairments.[11]

If symptoms aren't enough to determine if an athlete can return to play, what is the current gold standard? In 2016, the International Conference on Concussion in Sport brought together the world's leading experts to evaluate the state of the current concussion research. Based on the available scientific literature, they concluded the best method to determine full clinical (symptoms) and physiological recovery appears to be physical testing — comparing baseline norms to an athlete's output post-concussion.[12] If athletes are pretested when healthy, and if they do suffer a blow to the head, then medical staff can retest them post–head trauma and compare the results to the athlete's "pre-concussion" baseline. This process helps medical staff determine how well athletes are recovering, but what about protocols to accelerate recovery? Unfortunately, on that note the research is still sparse. At the moment, the overall consensus is that light exercise — below the symptom threshold — can improve recovery and should be initiated two to three weeks after a concussion.

Most athletes are used to taking anti-inflammatories or other painkillers after a blow to the head to reduce adverse symptoms. But unfortunately, there's limited evidence that these medications are effective at reducing the negative effects of the injury or accelerating return to play. The experts summarized this in the Berlin Consensus Statement on Concussion in Sport, saying: "There is limited evidence to support the use of pharmacotherapy in treating (concussion)." Adding to the murky waters, the use of medication can mimic or mask many of the symptoms of sports-related concussions. For example, the side effects of pain medications like gabapentin include dizziness, headache, memory problems, and anxiety, to name a few. Medications to treat depressive symptoms — common in athletes who've suffered from multiple concussions — can lead to impaired concentration, anxiety, dizziness, poor memory, and more. Drugs to treat inflammation, such as ibuprofen, can lead to intestinal upset, headaches, nausea, and the like. You can see how difficult it becomes to tease out concussion-related symptoms from the side effects of these drugs.

The benefit of using pharmaceutical interventions is that they tend to work quite quickly and can help to reduce important symptoms such as pain, fatigue, and the process of inflammation in the short term. The trouble is, targeting a single method of action doesn't typically resolve a complex condition, nor does it address the multifactorial underlying root cause of the condition. Side effects begin to mount, as does the potential for nutrient depletion. If these pharmaceutical strategies were evidence-based and proven to work, you could live with the side effects. Unfortunately, the efficacy has yet to be demonstrated, so you need to monitor how long you take medications, and weigh the cost:benefit ratio of such interventions.

## Suffering: The Other Side of Pain

In a recent interview, Dr. Bennet Omalu said the current conversation around CTE is shifting the focus in the wrong direction. The concern is not simply the pronounced end-stage of CTE, but rather the cumulative effects of impact trauma on the brain. Alarmingly, Dr. Omalu warns, "CTE is just one disease in a spectrum of many diseases caused by brain trauma. . . . At the professional level, 100 percent would have brain damage of some kind to some degree . . . whether or not their brains are found to have CTE." That's a powerful statement. Despite this clear warning, athletes continue to play. Why do they do it? Why do some get stuck in a downward spiral of taking pain medications and experiencing substance abuse while the majority do not? It's a complex question and nobody can say for certain, but often-cited theories include pressure for athletes to return to play, it's how they earn a paycheck, fear of getting cut by the team, coercion from medical staff or coaches (unfortunately still a reality in some sports), athletes not being informed of the potential side effects, and more.

Of course, there is another aspect to chronic pain and concussion management that too often gets completely overlooked. Athletes who struggle with chronic pain and repeated head trauma are not just trying to fight off the physical pain of the injury but are also trying to numb deep and persistent emotional suffering. Pain and opioid expert Abhimanyu Sud, MD, is quick to point out that suffering is very tightly intertwined with pain. The use of opioid drugs to treat pain has skyrocketed across the general population in the last decade, and Sud says, "Today we have more people dying of opioid-related deaths than [at] the height of the HIV/AIDS epidemic in the early 1990s . . . and we don't seem to be any[where] near the height of the opioid epidemic."[13] Experts estimate that half a million deaths over the next decade will be directly related to opioid use. This doesn't even include all the other negative impacts of overdose, lives affected by addiction, and all the people impacted by opioid use.

Opioids are a class of chemicals that are derived from the opium poppy or are structurally similar to the compounds found in opium used to relieve chronic pain. Examples include morphine, codeine, hydromorphone, oxycodone, and fentanyl. Opioids have powerful pain-relieving effects and have been used for thousands of years in medicine for a variety of pain-related conditions. Over the last decade, the growing incidence of chronic pain conditions — car accidents, bad backs, post-surgery, cancer, and the like — has led to large increases in prescriptions of opioids. An important phenomenon in relation to opioids is called tolerance, where you develop a tolerance to your initial dose and continually need larger and larger doses to exert the same effect. This gradual tolerance is one reason people develop a dependence. The new class of opioids was touted as "low addiction risk" by manufacturers; as a result, doctors across the country started prescribing them to treat chronic cancer pain in an attempt to reduce patient suffering. Tragically, this wasn't the case — the new opioids were still highly addictive. Many experts in the field believe this was the genesis of the opioid crisis.

This combination of patients quickly developing tolerance to opioids coupled with the fact that they're highly addictive has sparked the current opioid epidemic we're experiencing. Given the widespread use of opioids in the medical system, you would assume there is strong evidence-based research to support the claims that opioids relieve chronic pain and suffering. Shockingly, it's not the case. There are no long-term, placebo-controlled, randomized trials showing efficacy for opioid use to treat chronic, non-cancer pain. These drugs were given out to patients to treat non-cancer-related pain despite a complete lack of evidence of their effectiveness. In fact, when researchers compared opioid drugs to non-opioid drugs for pain management, the non-opioid group had better pain outcomes and far fewer harmful side effects.[14]

In sports, there is a big need for pain management strategies. This is even more pronounced in contact sports where pain management strategies are required throughout the season to help athletes fight off pain, be fit for competition, or to return to play after injury. In the not-too-distant past, opioids were considered an acceptable strategy for combating pain. It's no longer the case today, although the practice still continues. In fact, the list of players Nick Boynton references at the start of his *Players' Tribune* article — Steve Montador, Wade Belak, Derek Boogaard, and Rick Rypien — all had a common theme to their tragic deaths: the consumption of alcohol and opioids. The large number of prescription opioid deaths involve the combination of opioids with other substances, particularly sedating substances like alcohol or benzodiazepines, which are commonly prescribed to treat sleep and anxiety. This deadly combination is often the cause of opioid-related deaths in athletes. Binge drinking is actually seen at higher rates in athletes compared to the general population. When you combine regular or excessive alcohol use with increasing opioid doses, you're exposing yourself to massive risk of respiratory depression and death.

Opioids most definitely reduce pain, but unfortunately do very little to reduce patient suffering. It's often not the physical pain athletes are trying to escape, but the mental-emotional suffering that can become overwhelming. The greater your struggles with healthy relationships, emotional stability, social isolation, and the like, the more likely you are to seek out and abuse pain medications such as opioids to numb the mental-emotional suffering. However, there are other alternatives. New research on how the brain responds to emotions and pain is unlocking some new frontiers in therapeutic strategies. Researchers are now able to better understand how the brain and nervous system work together. They're able to distinguish between pain *intensity* and pain *suffering* and how different regions of the brain mediate these two distinct effects.[15] This novel finding has allowed experts to develop new methods to support the specific brain areas associated with pain and suffering without having to rely on high-dose pain medications. Incredibly, your *breath* plays a powerful role in this story.

Yes, meditation, in its various forms, is an effective evidence-based treatment for chronic pain. In fact, the evidence-base for meditation is of higher quality than that for pain medications.[16] Studies of long-term meditators, compared to junior and non-meditators, found experienced meditators had greater cortical thickness compared to non-meditators.[17] In clients suffering with chronic low back pain, the cortical area of the brain atrophies and is often found to be much smaller than it would otherwise be, providing further evidence that meditation (with its cortical-thickening effects) can be a valuable therapy for pain sufferers. How much does meditation help pain suffering? Meditation has been shown to reduce pain effects (suffering) via its impact on the thalamus area of the brain. The thalamus is a gateway of sensation; you can think of it as a processing center for sensation. In people with chronic pain, there is an increase in thalamus activity and total mass. In people who meditate, there is less activity and reduced mass in the thalamus, which suggests the potential impact of breathwork on improving pain outcomes.[18] Dr. Sud drives home this point, emphasizing that "meditation doesn't just change the brain, it changes the brain in ways that are specific to pain." What type of meditation works best? There are many different types of meditation, and Dr. Sud suggests finding a type that suits you and your personality. Just choose a practice that gets you into a relaxed state. He also suggests finding a great teacher to accelerate the process. (I'll discuss this in more detail in chapter 11.) The more we understand how our brains work, and how to distinguish between pain intensity and suffering, the better able we'll be to support athletes who are suffering from concussions.

Let's be honest: most high-level athletes are still going to play despite the risks. Some might even argue athletes from generations past knew there was some type of inherent risk. Regardless, every athlete who makes the decision to play should know what the risks are, as well as what they can do to potentially mitigate some of the risk and protect their brain. Is it possible to build up "brain resiliency" to accelerate recovery from concussion? It's very early days in the research into this, but we're starting to see signs of progress. Before discussing strategies to support brain health, it's important to understand common themes seen in people with cognitive decline and dementias. As Dr. Omalu found, the scans of football players with CTE are virtually identical to patients with Alzheimer's disease. Let's take a closer look.

## Dementia, Cognitive Decline, and Concussions

Alzheimer's disease (AD) is the most common cause of dementia. A recent UCLA study found that 47 million Americans have preclinical Alzheimer's, with the number expected to almost double to 75 million by the year 2060. The term *dementia* describes a set of symptoms that includes memory loss and difficulties with thinking, problem-solving, or language. The signs and symptoms of dementia from Alzheimer's disease are highly individual, but early symptoms often include memory lapses and difficulty recalling recent events and learning new information. Damage to the hippocampus area of the brain — which converts short-term memory to long-term memory — is thought to be responsible for these deficits. (Memories in early life are often unaffected during early stages of the disease.) As the condition worsens, you start to lose things easily around the house, struggle to find the right word in a conversation, forget recent conversations, get lost in familiar places, and the like. As Alzheimer's progresses to late stages, patients need help with all their daily activities and become much less aware of what is happening around them. This has left experts scrambling to find a way to slow the progression of the neuropathological changes that occur in dementia patients.

There are many different types of dementia, but Alzheimer's disease (AD) and vascular dementia are the most prevalent.[19] In chapter 3 I highlighted how people with type 2 diabetes are at increased risk of cardiovascular diseases, cerebrovascular diseases, and dementia.[20] Today, there is now strong evidence that type 2 diabetes increases the risk of cognitive impairment and some dementias.[21] A recent meta-analysis found diabetics have a 65 percent increased risk of Alzheimer's and 127 percent increased risk of vascular dementia, highlighting the fundamental role blood glucose control has in supporting brain health.[22] Moreover, 80 percent of Alzheimer's patients have either been diagnosed with diabetes or glucose dysfunction.[23] With an aging baby boomer population and over half of Americans struggling with prediabetes or diabetes, this has the hallmarks of an emerging epidemic. For athletes, potential solutions for the prevention of dementia might yield some crossover benefit for brain health and recovery from concussion, based on the shared pathophysiology of the conditions.

With both type 2 diabetes and dementias threatening to reach epidemic levels around the world, and with concussions on the rise across all sports, it's important to understand how glucose intolerance can lead to poor brain health. In Alzheimer's, glucose metabolism of the brain is severely compromised; there's effectively an energy crisis in the brain. Experts often refer to Alzheimer's now as "type 3" diabetes, because just like in type 2 diabetes, tissues in the body (in this case the brain) become resistant to absorbing glucose. Despite the excess consumption of glucose the brain is resistant to it, effectively starving for fuel. What does this look like at the cellular level? Rapid repolarization of the membrane potential occurs, which internalizes the GLUT3 (glucose transporter 3) receptors on neurons and compromises the GLUT1 transporters on the blood-brain barrier.[24] As such, the brain can't get access to the glucose. The blood-brain barrier also becomes "leaky," triggering an inflammatory cascade as a result. Inflammasomes sustain inflammation in the brain, impair healing, and alter glucose metabolism (such as NLPR3). This triggers the cascade of harmful secondary reactions and can quickly become a downward spiral. In fact, the progression is eerily similar to that of concussions.

Of course, these pathological events precede the clinical symptoms in people with dementia and athletes with concussion, making the discovery of a reliable biomarker for both conditions a hot area of research. A reliable biomarker would help flag the harmful cascades as soon as they start, and could help medical professionals to slow the progression of dementia or better identify concussion. For Alzheimer's, beta-amyloid plaques and tau protein are considered the most reliable biomarkers; however, these validated markers are massively limited in their practical application due to cost and invasiveness of testing. Genetic testing for the ApoE (apolipoprotein E) allele is a possibility, as this protein has also been shown to be a risk factor — in a dose-dependent manner — for earlier onset and more rapid progression of Alzheimer's disease.[25] For concussions, experts are in a race to find a validated marker, not just for athletes but for the millions of people who suffer from mild traumatic brain injury every year. Military personnel are at particularly high risk; it's estimated 11–23 percent of soldiers who served in Iraq or Afghanistan have a history of mild traumatic brain injury (concussion), and approximately 8 percent report post-concussion symptoms.[26] Furthermore, a history of concussion is associated with an increased likelihood of developing PTSD in both military and civilians.[27]

Using a simple blood test, researchers at UCLA have recently identified four biomarkers that could help diagnose brain trauma and mild traumatic brain injury (mTBI). The biomarkers are astrocyte cell proteins released from the brain into the bloodstream when the astrocytes' outer cell membranes rupture due to brain trauma or impact.[28] Currently, doctors use a standardized scoring system to assess the level of consciousness in an athlete who has suffered a blow to the head; however, this approach doesn't correlate very well to recovery and might miss milder brain injuries. Scientists are still searching for a "brain signature" to definitely diagnose concussion and identify when the harmful secondary effects are initiated (often long before symptoms are present). Ina Wanner, PhD, a neuroscientist at UCLA, found that astrocytes leaked substantial amounts of specific proteins after inducing injury. When Dr. Wanner studied patients who had suffered from mTBI, the same signature of astrocyte proteins were found.

New advances like this are very encouraging; however, there is still no gold-standard biomarker that experts can agree upon.

If we don't yet have a reliable biomarker to warn us about the underlying harmful effects of head trauma or cognitive decline, then perhaps a preventative strategy to support optimal brain health can help mitigate the detrimental effects. Can you build better brain resiliency? Can you supercharge your brain to bounce back more quickly from concussion? Looking back through evolution might provide potential areas of interest.

## Evolution of the Brain: Is Bigger Better?

Our big brains account for only 2 percent of our bodyweight, yet draw 20 percent of our total daily energy intake. In order to understand what our brains need from a nutrition standpoint to be healthy and resilient, it's important to understand how the brain evolved. The brain is an amazing feat of evolution, containing more neural connections than there are stars in the galaxy. Humans have the biggest brains in the animal kingdom, triple the size of our closest relative, the chimpanzee, despite the five-million-year head start they had before the genus *Homo* arrived on the scene. How did the human brain grow at such an unprecedented rate, while our closest primate ancestors effectively have the same brain mass today as five million years ago? It's an incredibly complex question and experts can only speculate, but there are a few leading theories: the expensive tissue hypothesis, omega-3-rich diets, and the advent of fire.

The human and chimpanzee genomes differ by only 1.2 percent, yet we've evolved very different characteristics that ultimately influenced the complexity and size of our brains. Most prominent among these differences is our digestive systems. The human large intestine makes up 20 percent of our gastrointestinal (GI) tract, and thus we have a limited capacity to ferment dietary fibers. Comparatively, the large intestine of a chimpanzee accounts for over 50 percent of their GI tract. (That's why they have those cute little potbellies!) The chimpanzees' fermentative gut transforms the high-fiber plant matter they chomp on all day into short-chain fatty acids (SCFA), which then fuel their brains and activity. Similarly, ruminants like cows get 70–80 percent of their calories from the fermentation of grasses via short-chain fatty acids. That's why cows, too, must spend the majority of the day constantly eating, face down in the grass, in order to meet their caloric demands. The gut bacteria of these ruminants convert this massive intake of fiber into calories to fuel the animals' daily energy needs.

Humans evolved differently — we have a hydrochloric-acid based digestive system. The animals we consume as meat have already extracted and synthesized these nutrients for us. Thus our GI tracts are predominantly made up of the small intestine, which winds its way back and forth across the abdomen in order to extract and absorb the maximum amount of nutrients from the food we eat. What does the size of our gut have to do with the size our brains? Everything. It might seem trivial, but the expensive tissue hypothesis put forth by expert anthropologists suggests we made an evolutionary trade-off between the size of our gut and the size of our brain, sacrificing the former to fuel the growth and development of the latter.[29] This trade-off allowed humans to evolve to the top of the food chain. But this wasn't always the case.

Before the Ice Age, we were surrounded by enormous megafauna — woolly mammoth, giant oryx, Irish elk, and so on — which anthropologists believe were approximately 50 percent fat by volume. This was a preferred food source of our *Homo erectus* ancestors, and the massive intake of DHA-rich fats helped accelerate the growth of our human brains. It seems the growth of our brains also spurred the growth of our bodies. Recently, postdoctoral fellow Mark Grabowski, PhD, at the American Museum of Natural History, presented data strongly suggesting that humans' large brains pulled along the growth of the body.[30] The study showed that the strong genetic selection bias toward increased brain size played a dual role, selectively increasing body size, and therefore genetically linking these two key factors. Grabowski summarizes his findings by emphasizing, "Brain size is solely responsible for the large increase in both traits that occurred near the origins of our genus, *Homo erectus*." In short, we needed bigger bodies to house our bigger brains.

What did our early human ancestors consume to build such impressive brain size? Professor Dr. Hervé Bocherens and his colleagues at the Senckenberg Center for Human Evolution studied the dietary habits of early modern humans by investigating the oldest known fossils on the Crimean Peninsula, from the Buran-Kaya caves in the Ukraine. Using an innovative new technology, they reconstructed their likely food options by assessing the percentage of stable carbon and nitrogen isotopes in the bones of these early humans and the local potential prey animals. What was on the "menu du jour" of our early ancestors some 40,000 years ago that could build such big and robust brains? The researchers concluded, "Just like the Neanderthals, our *Homo erectus* ancestors had mainly mammoth and plants on their plates."[31] Interestingly, the investigative team was "unable to document fish as part of their diet." Today, fish is widely considered the ultimate brain food, yet it's curious that at the peak of our brain size it wasn't anywhere to be found on the menu. This isn't to suggest that fish shouldn't be a part of our modern diet — it's obviously a wonderfully rich source of brain-boosting DHA — but if our ancestors didn't get their omega-3s from fish, where did they get it? Fatty red meat.

Even in the Mediterranean region, renowned for its heart- and brain-healthy diet, expert Marcello Mannino, PhD, from Denmark revealed these populations ate "medium to large herbivores" and not the fish-heavy diet they consume today. Unfortunately, the buffet of omega-3-rich megafauna disappeared with the Ice Age, which subsequently had a bizarre effect on our brains: they got smaller. Renowned anthropologist Christopher Stringer highlighted in *Scientific American* how our brains have been getting smaller over the past 10,000–20,000 years, stating, "It's energetically expensive [to maintain a bigger brain] and will not be maintained at larger [body] sizes unless it is necessary."[32] Examples of this can be seen in the animal kingdom, where domesticated animals have smaller brains than wild animals, likely because they don't need to hunt or evade predators. Humans are also becoming more and more domesticated, leading a sedentary lifestyle that is fueled by processed foods. So should we be worried about our shrinking brains? Stringer says it doesn't necessarily reflect a decline in our intelligence as a species, because smaller brains yield faster computations (so long as we keep exercising and feeding our brains appropriately!).

Sacrificing the size of our gut for the size of our brain and eating a diet rich in the long-chain omega-3 DHA appear to have been primary driving factors in the development of the sophisticated human brain. But there is more to the story. Recall from chapter 1 the observations of Professor Matthew Walker regarding our early ancestors' ability to use fire. Walker maintains that "the use of fire allowed our ancestors to make the transition from sleeping in trees to sleeping on the ground," thereby bathing the human brain in unprecedented amounts of REM sleep, rapidly accelerating the connections and complexity of our brains. Walker goes on to say, "REM sleep exquisitely recalibrates and fine-tunes the emotional circuits of the human brain . . . REM-sleep dreaming-state fuels creativity. . . . [It] helps to construct vast associative networks of information within the brain." It should come as no surprise, then, that there are interesting links between poor sleep and poor brain health.

## Sleep, Concussions, and Cognitive Decline

A growing body of research is finding poor and inadequate sleep as you age is a predictor of cognitive decline, dementia, and Alzheimer's disease. If you experience head trauma, you're also at increased risk of sleep disturbances. A recent meta-analysis of patients with mild to severe TBI (traumatic brain injury) estimated that 50 percent are affected by a sleep disturbance after the event, followed by insomnia (29 percent), hypersomnia (28 percent), obstructive sleep apnea (25 percent), periodic limb movement during sleep (19 percent), and narcolepsy (4 percent).[33] Another longitudinal study found 67 percent of concussion sufferers still had disturbances in their sleep-wake cycle three years after a mild to severe TBI.[34] In fact, 45 percent of patients in this study had no other associated psychiatric symptoms, such as anxiety or depression, which could have confounded the effect of concussion on sleep quality. This highlights the deep connection between sleep and brain health.

Circadian rhythms are also affected by concussion. Research in TBI patients commonly reveals dysfunctional circadian and melatonin rhythm. Interestingly, the use of high-dose melatonin has been shown to significantly attenuate trauma-induced neuronal death from concussion, as well as to reduce edema and blood-brain barrier permeability.[35] Does this research in animal models translate to humans? Unfortunately, there is not enough evidence yet to confirm.

## Brain Health Solutions: Sleep and Nutrition

Sleep is fundamental to brain health, but what about nutrition? Can nutrition slow cognitive decline as you age, or perhaps accelerate healing after a head trauma or concussion? It's difficult to say, but early research in animal models helps to shine a light on potential solutions. Researchers investigated the use of high-fat diets, caloric restriction, and standard diets on markers of healthy brain function. The caloric restriction group showed increased levels of BDNF (brain-derived neurotrophic factor), SIRT1 genes, and increased telomere length — all recognized markers of good brain health. The authors' findings noted that a calorie-restricted diet could potentially help create better "brain resiliency" to injury.[36] A follow-up study post–brain injury found short-term caloric restriction may improve cognitive dysfunction via "increasing the level of autophagy and suppressing astrocyte activation."[37] How did the high-fat diet stack up in the study? The mice consuming the ketogenic-like high-fat diet demonstrated reduced susceptibility to poor outcomes post mTBI (mild traumatic brain injury). In other words, it looks like a low-carb or ketogenic approach may also provide potential support. This all sounds exciting — diet improving pre-trauma brain resiliency and post-trauma recovery — but these studies are done in mice. (As one expert recently said, bluntly, "When my mouse has a concussion, I'll be sure to take this advice!")

What does the research tell us about humans? It's very sparse as it relates to concussions. However, there is a growing body of research that suggests the benefits of ketogenic diets in Alzheimer's and dementia patients. Of course, like everything in life, the challenge comes when trying to implement evidence-based findings (admittedly still in its infancy) and put them into real-world practice. If your athlete is sidelined for two weeks due to concussion, can you really completely overhaul their diets and achieve a therapeutic benefit? Would the athlete even comply with the advice given? It's complicated, especially when you consider the following: the higher the baseline levels of inflammation, the lower the threshold of microglia and astrocyte activation. (There may be a shortcut: ketone supplements, which I discuss in a following section.)

The ideal nutritional strategy for you is ultimately the one that keeps your blood glucose control on point. In chapter 3, you learned about the fundamental role of blood glucose control in overall health and how dysfunction can translate to low mood and cognitive decline. Earlier in this chapter, we explored the deep connection between chronic blood sugar dysfunction and dementias, as well as the striking similarities to the pathophysiology of concussion. Therefore, your first priority should be to establish healthy blood glucose control as measured by HbA1c, HOMA-IR, and morning fasting glucose upon rising. (Refer back to chapter 3 for more details.)

The rapid explosion of ultra-processed, hyper-palatable foods has led to a massive increase in caloric intake over the past 40 years and subsequent epidemic levels of type 2 diabetes, obesity, and dementia. In terms of brain health, processed foods are not only potentially damaging due to their high levels of sugar (and calories) but also because of the large concentration of pro-inflammatory fats they contain that may in turn spark the internal flames of brain inflammation. Today, for example, vegetable oils are ubiquitous in our food environment. The industrial revolution and human ingenuity led to the extraction of the oils from corn, rapeseed (canola), soy, sunflower, cottonseed, safflower, and rice bran, and they have been used in industry to make candles and waxes, to lubricate engines, and so forth. They were originally called industrial seed oils and were not intended for human consumption. But the need for shelf-stable foods to ensure adequate food availability in the mid-twentieth century led to the incorporation of industrial seed oils into packaged and processed foods. The name was changed to "vegetable oils" around the 1950s — despite that they're not derived from vegetables — when large food manufacturers began adding these oils to packaged and processed foods. Initially, it was a big help to areas where available food supply was short.

The processed food explosion over the last four decades has led to vegetable oils being added to virtually every processed and packaged food you eat: popcorn snacks, post-workout protein bars, dried fruit, almond milk, the list goes on and on. The overwhelming consumption of omega-6 fats has skewed the traditional omega-6:omega-3 ratio massively in the wrong direction. We now consume 10 times the amount of omega-6:omega-3 compared to our ancestors, who consumed a 2:1 to 1:1 ratio.

Why is this potentially problematic for a healthy brain? The PUFAs (polyunsaturated fats) in these processed and packaged foods, or the vegetable oils you might use to cook your dinner, are incredibly reactive and combustible. In a recent interview I did with Cate Shanahan, MD, she explained the main problem with a diet high in vegetable oils is that they're highly reactive, which puts a huge strain on your antioxidant defense systems. Dr. Shanahan said that "even a single meal of fries cooked in week-old vegetable oil can cause endothelial dysfunction lasting up to 24 hours . . . [and] vegetable oil consumption is followed by a form of diet-induced arterial aging." Earlier in this chapter I described how concussions can trigger damaging inflammation and oxidative stress. Because the brain is made up of 30 percent PUFAs by dry weight, these sparks of inflammation turn into a full-blown firestorm in the brain (like dropping a match in a tinderbox!). Excessive vegetable oil consumption can predispose you to similar patterns.

**TABLE 10.1.** Polyphenol-Rich Foods and Drinks, and Content per Serving

| POLYPHENOL-RICH FOODS AND DRINKS | PER SERVING (MG) |
|:---:|:---:|
| Blackcurrant | 1,092 |
| Coffee | 408 |
| Blueberry | 395 |
| Sweet cherry | 394 |
| Strawberry | 390 |
| Blackberry | 374 |
| Raspberry | 310 |
| Dark chocolate | 283 |
| Green tea | 173 |
| Pure apple juice | 168 |
| Red wine | 126 |
| Pomegranate juice | 99 |
| Black tea | 90 |
| Broccoli | 33 |

*Source:* J. Pérez-Jiménez et al., "Identification of the 100 Richest Dietary Sources of Polyphenols: An Application of the Phenol-Explorer Database," *European Journal of Clinical Nutrition* 64, Supplement 3 (2010), https://doi.org/10.1038/ejcn.2010.221.

Of course, the problem is compounded if your intake of antioxidants is also poor — without them, you can't put out the fire in your brain. For the typical American, 50 percent of their antioxidant intake is from the polyphenols found in coffee and tea, so if you don't consume either you may be playing from behind.[38] Next on the antioxidant list are vegetables and fruits, so ensuring an adequate intake is crucial for antioxidant defense (see table 10.1).

Your brain has a built-in antioxidant defense system, and antioxidant enzymes are your body's first line of defense against oxidative stress for snagging and snuffing out reactive oxygen species (ROS). Antioxidant enzymes require key minerals like zinc, copper, iron, or sulfur-based amino acids to do the job effectively. The quality of the food you eat supplies fat-soluble antioxidants, such as vitamins E and A; water-soluble antioxidants, such as vitamin C; and phytonutrients found in vegetables and spices, including sulphorophanes in broccoli, anthocyanins in dark berries, and cinnamic acid found in cinnamon. For example, if you have a low intake of dietary fat-soluble antioxidants such as vitamin E, then delicate PUFAs like DHA may be exposed to greater oxidative damage in the brain, which creates a heightened level of oxidative stress. A diet rich in vegetables and fruits provides an array of these powerful antioxidants to protect your brain and body. Ideally, most of your cooking should be done at low to moderate temperatures using healthy MUFA fats (monounsaturated fats), including extra-virgin olive oil, avocado oil, macadamia oil, and walnut oil, and minimal to modest amounts of omega-6 vegetable oils. When cooking at high temperatures, use moderate amounts of stable saturated fats, such as butter, ghee (clarified butter), beef tallow, or duck fat. (Note: although coconut oil is a saturated fat, it has a moderate smoke point of 350°F and therefore shouldn't be used at high temperatures.)

## Brain Health Solutions: Supplements

Sleep, blood glucose control, a diet rich in antioxidants, and limiting pro-inflammatory omage-6 fats are important pillars for brain health. But what about supplements? Clients post-concussion or those who are struggling with a chronic degenerative condition such as dementia are quick to ask if supplements could provide any benefit. Can supplements have a prophylactic effect, increasing brain resiliency and protecting it from the damage of head trauma? While the evidence-base is small, there is emerging evidence hinting at potential benefits from the following supplements: ketone esters, omega-3, creatine, and curcumin.

### KETONE ESTERS

Ketone researcher Brianna Stubbs, PhD, formerly of Oxford University, explains that since traumatic brain injury impairs glucose uptake to the brain, providing an alternate fuel source has major potential therapeutic benefit. Ketones are 25 percent more efficient than glucose as a fuel source in the brain, and incredibly, are taken up efficiently in Alzheimer's patients despite the patients' impaired ability to absorb glucose in the brain.[39] Following a concussion, the transporters that move ketones into cells increase by a whopping 85 percent, suggesting that our brains attempt to search for another fuel source during the "energy crisis" induced by trauma. Ketones have also been found to dampen free radical production via increasing mitochondrial function and antioxidant enzyme activity.[40] Ketone ester supplements have shown to be a benefit for improving insulin signaling, increasing neurotrophic factors such as BDNF (brain-derived neurotrophic factor) to promote nerve growth and repair, as well as supporting mitochondrial health and reducing inflammation.[41] These are all underlying traits in the pathophysiology of concussion and cognitive decline.

A key advantage of ketone supplements for concussions is that clients don't need to overhaul their nutritional regime and adopt a 100 percent keto diet to obtain the potential benefits. Nutritional ketosis can be a challenging and restrictive dietary pattern for athletes to follow; one can experience many adverse symptoms in the first few weeks of a very low-carb, high-fat diet, not to mention the effects that stem from a significant potential loss of important electrolytes (referred to as "the keto flu"). It's also easy to under-consume calories and fall into a low–energy availability state on a ketogenic diet. And while caloric restriction may be beneficial for brain health, athletes in-season typically need to maintain lean muscle mass in order to be ready to return to play. In terms of practical application, exogenous ketone supplements allow you to increase plasma ketone levels very quickly and easily without having to adopt a full ketogenic diet.

Expert researcher Dominic D'Agostino, PhD, neuroscience researcher and associate professor at the University of South Florida, believes this combination of compromised brain energy metabolism and neuro-inflammation is a driving factor behind concussions and the dangerous progression to CTE. At the moment, the most difficult thing with concussion diagnosis is that typical imaging methods like MRI or computed tomography (CT) are too crude to pick up subtle changes. Dr. D'Agostino prefers new molecular imaging techniques that examine functional processes within the brain, such as FDG-PET (fluorodeoxyglucose positron emission tomography) that can be used to measure glucose uptake in the brain and therefore detect small but significant changes after concussion. The FDG-PET scan is arguably the best predictor of patient outcome after a brain injury, as it is effectively measuring glucose metabolism in the brain. This further highlights the importance of glucose control as a pillar of brain health.

Just like expert pathologist Dr. Omalu, Dr. D'Agostino is quick to point out you don't need to have had a diagnosed concussion for the harmful secondary effects to play out. When you get your "bell rung" from a blow, fall, or trauma, you experience microtears in the arterioles and capillaries that feed the brain, which impairs key enzymes such as pyruvate dehydrogenase (PDH) and leads to an accumulation of lactate. In this scenario, FDG-PET scans show reduced imaging intensity, confirming impaired energy flow, mild ischemia, and neuro-inflammation brought on by astrocyte activation post-brain injury.[42] Even mild trauma (when you've not experienced a diagnosed concussion) can bring on these serious and harmful effects. This scenario is likely what ex-NFL players like Mark Rypien, Junior Seau, and Dave Duerson, and NHL enforcers like Nick Boynton, Wade Belak, and Derek Boogaard (and many others) experience after years of physical play and head trauma. The research clearly shows repeated brain trauma has a cumulative effect in the brain if it's not allowed adequate time to recover.

The FDG-PET scans also highlight the parallels between concussion and Alzheimer's disease. The scans of dementia and Alzheimer's patients reveal dimmer images, similar to the results obtained from athletes with brain injury. In deceased NFL players with CTE, their brains had the hallmark signs of advanced Alzheimer's. The use of ketone supplements may provide practical benefits for clients, as Alzheimer's patients can still absorb and utilize ketone supplements despite their brains' compromised ability to use glucose as a fuel.[43] D'Agostino points out that exogenous ketones also help to lower excitatory levels of glutamate and elevate GABA levels, helping to mitigate the hyper-excitability caused by concussion-driven release of excess glutamate. Ketone supplements may also activate glutathione to protect cell membranes from oxidative stress and suppress inflammasomes. All of these mechanistic findings make it seem like ketone supplements are a concussion and cognitive decline cure-all, but unfortunately the research is still in its very early days. The bulk of all this research is done in animal studies. Do the findings apply directly to humans as well? It's a gray area in the research, but one that is making rapid progress. It will be interesting to see what the future holds.

## DHA

Your brain is 60 percent fat. One-third of this amount is made up of the long chain omega-3 fat DHA (docosahexaenoic acid), which plays a critical role in supporting membrane fluidity and structure, cell signaling, inflammation cooling, and nerve growth (via BDNF) in the brain.[44] During fetal development, the long chain omega-3 fat DHA and the omega-6 fat AA (arachidonic acid) accumulate in the central nervous system, whereas only very small amounts of eicosapentaenoic acid (EPA) are found there. Experts assume these highly unsaturated fats are continuously exchanged throughout our lifetime, but very little is actually known about the transfer across the blood–brain barrier. In animals, supplementing with DHA increases the concentration of DHA in the central nervous system, and the supplemental omega-3 shows improved cognition, reduced neuronal edema, increased dendrite growth, and stabilization of brain energy levels.[45]

In Alzheimer's disease patients, low brain DHA levels are commonly seen, and studies show diets high in omega-3-rich fish are linked to a reduced risk of developing Alzheimer's and a delaying of cognitive decline.[46] High levels of DHA have also been correlated with a decreased risk of cognitive loss in normal aging and a reduced risk of dementias. In concussion, the research suggests omega-3 supplementation could lessen the harmful secondary cascade of effects post-concussion that elicit many of the symptoms.[47] A recent study on DHA supplementation in NFL players showed DHA increased plasma DHA levels in a dose-dependent manner up to 2 g daily and mildly reduced surrogate markers of concussion damage.[48] If 2 g shows neuroprotective effects, what happens if you double or triple the dose? The work of Michael Lewis, MD, founder of the Brain Health Education and Research Institute, has found supra-physiological doses in patients with mTBI to be highly effective in clinical practice. Dr. Lewis regularly uses large doses of DHA – 27 g daily divided into three doses – in the first week post brain-injury to accelerate healing. In a recent research paper, he stated: "Early and optimal doses of omega-3, even in a prophylactic setting, have the potential to improve outcomes. . . . With evidence of unsurpassed safety and tolerability, [omega-3] should be considered mainstream, conventional medicine."[49] This is a strong statement from an expert with decades of clinical experience. However, the research hasn't yet found a 4–6 g dose to be any better than 3 g of DHA. Concussion and cognitive decline are highly complex, making the research of these conditions incredibly challenging. While much more research needs to be done, relaying this information to your medical team director may be useful. Conventional doses appropriate after injury are 2–3 g daily for one month.

### CBD Oil for Pain and Anxiety

Cannabidiol, typically known as CBD, is one of over 60 canna-binoid compounds, and is most commonly found in cannabis. Tetrahydrocannabinol, or THC, is what produces the euphoric, psychoactive "high" from smoking weed; however, CBD doesn't affect the THC receptors in the body, and therefore doesn't produce the characteristic "high" of THC. In fact, the body produces its own endocannabinoids via an endocannabi-noid system (ECS) that also helps to regulate sleep, immune function, and pain. CBD activates or inhibits other compounds within the body's own endocannabinoid system. For instance, CBD blunts the absorption of anandamide, a compound as-sociated with pain regulation. Increased levels of anandamide in the bloodstream have been shown to reduce chronic pain, anxiety, and inflammation in animal models. These are com-mon symptoms in post-concussion clients, making CBD a hot area of research as a complementary therapy for brain trauma and anxiety. In fact, a key downstream effect of omega-3 is to interact with the endocannabinoid system, highlighting its important therapeutic effects. CBD is typically taken as an oil, and it's best to start with low doses and work your way up. Side effects of CBD use can include fatigue, loose stools, changes in appetite, weight gain, or weight loss.

### CREATINE FOR BRAIN SUPPORT

Creatine is a popular and potent evidence-based supplement for sup-porting athletic performance and recovery, but what often flies under the radar is its potential role in supporting the brain. Concussions cause an energy crisis in the brain, as you've learned in this chapter, and the addition of creatine helps to keep cellular ATP levels constant post-concussion when there is a large demand on ATP. Creatine can also help with concussion recovery by restoring membrane potentials and preventing the influx of calcium into the cell (a key secondary concern post–brain injury), reducing ROS, buffering lactate, and playing a direct role in reducing glutamate excitotoxicity.[50] The overlap between concussion pathophysiology and the beneficial role of creatine supplementation makes it an attractive option as not only a post-trauma strategy, but as a preventative support for athletes as well. Most sports with significant physical contact — football, rugby, hockey, MMA — put athletes at a greater risk of concussion and place large training demands to improve strength, power, and speed. This makes creatine supplementation seem highly appropriate (especially when you take into account its safety profile). Creatine supplementation also improves working memory, processing speed, and cognitive performance in both young and older people who are completely healthy and have never suffered a TBI.[51] For prevention, aim for 5 g daily for men and 3 g for women. However, if used post-concussion, the typical creatine loading phase (20 g daily in divided doses for 5–7 days) may provide added benefit, some experts speculate, due to the rapid increase in creatine levels.

## Curcumin

Curcumin is the active ingredient in the traditional Indian spice turmeric, and it has several brain-boosting benefits. It augments DHA levels in the brain by increasing the enzymes responsible for converting alpha-linoleic acid (ALA) into DHA, and it prevents the peroxidation of lipids. Both of these mechanisms are crucial for supporting recovery from concussion.[52] Unfortunately, just adding a powdered or juiced turmeric root to your food is not enough to get the job done. The turmeric spice contains approximately 5 percent curcumins by dry weight, so you would need to consume about 10 g to obtain a therapeutic dose of 500 mg. (That's a ridiculous amount of turmeric root!) Unfortunately, it's also not very bioavailable, making supplementation an attractive option. To date, the only human trial used a lipid-based curcumin particle developed by experts at UCLA, and researchers found a single dose was effective for improving working memory and focus. This study was done in older subjects, so it may be population-specific. High-quality curcumin formulas increase *bioavailability* (absorption from your gut into circulation) as well as *bioactivity* (the ability of your tissues to use the compound once absorbed).[53] Aim for 1,200 mg daily, in divided doses, in a formula standardized to contain 95 percent curcuminoids. The addition of dietary fat or black pepper dramatically increases the bioavailability of curcumin, though clients with active ulcers should avoid doing this.

————

Finally, do you recall from Part Two: Fuel how the evidence-base for antioxidant supplementation was shaky at best? Well, acute-phase brain trauma may be the exception. A recent paper in the *Journal of the American Medical Association* states that "the administration of effective antioxidants has the potential to significantly limit the spread of damage and inflammation if given soon after brain injury."[54] The brain has a greater need for antioxidants post-injury, particularly in the acute phase. A systematic review suggests "clinicians can help attenuate the oxidative posttraumatic brain damage and optimize patient recovery . . . by incorporating antioxidant therapies into practice."[55] In a real-world scenario, the athlete will not be training post-concussion, and thus the worry of blunting training-induced adaptations is less or no longer relevant. Concussion is a scenario where supplemental antioxidants could play a supportive role in recovery.

Mental-emotional health is an important pillar of the new science around peak performance. Supporting brain health via optimal sleep, digestive-inflammatory-immune health, and blood glucose control may help to increase brain resiliency. If you play a sport with physical contact, ensuring that these fundamentals are in place and being proactive in your plan are crucial. Mental and emotional health is more than biochemistry; it's also about emotions and mindset. In the next chapter, let's explore how they may impact athletic performance.

# CHAPTER 11

# Emotions and Mindset

I t happened in an instant. It was 2006, and France and Italy were dead-locked at 1–1 in overtime of the World Cup final when all-time great footballer Zinedine Zidane exchanged words with Italian defender Marco Materazzi. Zidane and Materazzi had already scored a goal apiece and were barking back and forth at one another throughout the game. Now, at a pivotal moment in the game, they were staring each other down in the center of the field like two cowboys ready to draw. That's when it happened. Zidane lost his temper and unthinkably head butted Materazzi like a battering ram directly in his sternum. Materazzi fell dramatically; Zidane was given a red card and was immediately ejected from the game. The hopes of Les Bleus were sealed as Zidane walked through the tunnel while the overtime period continued (they would lose 5–3 in penalty kicks). Zinedine Zidane's illustrous career ended with this incredulous head butt heard around the world, coaxed into a reaction by the taunting words uttered by Materazzi. In the blink of an eye, Zidane went from hero to goat in his last match ever as a professional player. But why? How could someone lose control in such a key moment of the game? There's a reason: it's called the amygdala hijack.

Are you an emotional person? You may not think so, but the reality is you are. You're emotional because you're human. Have you ever felt butterflies in your stomach before a big game? Has your heart rate ever picked up in anticipation of an important moment? Have you ever experienced anxiety or irritability when confronted with a difficult new task? How about uneasiness late at night in a strange environment? These are physiological effects of your emotions. Emotions drive your behavior, your decision-making, and your relationships (whether you realize it or not). Fail to channel them in the right direction and not only will your performance plummet so will your health. Today, 75 percent of all doctor's visits are stress-related, costing the health care system a staggering one billion dollars a year.[1] Chronic stress increases the likelihood of experiencing everything from the common cold, to cardiovascular disease, to depression, to even premature death. Long days at the office and today's culture of constant connectivity leads to a perpetual stressful state of being "busy" or "on the run" — regardless if you're an athlete, business person, or raising kids — and this constant state of fight or flight heavily taxes your brain, resiliency, and emotional stability.

Constant stress fundamentally impacts your brain, literally changing how it works. Research in people working over 70 hours per week and faced with constant daily stress reveals an enlarged amygdala — your brain's radar center for threat — and weaker connections between the prefrontal cortex and amygdala that are responsible for quieting the intense emotional responses during stressful moments.[2] The stressed-out workers were unable to down-regulate their emotional reactions; their brains were stuck in a constant state of stress-response overdrive. If you're training or working countless hours in the day (or both as is common for athletes!), the inability to control mental and emotional stress can easily push you over the recovery edge and compromise your ability to train and perform.

Harnessing the power of emotions can be a powerful weapon. Any high-level athlete or coach will attest that emotions are crucial for elite athletic performance. John Sullivan, PsyD., an expert sport psychologist and neurophysiologist who has 14 years of experience working with the NFL, EPL, and NCAA, says that "the fastest way to connect with an athlete is through emotions." Why? Your emotional brain responds to events more quickly than your thinking brain, making emotions a potentially powerful performance enhancer if harnessed skillfully. However, if you lack these skills, then emotions can shackle your performance and stifle your growth as an athlete (and as a person). Dr. Sullivan notes that the emotional system in the brain is the first to develop, steering us away from danger, and sometimes toward it if necessary. From an evolutionary perspective, this emotional system enabled us to survive and thrive. Emotions connected individuals with others, ultimately helping them find a mate and reproduce.

But what exactly *is* an emotion? While there are many scientific definitions across disciplines, Dr. Sullivan says the experts in the field generally agree to the following: "An emotion is a complex psychophysiological state that has three components: a subjective experience, a neurophysiological response, and a behavioral or expressive response." For example, when you feel the pressure of the big game, you experience neurophysiological responses like a rise in heart rate, respiration rate, and adrenaline levels, and then you react. High-level athletes will typically thrive in this scenario, but when the stakes are highest, many others will not. "How you react to your emotions," says Dr. Sullivan, "and channel them to support your performance (rather than sabotage it) is key to unlocking your performance potential."

Of course, stress is not a bad thing, both in training and in life. Kelly McGonigal, PhD, expert health psychologist and lecturer at Stanford University, says, "Stress is your friend!" Her work revealed people who experienced high stress, but who didn't perceive stress as being harmful, experienced none of the harmful health risks of stress, and even had the lowest risk of premature death. She highlights simply *believing* stress is bad for you worsens your health and increases your risk of dying prematurely. Also, as Dr. McGonigal is quick to point out, feeling pressure isn't a bad thing. She says it reveals two very important things: that you care and that you feel like you can make a difference. This is important to remember when the pressure mounts. Renowned sport psychologist Peter Jensen, PhD, who has supported Canadian Olympic teams over the last 10 Winter and Summer Olympic Games, agrees, stating that pressure is a privilege. He recounted the story of legendary hockey coach Mike Babcock, who said in the lead-up to Team Canada's 2010 Olympic hockey finals game, "100 percent of the players *not* in this room don't have any pressure." Coach Babcock was implying if you weren't good enough to be in the room (on the team), you've got no pressure on you. Dr. Jensen emphasizes to his athletes, "The only reason you have pressure is because you have a chance." Pressure is a privilege. It's what gives a basketball its bounce, and Jensen believes it's also what gives people their bounce. How you manage your emotions and energy are crucial for striking the balance between too much or too little.

Emotions don't just impact your day-to-day performance, but also how you respond to challenges along the training journey and the roadblocks in your athletic career. Progress isn't linear; there will always be ups and downs. At some point your progress will plateau; you won't always be hitting personal records (PRs) or be the best athlete on the field or in the gym. This is when your emotional intelligence and mindset can be a secret weapon to overcoming challenges and succeeding. How important is the brain in performance? Last year, I sat in a conference room at the Directors

Forum for the Leaders in Performance conference — a gathering of professional sport directors from the MLB, NBA, NHL, NFL, and others — and the overwhelming consensus was that the next frontier in human performance was the brain. Humans connect via emotion, be it athlete to athlete, coach to player, and practitioner to patient. The ability to motivate, learn, teach, and lead depends tremendously on your emotional intelligence.

But what is emotional intelligence? Daniel Goleman, PhD, expert psychologist, author of *Emotional Intelligence*, and pioneer in the field of mindfulness and meditation, describes an emotionally intelligent person as "someone who can recognize the emotions they're feeling, manage them, and avoid being overwhelmed."[3] An emotionally intelligent person demonstrates a high level of motivation. An emotionally intelligent person recognizes the emotional response of others. An emotionally intelligent person then uses this awareness to effectively manage relationships. This last point may be the most salient for athletes, coaches, and practitioners. Sounds easy, right? Unfortunately, the bulk of your emotional intelligence (EI) is formed in childhood. It takes root long before you realize its tremendous importance. You can't go back in time and reboot your EI formation, but the good news is you can train it — an excellent opportunity to set yourself apart from the competition.

Sport is emotional. If you struggle to deal with negative emotions, you'll struggle to succeed at the highest level. If you fail to effectively channel negative emotions, you'll never achieve your full potential. In short, if your emotional abilities are not in hand, if you don't have self-awareness, if you're not able to manage distressing emotions . . . then no matter how smart you are, you are not going to get very far. Dr. Sullivan perhaps sums it up best: "It's not about suppressing your emotions but rather channeling them to support your goal." This insight applies to life just as strongly as to sport. In order to build a champion's mindset, it's important to appreciate what's happening in your brain when you experience an emotion. Then you can fully appreciate how strategies to build empathy, self-compassion, and gratitude transfer to success.

## Emotions and the Evolutionary Brain

The emotional center of your brain is called the limbic system. It consists of three main areas: the hypothalamus, hippocampus, and amygdala. The hypothalamus is like the master conductor of an orchestra, directing your response to your emotions. The hippocampus regulates your metabolism, hunger, thirst, body temperature, and so forth, and it plays a key role in supporting sleep. It also acts like a storage warehouse for memories, but it has a limited capacity, so when you're sleeping it uploads them to the cerebral cortex for long-term memory and integration. Finally, as described previously, the amygdala is a fundamental part of your ancestral subconscious brain; it is responsible for your primal response to danger and threats with emotions like fear, anger, or aggression (as well as positive emotional responses to such things as love and tenderness).

Your brain doesn't work alone in creating and expressing emotions; your heart and gut are intricately linked. This ancestral connection occurs via the vagus nerve rooted in the brain stem (and cerebellum), which travels down to the heart (and other major organs) before terminating in the gut. The vagus nerve acts as a feedback loop between your brain and gut, constantly surveying your emotional and physiological state, as well as the external environment. Your heart and gut play key roles in this process, both acting like a second brain to interpret information and relay it to the brain to act on.

Mental and emotional health is the final crucial pillar of the new science around peak performance. Lack of sleep, poor blood glucose control, and digestive disturbances (and the resultant inflammatory and immune responses) all deeply impact how you think, look, and feel. In chapter 1, you learned that getting less than 7 hours of sleep per night can significantly impair your immunity, worsen blood sugar control, and harm your memory and executive brain function. A recent study found a lack of sleep *also* impairs your ability to disengage from negative thoughts.[4] Think of a baseball player struggling in a batting slump, a basketball player not hitting their shots, or an Olympic lifter constantly missing attempts at a new personal best: Are these failures technical in nature, or do they come from the brain's inability to disengage from negative thoughts? Dr. Sullivan clearly highlights the importance of emotions in his book *The Brain Always Wins*: "Emotional health is the primary driver of all beneficial changes in our brain and in all other parameters of health." Your emotions are the gateway to unlocking your fullest athletic and performance potential. Unfortunately, they can also be a trapdoor that sabotages success. It's one thing to acknowledge that negative thoughts are a performance limiter, but it's quite another to develop effective strategies to battle through them and succeed.

## The Power of Positive Self-Talk

Serena Williams is arguably the greatest female tennis player of all time. Serena's physical strength, power, and quickness combined with her elite technical and tactical skills has made her a favorite in virtually every tournament she entered. But that's not only what made her a champion. Serena spent long hours harnessing the mental aspects of the game in order to consistently defeat her opponents and win major tournaments. At every match Serena plays, the opposing player brings extra motivation to knock off the champion. When you're the best, every opponent brings their A game against you. It's a daunting task that Hall of Fame tennis players like Serena must endure, and physical prowess alone doesn't lead to the ability to consistently win year after year. Serena uses positive self-talk and "power thoughts" to dial in her focus and keep her confidence high during tennis matches. A few years ago, Serena could be seen during the game change-overs in her matches reviewing a small notebook in her lap:

> "You will move up"
> "You will add spin"
> "You are #1"
> "You will win Wimbledon!"

If one of the greatest female tennis players, and arguably the greatest female athlete in any sport, needs regular mental practice to be the best, what does it say for the rest of us? The brain naturally defaults to negative thoughts, and if you don't harness and steer those limiting thoughts, you'll be hard-pressed to beat your opponents and win consistently. Most tennis experts agree her mental game is what separates Serena from the competition, not simply her physical gifts. Positive self-talk can be a powerful weapon.

Will Hart, PhD, renowned professor at the University of Alabama, uncovered how the language you use to describe your situation — in sport or in life — determines how you actually see it, experience it, and participate in it. Positive self-talk is a proven strategy for boosting confidence, mood, and productivity.[5] It sounds simple, but overcoming negative self-talk is a major hurdle for even professional athletes. Negative self-talk can quickly turn small problems into big ones; it can crush mood, motivation, and as every athlete has experienced at some point... performance. Every athlete, no matter how great, has had negative self-talk impact the outcome of a competition. What separates the best from the rest is the elite athlete has the ability to steer their inner monologue in the right direction and wrestle it away from the doubtful subconscious mind. The best athletes can reframe things; they have short memories for poor plays or performances. They get over things quickly.

The difficult part for most athletes is committing the time, and developing the skills, to change their inner voice. The greatest athletes, of course, didn't develop their killer serve, quick first step, or effortless Olympic lifts overnight. They practiced. Over and over and over again, they practiced. You need to apply the same level of commitment to your mental game. The godfather of modern psychology, Albert Ellis, found that how you talk (and think) about your experiences has a major influence on how you perceive them. Your thoughts are tightly linked to your emotions. Subtle things like, "This is too hard, I'll never get it" leave you in an anxious or worried state of mind that hinders performance. You probably think this just affects you in the short term, but your self-talk sinks deep into your subconscious. If you begin to internalize negative self-talk, it can become a huge performance roadblock.

Think of the tennis player who seems to always double-fault in crucial moments. They work hard, practice their second serve religiously, yet it still rears its ugly head at the most critical moment of a big match. Is this really a technical problem, or simply a mental block? Similarly, a weightlifter struggling to hit new personal-best lifts in competition will likely have a very different inner monologue over these attempts during an event compared to training sessions. Why can some athletes perform effortlessly in practice, yet when the lights shine brightest, cannot deliver the same quality performance? Mindset has a *huge* role to play.

The best sport psychologists will quickly tell you problems are not problems, they're opportunities. You need to be assertive in your self-talk: "I am . . . I will . . . I embrace . . ." Once you find yourself using the word "but," you're turning yourself into the victim. To develop a champion mindset, *you cannot be a victim*. As the well-known Roman philosopher Epictetus said, "Circumstances don't make the man, they only reveal him to himself." You can't control what happens to you, but you're 100 percent responsible for how you react to those events. What you do once the dust settles is entirely up to you. Stop blaming your coach. Stop blaming your teammates. Stop blaming your parents. Be willing to make the change. When you draw a line in the sand and say, "I am willing. . ." you transform your circumstances from

### Supercharge Your Self-Talk

Many terrific scholarly books are dedicated entirely to the topic of self-talk. I stumbled upon one that has been a surprising winner with many of the athletes I've recommended it to. The book, from personal development coach Gary Bishop, is called *Unfu\*k Yourself*. It's highly practical and engaging, and it's an easy read that can help clients start to build more positive self-talk. Try repeating one of the following mantras to yourself every morning when you get up, or paste it on your mirror so that you can read it every day:[7]

"I am willing . . ."
"I expect nothing. I accept everything . . ."
"I embrace uncertainty . . ."

OR

"I am resilient . . ."
"I am not my thoughts, I am my actions . . ."
"I am wired to win . . ."

Feel free to create your own mantra that's in line with your goals and core beliefs. The repetition of positive self-talk is a powerful tool that can sharpen and supercharge the athlete mindset.

pitfalls to possibilities and potential. Bruce Lipton, PhD, a world-renowned stem cell researcher, has found 95 percent of what we all do, every single day of our lives, is controlled by our subconscious.[6] Your deepest thoughts, unrecognizable to you on the surface, are driving the path you follow in performance (and life). Positive self-talk is a good start, but the confidence it builds is not a panacea. It also presents its own set of obstacles.

## The Problem with Confidence

Elite athletes are confident. When you think of Michael Jordan, Wayne Gretzky, Tom Brady, or Cristiano Ronaldo, you think of complete and total confidence. It comes with the territory, as a result of years and years of success. Almost every high-level athlete will tell you confidence is crucial in sport. If you don't have enough confidence, you can get crushed by the tidal wave of doubt and lose your edge. Eric Barker, author of the terrific book *Barking Up the Wrong Tree*, was quick to point out in my interview with him, "Nobody writes books about having too much confidence. We treat it like a limitless quality with ever-expanding benefits."[8] You need confidence to win in sport, but there is another side to the coin.

It's easy to be confident when you're performing at your best. When you're making shots, scoring touchdowns, or continually hitting new personal bests, you feel on top of the world and you don't think twice about confidence. You *know* you can do it. You know you can beat the best; it feels easy and effortless. Then one day, all of a sudden and seemingly out of the blue, it vanishes. You can't make a shot. The bar feels inexplicably heavier. You're slow on your starts and runs.

At the extremes of confidence you have hubris. Not only do you become overconfident, but you become more self-centered and narcissistic. Even worse, too much confidence makes you less likely to take advice, be it from coaches, teammates, performance staff, or others. In today's generation of Instagram and Twitter stars who are famous before they've accomplished much, this can easily be a major trap. Ultimately, the research shows the problem with confidence is that it's either *delusional* or *contingent*. Delusional confidence is thinking you're better than you actually are. Of course, that's not always a problem. In fact, in elite sport it's normally a good thing. Matching up against NBA legend LeBron James, international soccer star Cristiano Ronaldo, or former MMA champion Conor MacGregor and doubting yourself is not a good recipe for success. You can't kick a game-winning field goal or sink a putt to win the Masters for the first time thinking, "Don't miss." Similarly, in the business world, you can't give an impassioned talk to your team or an audience at a conference if you aren't confident. Convincing yourself you're better than the competition — even if you might not actually be — can be crucial for success in sport (and life). However, if your confidence is all rolled up into this exaggerated form of yourself, then what happens when LeBron James dunks on you, Ronaldo scores the game-winner against you, or MacGregor knocks you out? What then? Delusional confidence can quickly come crashing down on you after you've failed or after you've hit a few bumps in the road. For example, in

## A Lesson in Confidence from the
## Worst Free-Throw Shooter in the NBA

Andre Drummond is the worst free-throw shooter in the NBA. In his first five seasons, Andre averaged 38 percent shooting the uncontested 15-foot shot, the worst percentage in the league every year, and remarkably lower than the 75 percent NBA average.[9] A free throw in basketball is a rare moment in sport where a player can attempt to score without any defensive pressure. It's a very different type of shot compared to any other in the game. Once fouled in the act of shooting, the play stops, and the player goes to the free-throw line to shoot. Why is this shot so difficult for Andre Drummond (and many others)? The fluidity of the game is halted. Everyone is watching. The player has all the time in the world to think, to overthink, and to fear failure. "Imagine standing in front of 20,000 people that either really want you to be successful, or really want you to fail," says Dave Love, shooting coach for the Orlando Magic; "It is really the only time in the game the players become aware that everyone is watching them, and them alone." How would you feel if you were the worst free-throw shooter in the NBA? Despite the fact Andre could make his free throws in practice, he was horrible in game situations when everyone was watching. Worse yet, at the end of games, teams would intentionally foul Drummond because they knew he would miss — thus they could get the ball back and hopefully pull away for the win. It got so bad that the Detroit Pistons would remove Andre, their best player, at the end of games. Not surprisingly, Drummond was afraid to go to the foul line, and despite endlessly trying to fix his technique, nothing seemed to help. Then all of a sudden in 2018, something shifted. Andre Drummond was shooting 75 percent from the free-throw line for half a season, and he finished the year shooting 20 percent better than his career average. How did he achieve such a monumental turnaround? The answer was between his ears. Drummond reignited a relationship with an old coach and shifted the focus away from technical skill and toward his mindset. Drummond used to feel tense at the line. He would stare at the rim after missing or take long walks to half-court. His coach helped Andre bring the emphasis back to a state of attention and focus on the present, allowing Drummond to relax and get out of his "thinking" brain. Drummond said, "I took the time to really find what keeps me at peace while I'm at the line. Even if I miss a shot I think back to that thing that keeps me positive . . ." He no longer takes a long walk to center court to review his strategy. He stands at the line, stares at the basket, takes an exhale to relax, and then shoots. Clear mind, clear strategy. Drummond's performance boost wasn't the result of more hours of deliberate practice (he had already done that and failed). Instead, he explored his emotions. Andre's confidence is no longer contingent on making shots, and remarkably, he makes a lot more than ever before.

youth sports today, elite athletes become immediate social media stars with tens of thousands of followers. The hype can quickly take over reality, building a player up to levels that are much higher than their ability. Then once they get exposed in college or the pros, their confidence plummets. A little bit of delusional confidence is probably a good thing, but too much can easily set you up for failure. In elite sport, you will get exposed at some point (that is for certain), so how will you respond?

If your confidence isn't delusional, it's likely *contingent* on something. This is when your sense of self-assurance is dependent on something in particular. In elite athletes, it's typically the fact that they are the "all-star" and everyone around them recognizes them as such. Eric Barker warns about the perils of having your happiness so tightly tied to your performance, saying in my interview with him, "You wake up every day having to slay the dragon to feel good about yourself. But some days, you won't feel the best and you won't slay that dragon. What then?" In elite sport, this is probably more days than athletes care to admit (and good coaches are quick to point out). If your confidence is contingent, it's difficult to regain your form and get consistent results.

Most athletes don't realize how closely linked their performance is to their sense of self-worth. Sport is their identity. Jeff is the all-star basketball player, Isabel is the champion Olympic lifter, Jermaine is the all-world track star. But what happens when you're no longer the best? Who are Jeff, Isabel, or Jermaine then? It sounds abstract, but if your self-worth is tied up too tightly in your performance, it will eventually take a hit and you may not be able to absorb the blow. For instance, imagine you're a first-round draft pick in the NFL. You've made it all the way to the pros, and you're getting all the accolades from friends, peers, and fans. Then your first season starts and the transition to the next level is a bigger jump than you imagined. You struggle. You fail to perform. You get criticized by fans and media. Before you know it, one or two seasons pass, and all of a sudden the team releases you. You have to start over again. Only this time, you're not the superstar protégé. You're stuck at the end of the bench with no hype, no playing time, no confidence. Because your self-worth is too tightly bound to your performance, your confidence is rock-bottom. How can you escape this cycle? Is it possible to develop skills to help you bounce back from such lows? Regardless if you're a high school, collegiate, professional, or high-level recreational athlete, this pitfall is very real and deeply impacts not only your athletic success but your happiness in the rest of your life. Does this mean you shouldn't be confident? Definitely not. You need confidence to perform at any level. But there is a middle ground that offers all the benefits of confidence while buffering against the pitfalls of delusional or contingent confidence: *mindfulness* and *self-compassion*.

## Mindfulness and the Little Red Dot

In general terms, mindfulness is the ability to place your full attention on what is happening in the present. In today's world of never-ending social media streams and information overload from smartphones, mindfulness is an increasingly important skill to have. We live in a generation with a wealth of information and poverty of attention. You can either receive a wealth of information or you can focus on one specific area; the experts say you cannot have both. Constantly being exposed to updates on Facebook streams, Twitter posts, and Instagram pictures depletes your "attention" resource and ultimately your focus. We get five times more information today than a generation ago — which sounds great, but this has created an epidemic of absence of attention. Mindfulness enhances your ability to maintain attention.

Today, our collective absence of attention is almost expected. In terms of social norms, attention has taken a monumental shift in just a generation. Observe a couple sitting across from one another at a restaurant; they're likely focused primarily on their phones. Watch a group of young athletes interact; they all have their heads down, engrossed in social media. This new form of being 50 percent present, of listening while also interacting on your phone, is a deficit of attention. Regardless of whether you're trying to do your best on the playing field, in the boardroom, or at home with your kids, attention is crucial to your ability to perform.

Incredibly, even when you're doing nothing your brain is very active. It's actually more active than when you're engaged in a complex task. Why? The work of neuroscientist Marcus Raichle, PhD, at Washington University attempted to answer this perplexing question. Your brain uses about 20 percent of your body's metabolic energy, and that doesn't change, regardless if you're sleeping or solving a complex math problem. Dr. Raichle identified the default mode network — areas of the brain that calm down during a precise task when the brain is focused, but then ramp back up once the mental task is finished. In his research, when he asked participants what they were thinking about when they were doing nothing, they reported their minds were ablaze with all sorts of thoughts.[10] "Am I doing this task correctly?"; "I wonder what they're trying to figure out about me?"; and so forth. Raichle discovered that when the mind wanders, it wanders to something about "myself": my training, my nutrition, my Instagram post, my stress, my life. This default mode frames everything in terms of how it impacts "I" or "self," effectively making you the center of your own universe. A recent Harvard study found that 50 percent of the time our minds are wandering, which means this default mode is constantly running, putting ourselves on center stage as the star in our own movie.[11]

What's the problem with being the star of the show? Unfortunately, as mindfulness experts all seem to agree, a wandering mind is an unhappy mind. Making matters worse, we seem biologically driven to think about threats. Our brains default to the bad stuff that happens to us rather than the positives, which can be a major performance roadblock for athletes. The golfer always remembers her poor shots, not her best. The basketball player remembers his missed free throws, not his made shots. The Olympic lifter tries to fight off flashbacks of missed lifts, rather than effortlessly remembering PRs. Practicing mindfulness increases your cognitive control, helping you build the skill of maintaining attention, thus preventing the wandering mind and its negative thoughts from filtering into your subconscious. Dr. Goleman says people need to "strengthen the muscle of the mind . . . which is attention." Meditation is a tool to help build your capacity to hold attention. During meditation, your mind wanders and your attention loosens (and when you're a beginner, it feels like *all* it does is wander!). The practice of meditation helps you to bring it back.

Mindfulness also helps to increase working memory and transform short-term memory to long-term memory. Players in sports such as football, with complicated playbooks or tactics, or athletes whose skill development is learned over a long arc, would all benefit from supporting the brain's ability to be mindful. Studies show students who practice mindfulness do better on their SAT tests as well, demonstrating its impact on learning and the benefit it has for balancing rigorous training and the academic requirements of the student-athlete.[12] Unfortunately, the stigma of meditation being "too boring," "too slow," or "too weird" is still very real in athletic circles. It prevents many athletes from maximizing the ultimate performance resource: the brain. The future of human performance is in unlocking the power of the brain, and mindfulness is a gateway to this potential. It's time to start training your brain like you train your body to maximize your athletic potential. The "little red dot" is a quick lesson in mindfulness.

In 2010, one of the greatest displays of golf under pressure the world had ever seen was on full display. A talented young golfer was destroying the field in the British Open major championship at historic St. Andrews Golf Club in Scotland. It wasn't Tiger Woods, Phil Mickelson, or Rory McIlroy, but an unknown South African named Louis Oosthuizen. For the first 3 days, Oosthuizen played brilliantly and had a four-shot lead going into the last round of The Open. The challenge in individual sports such as golf is the immense pressure players feel, and the pressure is enormous in the final round of a major. Almost every time, seemingly without fail, the inexperienced leader cracks under the pressure and succumbs to the charging superstar further down the leaderboard. It happens time and time again. So how did Oosthuizen accomplish the rare task of holding off the field on Sunday and win by one of the largest margins in British Open history? The little red dot. In the lead-up to the British Open championship, Oosthuizen had been playing very well but couldn't quite get over the hump and into the winner's circle. In the most crucial moments, negative thoughts crept into his mind and he failed to pull off the winning shots (the same shots he effortlessly hit in practice sessions). Oosthuizen decided it was time to hire a sport psychologist, and he teamed up with the renowned Dr. Karl Morris to help him take his game to the next level. Dr. Morris suggested a very simple strategy. He had Oosthuizen place a little red dot, made with a Sharpie pen, on his golf glove at the base of his thumb. Before every shot, Morris instructed Oosthuizen to focus his complete attention on the little red dot. Nothing else mattered: all attention was on the red dot. Remarkably, Oosthuizen used this technique to clear his mind of negative thoughts and maintain laserlike focus in the last round of The Open, propelling him to a historic seven-shot victory over the best golfers in the world. The ability to maintain focus — the little red dot — earned Oosthuizen his first major championship.

## Losing Your Cool: The Amygdala Hijack

Have you ever had a fight with your teammates or coach and said a few things you regretted later on, like Zidane's episode described at the start of the chapter? How about your partner or spouse? Most of the time, when the dust settles, you feel embarrassed about the things you said. This is your brain's evolutionary response to danger or threat that has run amok in your modern life. The amygdala is the brain's alarm system for threat, and it scans the body for danger (or safety) via immediate input from all of your senses. It also responds to anything we need to pay attention to (important or not). This dual connection in the brain's circuitry to both intense emotional reactions and intense focus explains why you can be highly distracted by whatever you feel is a threat to you.

If the brain perceives a threat, the amygdala jumps into action and triggers a rush of adrenaline, cortisol, and the fight-or-flight response. This paralyzes the prefrontal cortex area of your brain that is responsible for executive control and determining appropriate behavior. It's the part of your brain that stops you from yelling "asshole" (even though you may want to) at the referee who just made a bad call or someone who cuts in front of you on the highway. The amygdala inhibits the action of your "thinking" brain when you perceive a threat or you feel like you've been treated unfairly. You fixate on the threat and effectively become mindless for an instant (just like

Zidane was in response to Materazzi's personal taunts). This is called the amygdala hijack.

Interestingly, while the amygdala is fully developed at birth, the prefrontal cortex isn't fully develop until your mid-20s, which explains why teenagers and young adults react more strongly and emotionally than adults. Inhibition of the amygdala also impacts your memory hierarchy, altering how you organize memories and shift your focus on the present. What's impacting you right now is all your brain cares about. This memory shift blocks out longer-term, deeper beliefs. You can see how this could be a major problem during conflicts with coaches or teammates, or when you feel your position on the team is threatened. The result is you react in ways you'll likely regret. To improve your capacity to cope with adversity, you need to cool down your amygdala. A recent study at Emory University found that the practice of mindfulness reduced amygdala activity in response to stressful stimuli.[13] Mindfulness is also a proven strategy for relaxing the amygdala hijack response, making it less "hyperreactive" and less likely to inhibit rational and effective decisions.

## How to Build Mindfulness

Building mindfulness and cultivating the moment-to-moment awareness of your surroundings helps you cope with negative thoughts and feelings that cause stress and anxiety. Practicing mindfulness helps you harness the energy of your emotions toward your goals, which helps prevent you from being the victim of negative self-talk and self-sabotage. Creating a clear, calm, and assertive mind through mindfulness practice will help you overcome whatever challenges are thrown your way. The following are three simple techniques to try: mindful breathing, mindful awareness, and mindful immersion.

*Mindful breathing* is a simple and highly effective strategy that a lot of coaches have brought into their training programs. It's a great strategy to use during a warm-up or cooldown period. Here is how it goes:

1. Lie on the ground with your knees bent and feet on the floor.
2. Place your hands on your abdomen (or use a small weighted object).
3. Breathe in, focusing on your belly rising up to the sky as you inhale.
4. Breathe out, feeling your belly move down toward your spine as you exhale.
5. Aim for 2–4 seconds per inhale and exhale.

This practice helps to develop attention and mindfulness, and is age-appropriate for young athletes, too. Mindful breathing can also be done while walking: inhale for 3–4 steps, then exhale for 3–4 steps. Focusing on your breath and maintaining the breathing rhythm is a great way to build mindful attention. Finally, in stressful situations, such as before a big game or presentation at work, you can borrow a highly successful tactic from the Navy SEALs playbook, the 4-minute drill. It's simple: Inhale for 4 seconds, then exhale for 4 seconds, and perform for a total of 4 minutes. It's a great strategy to curb anxiety and direct attention when the pressure mounts (or in the case of the Navy SEALs, when dodging bullets!).

*Mindful awareness* is the practice of clearing your head of negative thoughts. Sit in a comfortable position for 10 minutes and just let your thoughts appear. If negative thoughts crop up, label them as such, and picture yourself discarding them in the garbage. Detach yourself from the negative thoughts. I find performing this meditation sitting cross-legged helps because it creates a level of discomfort in my hips and back. I start thinking "my hips ache" or "my back is tight," and as I sit silently during the meditation I shift the focus to "there is discomfort in the hip" in an attempt to remove myself from the focus of attention. The level of discomfort typically ratchets down the more skillful you become.

*Mindful immersion* is simply relishing mundane tasks. Such tasks can be an opportunity to "turn off" the default mode of your brain and actually sink your focus deep into the chores you're doing, be it washing the dishes, folding clothes, or preparing your food for the next day. Just like the Karate Kid "waxing on and waxing off," mundane tasks allow you the opportunity to dial in your attention. (Interestingly, it actually makes the task much more enjoyable too!) There are countless different methods to incorporate meditation and mindfulness into your day; the trick is to find the one you enjoy and try to adhere to it for 8–10 consecutive weeks to maximize the benefit.

## All-Stars, Self-Compassion, and Psychopaths

Mindfulness — the ability to maintain attention and laserlike focus under pressure — is a characteristic shared by many legendary athletes, including Michael Jordan, Kobe Bryant, Tiger Woods, Tom Brady, Clayton Kershaw, Roger Federer, Serena Williams, and Cristiano Ronaldo. It's also a common characteristic in a much less desirable group: psychopaths. Professor Kevin Dutton, PhD – psychologist at Oxford University and author of the frightfully fantastic book *The Wisdom of Psychopaths* – observes how elite athletes, CEOs, top executives, and yes, psychopaths, share a collection of specific traits. They have the ability to maintain focus (that is, mindfulness), are ruthless competitors who want to win at all costs, have the mental toughness to come back from adversity and the brink of losing, exhibit fearlessness to take on any opponent, have the ability to always stay focused at the task at hand, and are always able to spring into action at the most critical moments. Although we all have these abilities to some degree, these characteristics are displayed to much greater degree in elite athletes and high achievers, and they are highly praised by coaches and fans.

From an evolutionary perspective, a genetic component is likely responsible for violent competitive and psychopathic behavior. Kent Bailey, PhD, emeritus professor in clinical psychology at Virginia Commonwealth University, believes that "some degree of predatory violence was required in the seek and kill aspects of hunting large game animals."[14] These individuals, referred to as "warrior hawks" in scientific literature, would have been pretty useful when trying to fight off foreign invaders or tracking down dangerous prey. Ironically, their insensitivity or lack of caring of what others thought most likely allowed them to excel in situations of uncertainty and danger. It brings to mind the famous quote by Richard Grenier: "[P]eople sleep peacefully in their beds at night only because rough men stand ready to do violence on their behalf."

Of course, during peaceful times these traits would backfire. Psychopathic traits of insensitivity and a propensity for violence would rear their ugly heads within one's own tribe. With no adversaries or threats to fight off, the warrior hawks would inflict irrational and unthinkable harm on their own people, the ones they were responsible for protecting. In short, they behaved like psychopaths.

Although today we're led to believe psychopaths are pure evil (and no doubt their acts most definitely are), the scientific truth seems to be much more nuanced. There is a spectrum of characteristics that make up a psychopath, and many of those traits are not inherently bad. In fact, many are the reason you perform at a high level in elite sport or get hired by a Fortune 500 company. Not convinced? Researchers Belinda Board, PhD, and Katarina Fritzon, PhD, of the University of Surrey in England performed an experiment to find out exactly what made business leaders so successful. They wanted to identify the personality traits and characteristics they possessed that allowed them to rise above the rest. The findings of their study revealed top businesspeople had a great deal of charm, were egocentric, persuasive, independent, highly focused, and lacked empathy . . . all common traits of psychopaths.[15] In his book, Professor Dutton shares the story of Jon Moulton, a highly successful venture capitalist in London, England, who outlined his three most important characteristics for success: curiosity, determination, and insensitivity.[16] The first two seem obvious, but how does insensitivity help performance? Moulton was quick to point out "the great thing about insensitivity is that it lets you sleep at night when others can't." These characteristics seem eerily similar to the GOATs (greatest of all time), including Michael Jordan, Serena Williams, Tom Brady, and Tiger Woods. Experts in the field now believe the traits of psychopaths are on a continuum, not all are negative, and they are far more widespread than we'd like to think.

If some of the traits of psychopaths are shared by elite athletes, and thus beneficial for elite performance, the obvious question is: How can you maximize the beneficial traits of psychopaths while minimizing the negative traits — like narcissism, insensitivity, and lack of empathy (and of course, the really bad ones like propensity to sudden violence!)? Professor Dutton uses the analogy of a DJ's mixing desk, with all its various knobs and dials. "Think of psychopathic characteristics as dials on a mixing desk," says Dutton. "[C]rank them all up to ten and you're borderline psychotic, but dial them all down to one and you'll likely be depressed." (Interesting note: Psychopaths rarely ever suffer from depression.) The key is finding the right balance, the correct amount to turn each dial, so as to maximize the benefit for you. If you apply the right amount of ruthlessness, focus, mental toughness, fearlessness, mindfulness, and action in your training, you can respond to adversity and overcome challenges. They can propel you to victory so that you're not stuck in the middle with the rest of the pack.

Of course, the real question is, how can you do this without turning into a narcissistic villain? If you can somehow be a ruthless killer on the playing field, yet be an open-minded, humble and respectful person off of it, then you'll have found an elite-level winning formula. While this quality may be innate in world-class athletes — such as Roger Federer, Serena

Williams, Tom Brady, Michael Jordan, Tiger Woods, and the like — it may not be innate for you. However, there may be something you can do to attempt to build this attribute in yourself. The answer may lie in *self-compassion*.

Compassion seems to be a universally admired trait. It's an umbrella term for commonly admired qualities, such as kindness, sympathy, understanding, empathy, and wanting to support others (basically, the opposite of all the psychopathic traits!). Ironically, pioneering self-compassion researcher Kristin Neff, PhD, of the University of Texas at Austin says a complete U-turn occurs when we put *self* out in front of compassion. The term "self-compassion" seems closely related to negative qualities like self-pity, self-indulgence, or self-centered, which all trigger associations with selfish qualities. Dr. Neff has been studying self-compassion for over a decade and says it is none of those things. While she does admit the term doesn't sound very tough — it doesn't have the same ring as "no pain, no gain" — the research on self-compassion is impressive. It seems that self-compassion helps build resiliency, fights off the "poor me" mentality, and is an even more powerful intervention than positive self-talk.[17]

Self-compassion is also essential for building a solid foundation of emotional intelligence: recognizing the emotions others are feeling, managing them, and avoiding being overwhelmed; demonstrating a high level of motivation; and recognizing the emotional response of others and using this awareness to effectively manage relationships. These skills are crucial for athletic (and life) success.

Unfortunately, self-compassion often gets dismissed in elite sports. You don't see many football, rugby, or hockey coaches rounding up their players for a breakout session on self-compassion. Ironically, it's often the antidote many athletes need to fight off performance pitfalls. For instance, confidence and narcissism are highly correlated, and they have the potential to blunt athletic and personal development. Compassion doesn't sound tough, but looking at the world realistically and allowing yourself to fail means that you won't run away from challenges when things get difficult (and in elite sport, things will get difficult at some point, guaranteed). When your self-esteem is not tied to your achievement, you can listen to people, you're more easily able to learn, and thus you're more coachable. Being more coachable helps you, your team, and your coach achieve the ultimate goal.

The most common myths associated with self-compassion, identified by Dr. Neff, that prevent people from taking action have to do with equating self-compassion to weakness, self-pity, and complacency.

### 1. SELF-COMPASSION EQUALS WEAKNESS

The overwhelming reaction from coaches in response to self-compassion is an immediate facial expression that screams . . . "weakness!" It sounds like everyone will be sitting around, holding hands, and singing "Kumbaya." It evokes the famous quote from the character played by Tom Hanks in the baseball movie *A League of Their Own*, "There's no crying in baseball!" Once again, our inherent and deep-seated biases are playing against us. All coaches praise resiliency, and research shows that self-compassion is one of the most powerful tools for building resiliency.[18] You're going to face obstacles and roadblocks in your sport (and in your life), and how you treat yourself during these difficult times has a major impact on your ability to persist, overcome, and ultimately succeed. When you constantly self-criticize, you lose faith in yourself, your ability to take on new tasks, and you increase your risk of depression. We love the illusion of perfection in sport, but it's not realistic. It's not attainable. If you constantly need a whipping or harsh self-criticism to succeed, you'll soon find out that it's a limited resource. Self-compassion is self-acceptance, and it's the quickest path to resiliency.

### 2. SELF-COMPASSION EQUALS SELF-PITY

Self-compassion sounds like you're having a pity party — and let's be honest, nobody likes that. But actually, the exact opposite is true. If you're self-compassionate, you're actually less likely to get caught up in the negative emotions from poor performances, a season mired in injury, or life struggles. Research by expert Filip Raes, PhD, at the University of Leuven found that students who exhibited higher rates of self-compassion tended to brood less about their misfortune.[19] Can you think of an athlete or client who is moping about poor performance or lack of progress? Self-compassion isn't blowing things off, but rather it's seeing yourself more clearly.

Rather than being overly dramatic in your response or body language, self-compassion says, "It's hard for all of us out here," rather than simply, "Poor me." Don't ignore the poor performance, but don't get swallowed up in your misery and over-exaggerate it either. Self-talk can get extremely negative as well. It can be downright shocking the things you say to yourself in your head and how awful you can be to yourself during periods of poor performance. You would never say those words to a teammate or friend, so why would you bludgeon yourself with this mental hammer? If your confidence is contingent on you always slaying the dragon, you'll be crushed by poor performances. Many elite athletes don't ever recover.

### 3. Self-Compassion Equals Complacency

When you hear the term self-compassion, you may conflate it with a level of complacency. In sport, complacency is a first-class ticket to the bottom of the leaderboard. Any performance director, coach, or athlete can tell you about a time when "the team got complacent," quickly followed by a negative outcome. Nobody wants complacency on their team, nor for that matter the whiff of anything that smells like complacency. For elite athletes the common refrain is: If you don't beat yourself up over a poor performance, then you'll get complacent and lose your edge. Sound familiar? Inside your head you're beating yourself up for failing to meet your expectations. For example, "I always miss when the game is on the line" or "I can't close out games in the last few minutes" or "I'll never make it." You always assume you're not trying hard enough, yet for elite performers that's rarely the case. Research at the University of California found that students who demonstrated self-compassion about a recent transgression (written as a note to themselves) outperformed positive self-talk and positive mood for strengthening personal accountability.[20] Coaches at all levels praise accountability as a key driver of success, and head offices are quick to point to accountability as a major player in establishing a winning culture, yet rarely is self-compassion mined for its performance-enhancing benefits.

There is also an inherent wisdom in self-compassion. Self-compassion says we as humans are all flawed, and that hardship and struggle are embedded in the human condition. This is often overlooked in performance when you strive for perfection, when your confidence is contingent on new PRs every month, or when you insist on being the star of the game every night. Mindfulness is not self-compassion, but it's an ingredient. What separates self-compassion from mindfulness is that it takes you a step past accepting your experience and adds something integral: *you*!

## Build Self-Compassion and Supercharge Your Brain

Every athlete is training hard. Every athlete is working on their technical skills. Every athlete is now thinking about their nutrition and sleep. However, how many are developing a supercharged brain and mindset? Emotional intelligence, mindfulness, and self-compassion are pillars of strong mental and emotional well-being. The following techniques were developed by expert Dr. Kristin Neff, PhD, and I've adapted them over the years to suit my athlete client base. The next time you face a challenge in your sport or life, something that causes you stress, try one of these exercises:

The **Stopwatch Challenge.** Set a timer for 3 minutes on your phone and repeat the following three phrases with your eyes closed until the alarm sounds: "This hurts." "Other athletes struggle, too." "Be patient . . . I am strong."

**"Supercharge" Journal.** Journaling is a fantastic way to increase your mental and physical well-being. Get out a pen and paper, set aside 5 minutes and write down something you judged yourself for in practice today, a recent game, or in everyday life. It may be a difficult situation that causes you pain or something you feel bad about. Dr. Neff emphasizes the importance of noting how you felt (sad, embarrassed, ashamed, and so forth) and why you felt that way (what do you think was the underlying root cause of those symptoms?). Then finish with a sentence containing words of comfort (something like: I messed up, but next time . . .).

**Criticism Crusher.** Relying on criticism as a motivator — the constant cracking of the whip — is not an efficient means of motivation. Use the following technique to apply a more constructive approach to motivation: Think about the ways in which you criticize yourself or your performance. How does that make you feel? Next, how could you rephrase the self-criticism to use a kinder tone to highlight unproductive behavior? Finally, catch yourself when you revert to old patterns and reframe a more encouraging inner dialogue with your new phrase.

## Emotions and Mindset Solutions

Humans evolved to see and feel first and then to think. As Dr. Peter Jensen points out, "Emotion and imagery change people, logic does not." Imagery is the first language we're all exposed to. We're driven by images and emotions. Dr. John Sullivan, who is in agreement, expertly summarizes, "Emotions run the show in sport and life." Unfortunately, most athletes are taught to ignore emotions. Illusions like mental toughness and grit fail to take into account your complex neurobiology and ignore the interconnectedness between your health and resiliency. "We are wired to survive," says Dr. Sullivan; "It gets no tougher than that, no grittier than that. Our first major survival tool is emotion."

Allow your athletes to show purpose, and return it in kind. Connect with people; let them be heard. Dr. Jensen says, "Your ability to build relationships and connect with people is critical to your success." The exploration into emotions and mindset, and the tools I've outlined in this chapter — positive self-talk, mindfulness, and self-compassion — will allow you to start to identify your emotions, manage energy, and utilize them to your advantage. If you can't identify your emotions, you'll blunt them, and you'll fail to maximize your health and performance. Mastering emotional management will help you to become a better leader, a topic I'll dive into in the final chapter.

# CHAPTER 12

# Leadership and Great Coaching

I t was Game 7 of the 1957 NBA Finals. The Boston Celtics were leading by one point over the St. Louis Hawks, and rookie Bill Russell had just missed a dunk with 40 seconds left to play that would've likely sealed the win. The Hawks quickly inbounded the ball to Jack Coleman at midcourt, who had a clear path to the basket to give them the lead. Still underneath his own basket, Russell took off in pursuit of Coleman as the crowd and his teammates looked on. Russell covered the entire length of the court and chased Coleman down, making one of the most incredible and spectacular blocks in Finals history. The Celtics went on to win in double overtime over the Hawks. It was Bill Russell's first of 11 championship titles in his 13 playing seasons with the Celtics. Perhaps most impressive is that the Celtics never lost in 10 out of 10 Game 7 "do-or-die" playoff matches, despite never having a player lead the league in scoring or dominating in any statistical categories. Russell had immense talent, but so did other great players at the time. What set him apart? The most obvious trait is the extent to which Russell emphasized *the team* over individual awards. He famously turned down an invitation to his own Hall of Fame induction ceremony because he felt it was only an individual accolade. Russell believed his career was a symbol of team play. The "Coleman Play" marks the beginning of the Celtics's and Russell's dynasty, and paved the way for Russell to become arguably the greatest leader in team sports.

It raises the question, are great leaders destined for greatness from birth, genetically hardwired to lead? Or is a great leader developed over time, a product of environment and experience? It's an age-old question: nature versus nurture. A quick glimpse into what elite leaders in the world of sport think at the Leaders in Performance conference in London, England, high-lights the complexity of the questions. For example, legendary former player and Liverpool FC football manager Gérard Houllier believes "you need to have an innate quality." However, not everyone believes great leadership is innate. David Blitzer, owner of the Philadelphia 76ers and New Jersey Devils says, "I don't think there are born leaders, I think they're made." Which is it — are great leaders born or made? Well, good news: There is a third op-tion. Sir David Brailsford, director of performance at Team SKY and winner of countless Olympic gold medals and Tour De France championships, says it best: "Both!" It's a difficult question to answer, even for the best sport scientists, coaches, and management in the world. If you are born with it, then you're very lucky, so be sure not to waste your gift. The good news for everyone else — coaches, athletes, practitioners, entrepreneurs, parents — is that leadership development also seems highly dependent on environment.

But what exactly makes a great coach, team captain, or leader? The abil-ity to inspire and motivate? How well they communicate with teammates or staff? Their ability as a tactician and strategist? Are the skills of a great leader built around abstract thinking and intelligence — an approach that most CEOs and top executives gain from attending elite business schools — or are these skills the result of life experience and ability to engage and interact with people? Intelligence versus wisdom — another age-old question. In today's tech-centric "cure-all" smart solutions, where does intuitive wisdom fit into the picture? Ultimately, since sport is about *people*, understanding the human condition can make all the difference in performance.

## Intelligence versus Wisdom

Intelligence is defined in the Oxford dictionary as the ability to acquire and apply knowledge and skills. When you think of legendary coaches, such as the NBA's Gregg Popovich, the NFL's Bill Belichik, or MLB's Joe Maddon, you think of expert tacticians who can skillfully adjust and outsmart the opposition. No doubt there is tremendous need for intelligence to be a skillful coach, but it's not a zero-sum game: intelligence may have a down-side. Wisdom is the quality of having experience, knowledge, and good judgment. A great coach must also be able to connect with athletes and see things from their perspective in order to communicate and motivate in the most effective manner, thereby guiding them toward the ultimate goal (and often resolving conflicts along the way).

You can be highly intelligent without wisdom. However, the opposite is not true. You cannot have wisdom without intelligence. Not convinced? New research is shifting the balance of how behavioral psychologists look at wisdom. A groundbreaking new study by social psychologists Igor Grossmann, PhD, and Justin Brienza, PhD, from the University of Waterloo in Canada uncovered that "intelligence may come at a great cost, our ability to make wise decisions." Over a two-year span, Grossmann and Brienza recruited over 2,000 people in the United States to fill out an online survey. Participants were asked to recall a recent argument or conflict with a friend or spouse and answer 20 questions relating to the episode. Sample questions included: "Did you ever consider a third-party perspective?"; "How much did you try to understand the other person's point of view?"; and "Did you consider you might be wrong?" The participants were then assigned a wise-reasoning score based on how they answered the questions, as well as a score for their social class. When Grossmann analyzed the results, he was stunned; the people in the lower social class (less education, less income, and more worries about money) scored almost 100 percent better on the wise-reasoning scale compared to the participants from the higher social class.[1] The results were incredibly compelling, especially when you consider the study didn't include the very rich or very poor.

In the field of behavioral psychology, experts traditionally think of intelligence as a characteristic of higher learning or higher social class. Many still believe lower-class social environments promote inferior reasoning, postulating this is likely due to limited resources and the greater uncertainty in day-to-day living as compared to higher social classes.[2] However, Grossmann believes growing up in a working-class environment has advantages for interpersonal conflict resolution, as people have to rely more on shared or communal resources compared to those in the middle class. In the lower-class environments, there are more opportunities to develop the skills to resolve conflicts with peers, whereas in many middle-class environments the focus tends to be on IQ and less so on conflict resolution. Another key finding from Grossmann and Brienza's work is that a person is less likely to reason wisely when the other person involved in the conflict is of lower social status than they are themselves. Think about how this could impact coach-athlete or teammate-teammate relationships.

In the second part of the experiment, Grossmann and Brienza conducted a series of live interviews. They recruited 200 people and asked them to take an IQ test, as well as to read three letters from a "Dear Abby" advice column in a local newspaper. The participants were then asked to share with an interviewer their thoughts of how the scenarios they had just read would play out. The responses were scored by a panel of judges with respect to their wise-reasoning capacity (using a validated scoring method). The more the participant considered how a third party or an outsider might view the situation, the more "wisdom points" they were awarded. No points were given to participants who simply relied on their own perspective. Once again, participants in the higher social class showed a markedly lower capacity to reason wisely about the interpersonal conflicts encountered in the scenarios. It seems the participants in the lower social class had much greater pragmatic reasoning (more reflective of wisdom) compared to the abstract reasoning we associate with intelligence. In short, wisdom won over intelligence.

What exactly is *wise reasoning*? The concept has emerged in behavorial sciences over the past few years, and it effectively highlights the importance of combined cognitive strategies when people navigate uncertain situations in their lives.[3] In practical terms, it means thinking of the broader context rather than just the immediate issue, looking for compromises between conflicting points of view, and having a sensitivity to how personal behavior impacts relationships.[4] The central aspects of wise reasoning include intellectual humility, recognition that the world is constantly changing, and the ability to take different contexts into account (besides your own). All of these factors are strongly associated with handling conflict wisely. From an athlete standpoint, it's a skill that most successful team captains have for navigating the challenges of a difficult game, a difficult coach, or a long and grueling season among teammates. For coaches and practitioners, it provides the mindset for the most effective teaching strategies. If you can't see things through your athlete's eyes, you'll struggle to propel them to their performance potential. It's no doubt a shared trait by many of the legendary coaches who were able to motivate men and women from different backgrounds and social classes toward a common goal.[5]

Grossmann's findings are consistent with the specialization hypothesis in ecological and evolutionary psychology, which suggests that the propensity for thinking about yourself versus the group reflects how people are currently adapting to their different environments.[6] Working-class people display more wide-ranging attentional focuses and have enhanced sensitivity to contextual cues, which are well-established adaptive strategies when environments are threatening or resources are limited.[7] "They're more likely to focus on close relationships and cooperation within groups, helping to promote survival and success in environments with limited or poor resources," says Grossmann. He summarizes, "The higher your class, the less likely you are to reason wisely in interpersonal situations."[8] This view is supported by past research that demonstrates wise reasoning can occur independently from abstract cognitive abilities.[9]

If wisdom is crucial to successful leadership in sport and in life, how can you develop this high-impact quality? I asked many of the experts quoted in this book about gaining wisdom, and virtually all responded with the same advice: experience. You don't become wise from a textbook and you can't develop wisdom from an online course. Intelligence alone doesn't make you wise. Experience is the best teacher.

Unfortunately, experience can take a while to accumulate. What happens if you want to fast-track your ability to develop wise-reasoning skills? Is it even possible? While the research isn't clear, Grossmann's advice is to use third-person language when thinking about conflicts. During your next conflict situation with an athlete, client, coach, or practitioner, mentally address yourself by name (and the person with whom you're having the conflict). For example, rather than saying, "I think you need to put more work on his nutrition," you would say, "Mark believes John should put more focus into your nutrition." This simple technique makes you more likely to see the situations like a third person might see it, rather than through your own personal lens.

This can be a powerful weapon in dealing with the dynamics of a high-performance environment. For example, a new team strength coach may be striving to justify his position in the performance team (consciously or unconsciously) by focusing on getting the athletes as strong and powerful as possible at the expense of potential injury or reduced time devoted to movement quality, technical, tactical, or psychological practice. The experienced performance director would probably take the new strength coach aside, reiterate the team goals and philosophy, and ensure the strength coach knows their role in achieving those goals and how valuable they are in the process. In this scenario, the performance director's ability to see things from the third person's point of view allows them to understand why another member of the team is focused in a certain direction, and can then diffuse tensions and recalibrate that team member's focus in a supportive manner. It seems obvious, but too many practitioners in all areas — trainers, therapists, doctors, nutritionists — struggle with putting aside personal gain and seeing the bigger picture. Another great strategy Grossmann suggests is exposing yourself to situations where you can't rely on your own past experiences for guidance, or where your own expectations aren't front and center. For example, Grossmann suggests going to a multicultural event or volunteering at a homeless shelter — scenarios that force you to get out of your own comfort zone and see things from a third-person perspective. Intelligence is no doubt an asset, but building wise-reasoning skills will amplify your ability to make a difference with your team or athletes.

## The Dangers of a "Me First" Attitude

You often hear that young people and athletes today are more selfish and self-centered than in generations past. Is this true? Is social media and the "selfie" making people more self-absorbed? A recent study in *Psychology Science* suggests people across the world are becoming more individualistic. While individualism is associated with greater self-reliance, it can also foster greater self-centeredness and narcissism. Researchers believe this "me first" attitude makes it harder for people to see things from another's point of view (that is, they lack wise reasoning).[10] Social media connects us to others, but it also creates an environment where the emphasis is "all about me," which can lead to greater narcissism and an unwillingness to cooperate with others.

But is this really something new? Aren't humans inherently selfish and self-absorbed? The work of Andrew King, PhD, expert behavioral ecologist from Swansea University in Wales, helped shed some light on the subject via his recent TEDx talk, *Simple, Selfish and Hungover*. "We're built to survive and pass along our genes," said Dr. King during our interview. His research into animal behavior and group dynamics revealed more than meets the eye.[11] For example, the flocking pattern of sheep seems like highly coopera-tive behavior, as the group seems to be working together to escape a com-mon threat. But this is very misleading. The sheep all come together to form a herd, seemingly in order to protect the collective group from the predator (or from Dr. King's research, the herding sheepdog). However, upon closer inspection, each individual sheep is trying its hardest to get to the middle of the flock. The center position is farthest away from the predator, and thus the position with the greatest likelihood of survival. The sheep are herding for *selfish* reasons; they're trying to survive. Another result of this behavior is that they're also subsequently putting another sheep closer to the predator and exposing them to more danger. This animal behavior is inherently selfish. It turns out humans respond in a very similar and predictable way. "Fundamentally, humans are selfish, too," says Dr. King.

The sheep flock for selfish reasons, but how do they do it? Are there any rules to how sheep, birds, fish, or humans move and interact within groups? Dr. King's research uses computer models to assess whether any common rules exist among animal and human interactions, and lo and behold, there are, in fact, simple rules of interaction. It works like this: If you're too close to an individual, you move farther away from them, but if you're too far away, you move closer and are attracted to them. Of course, these lab models assume every animal or person is the same. But just like people, animals have different personalities; some are shy and some are bold. The personality difference is crucial for how well (or not so well) animals, people, or athletes work together. It's well-established in ecology literature that the greater the difference between animals' personalities, the better the coordination between the two. One bold fish and one shy fish will swim happily along together, whereas two bold fish will struggle to agree on a direction, and two shy fish don't get very far.

Diversity allows for coordination. This is known as the "leader-follower" dynamic, which highlights that diversity can elicit complementarity in social roles and when solving problems. You can find leader-follower dynamics everywhere in nature, be it in fish, donkeys, baboons, and of course humans. Rock ants teach other ants how to find the nest by leading them along the way, while alpha-male baboons lead by example (rather than enforcement). When the alpha male moves, the rest of the group follows him because he has many more, and stronger, social ties than others. "These simple rules create group level behavior and leader-follower dynamics," says Dr. King. Does the same thing really happen in people? Dr. King uses the example of renowned American economist Harry Markowitz to illustrate how even brilliant minds fall back on simple rules or heuristics when presented with complex problems. In 1990, Markowitz won the Nobel Prize for his work in developing a highly complicated model for maximizing asset allocation. Based on his brilliant work, you would think he followed his own advice when investing his money, right? Wrong. He used the simple heuristic of dividing his assets evenly across multiple funds. Why would he do such a thing after painstakingly proving such a brilliantly sophisticated and successful model? In a complex world, even the most highly intelligent individuals default to simple rules; they're human, too, after all. Dr. King notes how these unconscious biases are "the result of hundreds of thousands of years of evolution; trial and error." It used to be highly advantageous to follow the strongest or tallest male of the group to ensure survival, and today our brain's default decision mode is still to follow the tallest person. Not convinced? The average height of US Presidential candidates over the past 100 years is taller than the population average, and the winners of presidential elections have been, on average, taller than the losers. In the absence of other information, humans still tend to follow the taller person. This happens all the time across many different domains, including sport.

Teams call it "culture," but it's effectively a leader-follower dynamic. When you've got the right leaders in sports, the culture moves in a positive direction, yielding dynasties like the Golden State Warriors and New England Patriots. Research in animal behavior confirms you only need a certain number of individuals to adopt something for the whole group to start doing it, too. This extends to team play, sharing the ball, and making the right play for the team. Unfortunately, it also works in the other direction. In baseball, a simple leader-follower heuristic is referred to as the "dickhead rule," used by management to maintain a healthy team dynamic. Made famous by the Boston Red Sox in the lead-up to their historic 2004 World Series championship, it implies that for every difficult personality on the team, you need at least four high-character players to avoid souring the culture. In rugby, the renowned New Zealand All Blacks mental skills coach Gilbert Enoka similarly introduced a "no dickheads" policy that the players themselves enforce. The All Blacks are the most successful international rugby team of all time. It only takes a few egocentric players with loud voices for others to get sucked into the negative vaccum, and once you lose control of the locker room it's difficult to regain it. Too many dickheads ruin the team dynamics. This is also seen in nature — it's why animal groups have evolved systems that favor survival of the group over the individual (and thus fighting to the death). A great example are meerkats, a species of mongoose that forcibly evicts members who aren't cooperating in order to cleanse the group of the damaging behavior. This approach sounds a lot like what leading organizations and teams attempt to accomplish by building "culture" within an organization.

It looks like humans are inherently motivated by self-interest and still rely on simple rules to get by. Dr. King refers to these unconscious biases as our collective "evolutionary hangover." This term describes how our brains are coping in a modern environment with evolution-hardwired heuristics. The real question is, are these characteristics a benefit or hindrance? Dr. King believes simple rules are still effective in highly complex environments, pointing out heuristics are on average "fast, and quite accurate." But you also need to be aware if your gut reaction is steering you in the wrong direction. "Know the situation you're in," says Dr. King, "and use the information at your disposal." Then you can begin to figure out the optimal dynamics for the group. This is an important consideration for coaches, athletes, and performance staff.

Analytics in sports is helping to put objective measures to previously subjective opinions of a player's value on a team. Some players are not best on the starting five or the first team, but by simply being on the field, their play makes everybody else better. Big Data has added advanced analytics like WAR (wins above replacement) ratings in baseball and Player Efficiency ratings in basketball (just to name a few). These metrics illustrate the ways in which data is influencing how coaches strategize and how front offices make out the roster. How a player influences the team dynamic, and thus indirectly influences wins, is information that used to be almost impossible to quantify in a traditional boxscore. Big Data is changing the playing field. Even though humans are inherently selfish and somewhat simple, the leader-follower dynamic is a crucial piece of the leadership puzzle. Is that all it takes to build a great culture in your team, among your athletes, or within your organization? Let's see what some of the top experts in pro sports do.

## Culture *Is* the Strategy

Every team says they want to build a "culture" within their organization, but from the outside looking in, not all of them seem to accomplish the task. But what *is* culture? In business and high-performance settings, Peter Drucker's famous quote, "Culture eats strategy for breakfast" rings true. In fact, it's frequently used to highlight the importance of environment over technical application. It sounds great, but is it really true? Toronto Blue Jays CEO Mark Shapiro, who has been working in a leadership position in professional baseball for over 25 years, believes the quote is actually a little misleading. For the Toronto Blue Jays, "culture *is* the strategy," says Shapiro.[12] He firmly believes instilling a sense of ownership into all team staff — from coaches to training staff to the front office — is a major driver of a winning culture. If staff feel like they have ownership of their duties, rather than simply and mindlessly completing tasks, then the quality of their performance will improve dramatically. "If you're rehabbing a 17-year-old pitcher in Dominican Republic," says Shapiro, "you're having a major impact on team performance. You need to feel as though your efforts are invested in the overall outcome." This attitude or culture of connecting every staff member to the success of the team is paramount for Shapiro; he believes getting an edge on the competition doesn't come from just one single intervention, but rather from a hundred incremental efficiencies. He also offers this advice to practitioners looking to break into professional sport: Know yourself, align yourself with like-minded leaders, and contribute to the team from day one. Great advice from one of the best in the business.

This principle of being driven by the collective goal rather than individual accolades is shared by former Los Angeles Clippers general manager David Wohl. He notes the limitations of having a transactional view of all your interactions. If you're a strength coach, therapist or practitioner working in high-level sport, it's easy to get lost in thinking about your own interests. Wohl says that thinking, "What can I get out of this?" doesn't serve the greater team purpose and ultimately won't serve you. He emphasizes the fundamental importance of a collective drive and focus, adding, "Ultimately as the team succeeds so does everyone connected with the team." Wise advice.

Instilling a sense of ownership in the team, being driven by a collective goal, and striking the right leader-follower balance all appear to be crucial for building a team culture. Culture is also synonymous with Team SKY racing and British cycling coach Sir David Brailsford. Under his guidance as the performance director for British Cycling, Brailsford led Great Britain to two Olympic gold medals in the 2004 Olympics in Athens, Greece — the first cycling medals for Britain in almost 100 years. British Cycling went on to win eight gold medals in both the 2008 and 2012 Olympics, leading all countries in cycling. In 2010, Brailsford took on a new challenge as the general manager of Team SKY — a then new British-based professional cycling team — with the goal of winning a Tour de France within five years. Team SKY won five out of six Tours from 2012–2017, an unprecedented feat. Brailsford's phenomenal success led to him being knighted in 2013. How were these teams able to succeed at such an incredible rate under Sir Brailsford's leadership? Success was born from failure.

## A Life Lesson from the Big Tuna

A leading performance director recently shared a story about an important lesson he learned early in his career, one it took him years to unravel and fully understand. The lesson was from legendary Hall of Fame football coach Bill Parcells. The performance director was just starting out in the business and happened to be attending a friend's wedding, where Parcells was also a guest. Parcells was quite jovial and loquacious that day and he decided he would give the young executive a piece of career advice. It was a simple message: "Nobody gives a shit." The young performance director was happy to hear the words of wisdom from the legendary coach; however, he was left a little confused by the remark. He thanked him, walked off, and figured that was the end of the story. Later that night, as he was leaving, Parcells shook his hand to say goodbye, leaned in real close, and enthusiastically repeated the same advice: "Remember kid, nobody gives a shit!" Shocked by his persistence, he wasn't exactly sure what to make of Parcell's life lesson. Many years later, when faced with a very difficult decision that would dictate the future of a franchise, he remembered Parcell's words. In the blink of an eye, it finally made sense. Don't do things to appease others; don't take the easy way out. At the end of the day, you need to do what you think is right (because ultimately . . . nobody gives a shit!).

Brailsford recounts that Team SKY was a total disaster in their first year. They had tried too hard to revolutionize cycling. After that first season, Brailsford realized they were focusing too heavily on the minutiae and were ignoring the fundamentals. Rather than pursue the next shiny new toy, Brailsford famously enacted the "marginal gains" moniker. The emphasis was to make as many incremental gains across the board as possible, rather than aiming for a big win in a few specific areas. The focus shifted to doing all the little things — the fundamentals — with elite, expert precision. Moreover, everyone on Team SKY was required to have an opinion. Top-down decision-making was out the window in favor of the wisdom of the collective group. Nobody was allowed to sit quietly and not share insights. Collective wisdom is an evidence-based phenomenon, as Dr. Andrew King's research in human behavior uncovered. When Dr. King asked individuals to estimate the number of jelly beans in a jar, he received all sorts of answers well above and below the actual count. However, if he asked enough people, eventually the scores averaged out to almost exactly the number of jelly beans in the jar. Elite performance is about improvement and evolution. To evolve requires change, and change requires action. The line between success and failure in elite sport is incredibly thin. Sir Brailsford highlights this best, saying, "Try quickly, fail quickly, and try something else."

## Thinking Outside the Box:
## The Three Lions Pick and Roll

When you're trying to solve a complex problem and uncover an innovative solution, looking outside your sport or industry is a wise decision. Most great leaders do this. Albert Einstein famously said, "We can't solve problems by using the same kind of thinking we used when we created them." Looking at a problem through a third party's viewpoint can enlighten you and improve your ability to be innovative. That's precisely what Gareth Southgate, England's manager at the 2018 World Cup in Russia, decided to do to ensure his team had an advantage over the competition on set plays, where most of the goals are scored. Southgate learned how to upgrade the quality of his set pieces by borrowing a little strategy from the NBA. Sitting courtside at a Minnesota Timberwolves NBA game earlier that year, Southgate was intrigued and impressed by how NBA players created space around the basket. Thinking the basketball tactics could help his England players on set plays during the World Cup, he reached out to the Timberwolves coaching staff. Southgate went on to use a play taken straight out of an NBA playbook to open up space for his players in a game against Sweden in the knockout phase of the World Cup. The innovative strategy worked brilliantly, propelling England to an early goal and a win to advance to the semifinals. In fact, England's set play success also helped them make history by winning their first-ever World Cup penalty shootout and their best World Cup finish since 1966.

Southgate's successful strategy is something creative leaders across all industries do; they take an idea from one field and apply it to another. The scientific term is "association," the ability to connect ideas from unrelated fields. It's what separates good leaders from great leaders or entrepreneurs. Steve Jobs famously employed this technique when coming up with the design for the Apple stores, which is borrowed from luxury hotels like the Ritz-Carlton. Researchers also use this strategy to solve common problems, such as how to get people to wear safety gear to prevent injuries. In Europe, psychologists interviewed people from three completely different fields — carpenters, roofers, and in-line skaters — because they all shared this common problem. They also found staying stuck in your domain — in your same way of thinking about a problem — consistently stalled the creative process. The lesson is this: People who are more likely to look outside their specific field for innovative solutions come up with superior ideas. Southgate's use of a basketball bread-and-butter play, the "pick and roll," to create space for his players to succeed, was a brilliant move inspired by a leader who was confident enough (and wise enough) to adopt ideas outside his sport. This sort of mindset helps to create culture in a team or organization.

## Vulnerability, Authenticity, and Building Trust

Great leaders must be intelligent, wise, and attuned to the personalities on the team. They must also seek inspiration across all types of domains. But what about the work *between* the lines — the human aspect of inspiring players, motivating them, and ultimately building the trust needed to create a collective goal? Expert sport psychologist Peter Jensen, PhD, says, "The ability to build relationships and connect with people is absolutely crucial. Without it, you're sunk." It doesn't happen overnight; it takes time. In fact, it's an incredibly difficult thing to achieve: to have every member of the team completely bought-in and ready to lay themselves on the line for the ultimate goal. It's easy for experts to say, "You need to build trust with your athletes," but how can you actually do it? Expert psychologist Dr. Kristin Neff says you can't fast-forward trust; it takes time. But there are several strategies you can use to accelerate the process. The first is showing *vulnerability*. Getting on the same level as your athlete or teammate, seeing things from their perspective, is a great place to start. Circling back to the success England achieved at the 2018 World Cup in Russia, the psychology of the team played a massive role in their success. It wasn't simply Gareth Southgate's leadership that created an impact; behind the scenes, team psychologist Pippa Grange played a fundamental role in forging the tight bonds between players that catapulted them toward a collective mindset and common goal.

For decades, England had been burdened with heavy expectations. The roster was loaded with star players — the golden generation of Beckham, Gerrard, Lampard, and others — that were hyped to bring home the World Cup trophy. Unfortunately, too many entitled and surly stars compromised team unity, and cracks in the foundation grew wider as the team succumbed to the heavy burden of history and expectations. In 2018, the England squad came across as humble and hungry, and they were playing with joy and confidence. How did Pippa Grange manage to achieve such an impressive turnaround? It wasn't an overnight success — it took months to lay a foundation of trust in the team. Grange used a variety of strategies, all designed to allow players to show vulnerability, such as getting the players into small groups to sit down and share their life stories, experiences, and anxieties, in an effort for them to expose intimate truths about themselves and what really motivates them.[13] Grange said that the objective with these exercises (and showing vulnerability) was to build trust, "making them closer, with a better understanding of each other."

Another important factor in building trust is *authenticity*. In fact, Dr. Neff says authenticity is even more important than empathy, which can be faked. It's not about you saying to your athlete or teammate, "I feel what you feel," because in many instances you cannot. Are you struggling to earn a spot in the team or perhaps even pay the bills at home? Are you a minority? Are you a single parent trying to balance your work and athletic career while raising children? Perhaps not. Rather than empathizing, focus on acknowledging their challenges. Comments like "I can appreciate what you feel" allows space for both of you to gain ground. You can't rush trust. This is something Grange reinforces with the coaches she works with. It takes time.

What's different about Grange's approach is that rather than waiting for players to individually seek out the team psychologist, Grange has embedded activities into the team schedule. Everyone gets the opportunity to upgrade their mental game, not just players who feel they need extra support. (Because let's be honest, how many elite players actually reach out for help? Unfortunately, not many.) This is a revolution you can see cropping up slowly across elite sport. Rather than waiting for individuals to ask for help with nutrition, or sleep, or mindset, teams create an environment where the skills they want the athletes to develop are embedded in activities, drills, and day-to-day life. England's psychological transformation at the World Cup and Grange's influence on the team's mindset provide a great example

## The Power of a Smile

In 2017, elite marathoner Eliud Kipchoge attempted to run a sub-two-hour marathon in Nike's infamous Breaking2 marathon project. While Kipchoge's attempt wasn't at a sanctioned race (he was allowed to draft behind other runners), he did employ an unusual strategy. As the race got more difficult, he began smiling more and more. Was it a deliberate tactic? Could this actually impact his performance? Noel Brick, PhD, and his team at Ulster University had been investigating this question, and the results of their study were published in the journal of *Psychology of Sport and Exercise*. The researchers asked 24 runners to complete four 6-minute runs and assessed their running economy (how much oxygen they consumed at a specific speed), and perceived effort. Here is the best part: The runners were also asked to smile, frown, relax their hands, or think weird and bizarre thoughts during the test. How did smiling compare with frowning for running economy? It kicked its butt, improving running economy by 2 percent.[14] It might not sound like much, but this percentage is similar to the gains that can be made from doing four to eight weeks of plyometric or weight training. (The participants did have to hold their smile for 6 minutes — no easy task!) In 2018, Kipchoge smashed the world record at the Berlin Marathon with a time of 2:01:39, the first person to break the 2:02:00 mark. Did the power of a smile propel Kipchoge to history? Maybe. At the end of the day, it highlights how in sport — just like in life — there seems to be more potential upside with a smile!

for others in sport (and in life). Just remember, trust takes time. A great reminder comes from the Zen proverb, "When the student is ready, the teacher will appear." Showing vulnerability and authenticity help accelerate the trust-building process, but often both coaches and practitioners simply need to relax and let the process play out.

## Motivation, Habits, and Automaticity

Sam Walker is the founding editor of the *Wall Street Journal*'s prize-winning sports section and the author of *The Captain Class*. Walker spent years analyzing the greatest dynasties in the history of sport to determine whether these teams had any common traits. He analyzed more than 1,200 teams from 37 different sports around the world — cricket, football, basketball, baseball, Olympic team sports, rugby, and so on — and identified what he believed to be the 16 greatest teams in history. Walker had a few hypotheses around what might have made these teams great. The first centered on the coaches' intelligence and their abilities as expert tacticians. While these factors no doubt played some role, Walker didn't find these skills to be consistent across all the greatest teams in the last 100 years. Another was the coaches's abilities to inspire and motivate their teams.

Social media is awash in inspirational and motivational quotes, such as on #fitspiration, #instaquotes, #mondaymotivation (and to be fair, sometimes I do need some extra motivation on Mondays!). The Oxford dictionary defines *inspiration* as "the process of being mentally stimulated to do or feel something." Inspiration is a momentary spark in a willingness to engage. But, like lighting a match, unfortunately it fizzles rather quickly. You can't rely on constantly lighting matches to achieve your dreams. But inspiration can quickly lead to motivation, which Oxford says is a "desire or willingness to do something." Motivation is enthusiasm. It's a slower-burning form of inspiration that keeps you moving forward for a little while. But the embers of motivation inevitably burn out as well. You won't be inspired and motivated every day. Inspiration and motivation don't make great leaders; they don't pay the bills. Discipline does. Inspiration and motivation act as catalysts to help develop the discipline you need to show up every day, to train hard, to eat right, to prioritize recovery, to get your sleep, and to build the right mindset. Discipline is crucial to success in sport (or any domain), but it, too, is not a limitless resources. You don't have an endless supply of discipline (not even Jocko Willink has an endless supply!). If you always require discipline to show up to the gym or make it to late-night training sessions, you'd never realize your dream. But discipline helps you to build habits, and habits are where the difference is made.

In psychology, habits are defined as actions triggered automatically in response to contextual cues. For example, putting on your seatbelt (action) after you get into the car (contextual cue). Simply repeating this task over and over again in the same context leads to the action being triggered by simply sitting in your car. You don't need inspiration, you don't need motivation, and you don't need discipline; you've built a habit through associative learning.[15] It's just like brushing your teeth, washing the dishes, taking the dog for a walk, and what have you. If you can get to the point where an external cue is sufficient to trigger the action, you no longer need strong motivation or discipline to accomplish the task.[16] You just do it; it's automatic. It's also highly beneficial from a cognitive standpoint, because it frees up more space in your brain's "hard drive" to store more information.[17]

If you're depending on motivation to get you through, it's going to be tough sledding. Motivation comes and goes. Motivation is dynamic and constantly changing, like the weather. So what will you do to get the job done on cloudy and rainy days? (In sport and in life, there are lots of cloudy days!) Repeating a single action in a specific context is the ideal scenario for building habits. Habits ingrain automaticity; you just do it. For example, if every morning you get up and exercise, it becomes part of your routine. Eventually, you don't need motivation or discipline to get out of bed early to hit the gym; you just do it because you've always done it. Once you've achieved automaticity, it starts to feel strange or uncomfortable if you deviate from the norm. This is how great leaders and high achievers across all domains in life propel themselves above the rest.

The research confirms how habit-forming advice, paired with a small-changes approach, can help make new behaviors second nature. In one study, volunteers wanting to lose weight were randomized to a habit-based intervention — centered on diet, activity behaviors, and encouraging context-dependent repetition — or a no-treatment waiting-list control. After eight weeks, the intervention group had lost 2 kg compared with 0.4 kg in the control group. At 32 weeks, the intervention group had lost an average of 3.8 kg.[18] More important, the qualitative interview data revealed that automaticity had developed: behaviors had become ingrained. The authors noted how new habit-based advice "wormed its

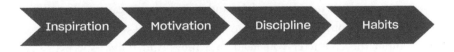

**FIGURE 12.1.** The Roadmap from Inspiration to Habit.

## Insights from the Best in the World

Elite strength coaches and practitioners are always thinking about problems from multiple perspectives and looking for expertise in other fields. Take, for example, experts Charlie Weingroff and Tim DiFrancesco. Weingroff has been working with elite and professional athletes in the NBA, NFL, MLB and more for almost two decades. He has learned a lot along the journey. What wisdom would he pass along to young coaches and practitioners? First, learn from observation. See how someone else does it successfully and learn from it. It's not enough to simply read about it or study it in-depth. Next, look to other areas of expertise to solve a problem, because you'll likely always default to looking at the dilemma through the lens of your profession. A strength coach sees a strength problem; a therapist sees a movement dysfunction; a nutritionist sees a deficiency. There may be an easier solution in another domain. Finally, don't be afraid to lose the battle to win the war. Weingroff's years of experience have taught him that he doesn't always need to win the day; rather, he keeps focused on the bigger picture so that the inevitable roadblocks along the way won't derail him from achieving his goal.

Tim DiFrancesco is the former head strength and conditioning coach for the NBA's Los Angeles Lakers. He's worked with NBA legends, including Kobe Bryant and Steve Nash, and has seen for himself the Hall of Fame-caliber work ethic, discipline, and authenticity these players brought to their teams. Tim offers three key pieces of advice to young trainers. First, be willing to take risks. You may have to sleep on your friend's couch for six months to take that unpaid internship, but if it gets you closer to your goal, it's likely worth the challenge. Next, understand you will make sacrifices along the way. Tim says bluntly, "You're going to have to eat some sh*t sandwiches in your career." That is, not all jobs and tasks are enviable or sexy, but that they help build the character you need to achieve and *sustain* success.

Finally, Tim emphasizes the power of always learning from every challenging scenario or hurdle in your journey. What lesson can it teach you so that it can help you now and when you're further along in your career?

Great perspectives and authentic answers from two of the best strength and conditioning coaches in the world!

way into your brain" so that participants "felt quite strange" if they did not do them. Actions that initially required motivation, that were difficult to stick to, became much easier to maintain. A larger randomized controlled trial is currently underway to test the efficacy of this intervention; it will be delivered in a primary care setting to a larger sample over a 24-month follow-up period.[19] Nevertheless, these early results indicate that habit-forming processes transfer to the everyday environment, and they suggest habit-formation advice offers an evidence-based strategy for promoting long-term behavior change.[20]

Of course, a lot of myths still exist when it comes to developing habits. Does it really take 21 days to form a habit? Nope. Strangely, researchers found this common myth stems from plastic surgery patients who typically need three weeks to adjust to their new appearance. Automaticity typically reaches its peak around 66 days, which means it takes just over two months to build a habit (although experts admit there is large interindividual variation).[21] The most important point experts hammer home is that as habits become more familiar and automated, they require far less motivation and discipline to continue doing them. This is the ultimate goal. No more waking up frantically looking for #instaquotes and #fitspiration. You've downloaded the habits onto your real hardware; you're good to go! This is highly reassuring to an athlete who is in the process of adopting a new nutrition regime, a weight-loss client who is struggling to achieve their goals, or a coach who is trying to develop new routines in the team. It also explains how so many elite athletes (or entrepreneurs, CEOs, executives, and parents) can wake up before the sunrise to get their training in; they're not always inherently motivated or disciplined to train, but they've logged enough hours that it's now programmed into their routine.

What common theme did Sam Walker find amongst the 16 greatest teams in sports history? Exactly one: the team captain. These legendary players developed the traits of great captains — extreme doggedness, willingness to do thankless jobs, ironclad emotional control, and the ability to motivate others with nonverbal displays, just to name a few — through decades of disciplined practice. Walker's research revealed the crucial ingredient in a team to achieve greatness was the character of the *player* leading it. Of course, a coach's ability to inspire and motivate is also important, and in fact can be truly life-changing.

## Why Great Coaches Matter

In 2018, big sporting events such as the Winter Olympics in South Korea and the World Cup in Russia brought a lot of attention to political divisions in the world and how sport can help bring people together. It's a common mantra: sport connects people. Nelson Mandela believed in the power of sport, saying, "Sport can create hope where once was only despair." Sport is heralded as an anticrime strategy, a public health policy, and an activity that boosts education outcomes. It's a wonderful narrative, but is it evidence-based? Unfortunately, if left in the wrong hands, experts have also found that sport can teach children, teens, and young adults to cheat, disrespect opponents and authority, and can exacerbate social divisions. This is what Greenhouse Sports, a charity-based organization in London, has learned after more than a decade and a half trying to change young lives through sport. The U.K. government ramped up funding for youth sports in the lead-up to the 2012 Olympic Games in an effort to boost participation in sport. Yet despite accomplishing this goal (and filling up the attendance in sport classes and camps) there was little long-term enthusiasm from the youngsters themselves. How was this possible? Doesn't sport inspire and motivate kids? Unfortunately, standing around waiting for an inattentive "coach" to tell kids what to do for an hour is hardly life-changing. Not surprisingly, reports from a leading think tank emerged suggesting the government was "funding sport for sport's sake."

Renowned journalist Matthew Syed of the *Times* (London) shed light on what really matters in shaping the lives of young people.[22] Turns out it's not the sport itself but the people leading them: the coaches. Syed tells the story of Sullivan Morris, a 13-year-old kid living in a low-income council flat in

## Take Care of Coach, Too

Coaches, trainers, therapists, and other sport practitioners need to take care of themselves as they serve their athletes or team. It's not just the players who must be healthy to perform their best; coaches, too, must be healthy. But the stress and rigors of coaching professional sport can make this incredibly difficult. Former NBA head coach Steve Clifford of the Charlotte Hornets found this out the hard way. In 2017, on a road trip to face the Toronto Raptors, Clifford was struck with an agonizingly painful headache. He had struggled with migraines for years, more or less controlling them with medications. But during the episode in Toronto, his head began pounding like it was going to explode. He couldn't sleep, he couldn't think, he couldn't even drive his car home from the airport after the long trip due to the unrelenting pain. Clifford hit his breaking point and finally went in to see a doctor. After consulting with an expert neurologist, he was told by the specialist, "Your body is saying enough is enough!" After 18 seasons of coaching, almost two decades of pushing the pedal to the metal, the doctor's opinion was that the migraines were a result of the massive stress on his body.[23] Clifford had been getting less than 5 hours of sleep per night for months, trading sleep for more hours analyzing game tape on the charter flights until the early hours of the morning. The doctor's solution for the migraines was simple: get more sleep and learn to relax. "Good nutrition and hydration are important, but nothing beats sleep," said the neurologist. He also advised Clifford to find another outlet in life. His brain needed the opportunity to relax; everything couldn't be about basketball. Extreme migraines are the body's way of saying, "It's time to make a change." The neurologist also noted that he saw the same thing in countless executives who logged long hours and traded sleep time for more time at the desk. Today, Clifford is the first to admit the problem. "I had to change not just my job, but how I live," he said. After taking a leave of absence from coaching the Charlotte Hornets, he resolved his chronic migraines. Clifford is now healthy and back in the NBA as the head coach of the Orlando Magic.

the west of London, who was about to be expelled from his local school for bad behavior. Then, out of the blue, Morris's attitude seemed to change; he was suddenly always on time for school, he was unexpectedly helpful and upbeat, and his work ethic increased dramatically. Syed wondered how a young man who seemed destined for prison could now be aiming for university. A local ping-pong project was credited with turning around his life, but Syed dug a little deeper and uncovered that "the real catalyst was his coach." Although Jason Sugrue was a skillful ping-pong coach, the sport itself didn't change Morris's life. "Sugrue was patient, charismatic, and had a wonderful ability to see the world through his student's eyes," says Syed. The coach taught his students to respect the rules, respect their opponents, and develop discipline. The coach strongly believed that discipline was required to build the right habits and to succeed. When Syed asked the students what made the difference for them overcoming obstacles in their life to achieve academic and life success, they didn't mention table tennis at all. "Coach made me believe in myself," they replied. Good coaches matter. In sport (and in life), people make the difference.

## Leadership Solutions

The ability to see things from the other person's point of view is essential for developing wise-reasoning skills and wisdom (despite a potential lack of experience). And while trust is an attribute of great leaders, it cannot be forced; showing vulnerability and being authentic are critical parts of the trust-building process. Successful cultures put team goals first and look for active participation from all staff and players. And great players, coaches, and practitioners don't wait for inspiration; they get to work and develop the discipline required to build automaticity and habits. So, in the end, we still wonder: Are great leaders born or made? Either way, it benefits athletes to improve communication, connection, and a culture of support to propel themselves toward unparalleled success!

# Conclusion

The evolution of high performance is where several paradigms meet. The overlapping areas of health, nutrition, training, recovery, and mental performance is where the leading experts are looking for the next big breakthrough in athlete performance. Upgrading your expert-generalist skills — even if you're already a specialist in a specific area — will help you build a robust foundation from which to support your clients, athletes, and teams. It will allow you to pull from their experience across multiple fields to make connections where others cannot. It will enable you to communicate in news ways to elevate your individual performance, and ultimately your contribution to the team. The expert-generalist studies widely across many different fields, understands the fundamentals and deeper principles that link them, and then applies these principles to their area of specialty. A century of specialization has yielded previously unthinkable rewards for human health and performance, but it's also left deep trenches between these areas of expertise that still need to be filled. Daring to be more of an expert-generalist provides the opportunity to bridge those wide gaps, communicate with specialists so as to connect isolated silos, and potentially unearth the next big breakthrough in athletic performance. An evidence-based brigade of athletes, coaches, and practitioners: This is the new frontier.

*Genius is one percent inspiration and
ninety-nine percent perspiration.*

— THOMAS A. EDISON, INVENTOR


*Without self-discipline,
success is impossible, period.*

— LOU HOLTZ, COACH


*Excellence is not an act, it's a habit.*

— WILL DURANT, PHILOSOPHER


*Wisdom is always an overmatch for strength.*

— PHIL JACKSON, COACH


*My ego demands — for myself —
the success of my team.*

— BILL RUSSELL, ATHLETE

# NOTES

## Introduction: The Revolution in Performance

1. Joseph J. Fins, "The expert-generalist: a contradiction whose time has come," *Academic Medicine* 90, no. 8 (2015), https://doi.org/10.1097/acm.0000000000000798.
2. Joseph J. Fins, "The expert-generalist."
3. David Oliver, "Celebrating the expert generalist," *BMJ* 354 (2016), https://doi.org/10.1136/bmj.i3701.
4. Scott Barry Kaufmann, "Creativity is much more than 10,000 hours of deliberate practice," *Scientific American*, April 2016.

## Chapter 1: Sleep and Circadian Rhythms

1. Shalini Paruthi et al., "Consensus Statement of the American Academy of Sleep Medicine on the recommended amount of sleep for healthy children: methodology and discussion," *Journal of Clinical Sleep Medicine* 12, no. 11 (2016), http://dx.doi.org/10.5664/jcsm.6288.
2. Nathaniel F. Watson et al., "Joint Consensus Statement of the American Academy of Sleep Medicine and Sleep Research Society on the recommended amount of sleep for healthy adult: methodology and discussion," *Sleep* 38, no. 8 (2015), http://doi.org/10.5665/sleep.4886.
3. Michael A. Grandner et al., "Mortality associated with short sleep duration: the evidence, the possible mechanisms, and the future," *Sleep Medicine Reviews* 14, no. 3 (2010), https://doi.org/10.1016/j.smrv.2009.07.006.
4. N. S. Simpson, E. L. Gibbs, and G. O. Matheson, "Optimizing sleep to maximize performance: implications and recommendations for elite athletes," *Scandinavian Journal of Medicine and Science in Sports* 27, no. 3 (2017), https://doi.org/10.1111/sms.12703; Andrew M. Watson, "Sleep and athletic performance," *Current Sports Medicine Reports* 16, no. 6 (2017), http://dx.doi.org/10.1249/jsr.0000000000000418.
5. Cheri D. Mah et al., "The effects of sleep extension on the athletic performance of collegiate basketball players," *Sleep* 34, no. 7 (2011), https://dx.doi.org/10.5665%2FSLEEP.1132.
6. Luke Gupta, Kevin Morgan, and Sarah Gilchrit, "Does elite sport degrade sleep quality? A systematic review," *Sports Medicine* 47, no. 7 (2017), https://dx.doi.org/10.1007/s40279-016-0650-6.
7. R. E. Venter, "Role of sleep in performance and recovery of athletes: a review article," *South African Journal for Research in Sport, Physical Education and Recreation* 34, no.1 (2012), https://doi.org/10.1007/s40279-016-0650-6.
8. Jonathan Leeder et al., "Sleep duration and quality in elite athletes measured using wristwatch actigraphy," *Journal of Sports Sciences* 30, no. 6 (2012), https://doi.org/10.1080/02640414.2012.660188.
9. Matthew Walker, *Why We Sleep* (St. Ives, U.K.: Allen Lane, 2017), 360.
10. Matthew Walker, *Why We Sleep.*
11. Nathan W. Pitchford et al., "Sleep quality but not quantity altered with a change in training environment in elite Australian Rules football players," *International Journal of Sports Physiology and Performance* 12, no. 1 (2017), https://doi.org/10.1123/ijspp.2016-0009; Andrew Watson et al., "Subjective well-being and training load predict in-season injury and illness risk in female youth soccer players," *British Journal of Sports Medicine* 51, no. 3 (2017), https://doi.org/10.1136/bjsports-2016-096584.
12. Christophe Hausswirth et al., "Evidence of disturbed sleep and increased illness in overreached endurance athletes," *Medicine and Science in Sports and Exercise* 46, no. 5 (2014), https://doi.org/10.1249/MSS.0000000000000177.

13. Charli Sargent et al., "The impact of training schedules on the sleep and fatigue of elite athletes," *Chronobiology International* 31, no. 10 (2014), https://doi.org/10.3109/07420528.2014.957306.

14. Charli Sargent and Gregory D. Roach, "Sleep duration is reduced in elite athletes following night-time competition," *Chronobiology International* 33, no. 6 (2016), https://doi.org/10.3109/07420528.2016.1167715.

15. Hugh H. K. Fullagar et al., "Sleep and athletic performance: the effects of sleep loss on exercise performance, and physiological and cognitive responses to exercise," *Sports Medicine* 45, no. 2 (2015), https://doi.org/10.1007/s40279-014-0260-0.

16. Haresh T. Suppiah, Chee Yong Low, and Michael Chia, "Effects of sport-specific training intensity on sleep patterns and psychomotor performance in adolescent athletes," *Pediatric Exercise Science* 28, no. 4 (2016), https://doi.org/10.1123/pes.2015-0205.

17. Hugh H. K. Fullagar et al., "Sleep and recovery in team sport: current sleep-related issues facing professional team-sport athletes," *International Journal of Sports Physiology and Performance* 10, no. 8 (2015), https://doi.org/10.1123/ijspp.2014-0565.

18. Ricardo Brandt, Guilherme G. Bevilacqua, and Alexandro Andrade, "Perceived sleep quality, mood states, and their relationship with performance among Brazilian elite athletes during a competitive period," *Journal of Strength and Conditioning Research* 31, no. 4 (2017), https://doi.org/10.1519/JSC.0000000000001551.

19. Lee Taylor et al., "The importance of monitoring sleep within adolescent athletes: athletic, academic, and health considerations," *Frontiers in Physiology* 7 (2016), https://doi.org/10.3389/fphys.2016.00101.

20. S. Hakki Onen et al., "The effects of total sleep deprivation, selective sleep interruption and sleep recovery on pain tolerance thresholds in healthy subjects," *Journal of Sleep Research* 10, no. 1 (2001), https://doi.org/10.1046/j.1365-2869.2001.00240.x.

21. Matthew D. Milewski et al., "Chronic lack of sleep is associated with increased sports injuries in adolescent athletes," *Journal of Pediatric Orthopedics* 34, no. 2 (2014), https://doi.org/10.1097/BPO.0000000000000151.

22. F. P. Cappuccio et al., "Sleep duration and all-cause mortality: a systematic review and meta-analysis of prospective studies," *Sleep* 33, no. 5 (2010), https://doi.org/10.1111/j.1365-2869.2008.00732.x.

23. P. von Rosen et al., "Multiple factors explain injury risk in adolescent elite athletes: applying a biopsychosocial perspective," *Scandinavian Journal of Medicine and Science in Sports* 27, no. 12 (2017), https://doi.org/10.1111/sms.12855.

24. Sheldon Cohen et al., "Sleep habits and susceptibility to the common cold," *Archives of Internal Medicine* 169, no. 1 (2009), https://doi.org/10.1001/archinternmed.2008.505; Aric A. Prather et al., "Behaviorally assessed sleep and susceptibility to the common cold," *Sleep* 38, no. 9 (2015), https://doi.org/10.5665/sleep.4968.

25. Sheldon Cohen et al., "Sleep habits and susceptibility."

26. Christine Benedict et al., "Acute sleep deprivation has no lasting effects on the human antibody titer response following a novel influenza A H1N1 virus vaccination," *BMC Immunology* 13, no. 1 (2012), https://doi.org/10.1186/1471-2172-13-1.

27. John D. Chase et al., "One night of sleep restriction following heavy exercise impairs 3-km cycling time-trial performance in the morning," *Applied Physiology, Nutrition, and Metabolism* 42, no. 9 (2017), https://doi.org/10.1139/apnm-2016-0698.

28. O. Azboy and Z. Kaygisiz, "Effects of sleep deprivation on cardiorespiratory functions of the runners and volleyball players during rest and exercise," *Acta Physiologica Hungarica* 96, no. 1 (2009), https://doi.org/10.1556/APhysiol.96.2009.1.3.

29. Samuel J. Oliver et al., "One night of sleep deprivation decreases treadmill endurance performance," *European Journal of Applied Physiology* 107, no. 2 (2009), https://doi.org/10.1007/s00421-009-1103-9.

30. Morteza Taheri and Elaheh Arabameri, "The effect of sleep deprivation on choice reaction time and anaerobic power of college student athletes," *Asian Journal of Sports Medicine* 3, no. 1 (2012), https://doi.org/10.5812/asjsm.34719.

31. F. Mougin et al., "Influence of partial sleep deprivation on athletic performance," *Science and Sports* 5, no. 2 (1990), https://doi.org/10.1016/S0765-1597(05)80210-2.

32. Melissa Skein et al., "Intermittent-sprint performance and muscle glycogen after 30 h of sleep deprivation," *Medicine and Science in Sports and Exercise* 43, no. 7 (2011), https://doi.org/10.1249/MSS.0b013e31820abc5a.

33. Namni Goel et al., "Neurocognitive consequences of sleep deprivation," *Seminars in Neurology* 29, no. 4 (2009), https://doi.org/10.1055/s-0029-1237117.

34. Kalina R. Rossa et al., "The effects of sleep restriction on executive inhibitory control and affect in young adults," *Journal of Adolescent Health* 55, no. 2 (2014), https://doi.org/10.1016/j.jadohealth.2013.12.034.

35. L. A. Reyner and J. A. Horne, "Sleep restriction and serving accuracy in performance tennis players, and effects of caffeine," *Physiology and Behaviour* 120, no. 15 (2013), https://doi.org/10.1016/j.physbeh.2013.07.002.

36. Benjamin J. Edwards and Jim Waterhouse, "Effects of one night of partial sleep deprivation upon diurnal rhythms of accuracy and consistency in throwing darts," *Chronobiology International* 26, no. 4 (2009), https://doi.org/10.1080/07420520902929037.

37. Gregory Belenky et al., "Patterns of performance degradation and restoration during sleep restriction and subsequent recovery: a sleep dose-response study," *Journal of Sleep Research* 12, no. 1 (2003), https://doi.org/10.1046/j.1365-2869.2003.00337.x.

38. Hans P. A. Van Dongen et al., "Systematic interindividual differences in neurobehavioral impairment from sleep loss: evidence of trait-like differential vulnerability," *Sleep* 27, no. 3 (2004), https://doi.org/10.1093/sleep/27.3.423.

39. Frank. A. J. Scheer et al., "Impact of the human circadian system, exercise, and their interaction on cardiovascular function," *Proceedings of the National Academy of Sciences of the United States of America* 107, no. 47 (2010), https://doi.org/10.1073/pnas.1006749107.

40. B. Drust et al., "Circadian rhythms in sports performance: an update," *Chronobiology International* 22, no. 1 (2005), https://doi.org/10.1081/CBI-200041039; Roger S. Smith and Thomas P. Reilly, "Athletic Performance," in *Sleep Deprivation: Clinical Issues, Pharmacology, and Sleep Loss Effects*, ed. Clete A. Kushida (New York: Marcel Dekker, 2005), 313-34.

41. Roger S. Smith et al., "The impact of circadian misalignment on athletic performance in professional football players," *Sleep* 36, no. 12 (2013), https://doi.org/10.5665/sleep.3248.

42. Michele Lastella, "Athlete chronotypes: performance and coaching implications," *Dr. Bubbs Performance Podcast*, Podcast audio, July 17, 2018, https://drbubbs.com/season-2-podcast-episodes/2018/7/s2-episode-28-athlete-chronotypes-performance-coaching-implications-w-dr-michele-lastella-phd.

43. D. W. Hill et al., "Effect of time of day on aerobic and anaerobic responses to high-intensity exercise," *Canadian Journal of Sport Sciences* 17, no. 4 (1992).

44. M. G. Figueiro et al., "The impact of light from computer monitors on melatonin levels in college students," *Neuro Endocrinology Letters* 32, no. 2 (2011).

45. J. Waterhouse, T. Reilly, and B. Edwards, "The stress of travel," *Journal of Sports Sciences* 22, no. 10 (2004), https://doi.org/10.1080/02640410400000264.

46. J. Waterhouse, T. Reilly, and B. Edwards, "The stress of travel."

47. Charmane I. Eastman and Helen J. Burgess, "How to travel the world without jet lag," *Sleep Medicine Clinics* 4, no. 2 (2009), https://doi.org/10.1016/j.jsmc.2009.02.006.

48. Brendan Kennedy, "MLB's exemption rate for ADHD drugs 'highly suspicious,'" *Toronto Star*, April 20, 2015.

49. Charles F. P. George et al., "Sleep and breathing in professional football players," *Sleep Medicine* 4, no. 4 (2003), https://doi.org/10.1016/S1389-9457(03)00113-8.

50. S. B. R. Fagundes et al., "Prevalence of restless legs syndrome in runners," *Sleep Medicine* 13, no. 6 (2012), https://doi.org/10.1016/j.sleep.2012.01.001.

51. Luke Gupta, Kevin Morgan, and Sarah Gilchrit, "Does elite sport degrade sleep quality?"
52. Maurice Ohayon et al., "National Sleep Foundation's sleep quality recommendations: first report," *Sleep Health* 3, no. 1 (2017), https://doi.org/10.1016/j.sleh.2016.11.006.
53. Derk-Jan Dijk and Simon N. Archer, "Light, sleep, and circadian rhythms: together again," *PLoS Biology* 7, no. 6 (2009), https://doi.org/10.1371/journal.pbio.1000145.
54. Amy M. Bender et al., "The clinical validation of the Athlete Sleep Screening Questionnaire: an instrument to identify athletes that need further sleep assessment," *Sports Medicine – Open* 4, no. 1 (2018), https://doi.org/10.1186/s40798-018-0140-5.
55. N. S. Simpson, E. L. Gibbs, and G. O. Matheson, "Optimizing sleep"; Andrew M. Watson, "Sleep and athletic performance," *Current Sports Medicine Reports* 16, no. 6 (2017), http://dx.doi .org/10.1249/jsr.0000000000000418.
56. Amber Brooks and Leon Lack, "A brief afternoon nap following nocturnal sleep restriction: which nap duration is most recuperative?" *Sleep* 29, no. 6 (2006), https://doi.org/10.1093/sleep/29.6.831.
57. Robert L. Sack, "Jet lag," *The New England Journal of Medicine* 362, no. 5 (2010), https://doi.org /10.1056/NEJMcp0909838.

## Chapter 2: The Athlete Microbiome

1. Mirjana Rajilić-Stojanović and Willem M. de Vos, "The first 1000 cultured species of the human gastrointestinal microbiota," *FEMS Microbiology Reviews 38*, no. 5 (2014), https://doi .org/10.1111/1574-6976.12075; Junhua Li et al., "An integrated catalog of reference genes in the human gut microbiome," *Nature Biotechnology* 32 (2014), https://doi.org/10.1038/nbt.2942.
2. Yang-fan Nie et al., "Cross-talk between bile acids and intestinal microbiota in host metabolism and health," *Journal of Zhejiang University-SCIENCE B* 16, no. 6 (2015), https://doi.org/10.1631/jzus .b1400327; J. K. Nicholson et al., "Host-gut microbiota metabolic interactions," *Science* 336, no. 6086 (2012), https://doi.org/10.1126/science.1223813; Hirosuke Sugahara et al., "Differences in folate production by bifidobacteria of different origins," *Bioscience of Microbiota, Food and Health* 34, no. 4 (2015), https://doi.org/10.12938/bmfh.2015-003; M. G. Marley, R. Meganathan, and Ronald Bentley, "Menaquinone (vitamin K$_2$) biosynthesis in Escherichia coli: Synthesis of o-Succinylbenzoate does not require the decarboxylase activity of the ketoglutarate dehydrogenase complex," *Biochemistry* 25, no. 6 (1986), https://doi.org/10.1021/bi00354a017; Catherine A. Lozupone et al., "Diversity, stability and resilience of the human gut microbiota," *Nature* 489, no. 7415 (2012), https://doi.org/10.1038/nature11550; G. Vighi et al., "Allergy and the gastrointestinal system," *Clinical and Experimental Immunology* 153 (2008), https://doi.org/10.1111/j.1365-2249.2008.03713.x; Lora V. Hooper, "Commensal host-bacterial relationships in the gut," *Science* 292, no. 5519 (2001), https://doi.org/10.1126/science.1058709; Jianxiong Xu et al., "Regulation of an antioxidant blend on intestinal redox status and major microbiota in early weaned piglets," *Nutrition* 30, no. 5 (2014), https://doi.org/10.1016/j.nut.2013.10.018.
3. Anastassia Gorvitovskaia, Susan P. Holmes, and Susan M. Huse, "Interpreting Prevotella and Bacteroides as biomarkers of diet and lifestyle," *Microbiome* 4, no. 1 (2016), https://doi.org /10.1186/s40168-016-0160-7.
4. Peter J. Turnbaugh et al., "An obesity-associated gut microbiome with increased capacity for energy harvest," *Nature* 21 (2006), https://doi.org/10.1038/nature05414.
5. Brian W. Parks et al., "Genetic control of obesity and gut microbiota composition in response to high-fat, high-sucrose diet in mice," *Cell Metabolism* 17, no. 1 (2013), https://doi.org/10.1016/j .cmet.2012.12.007; Elin Org et al., "Genetic and environmental control of host-gut microbiota interactions," *Genome Research* 25, no. 10 (2015), https://doi.org/10.1101/gr.194118.115.
6. Frances Collins et al., "A vision for the future of genomics research," *Nature* 422, no. 6934 (2003), https://doi.org/10.1038/nature01626.
7. Frances Collins et al., "A vision for the future."
8. David Zeevi et al., "Personalized nutrition by prediction of glycemic responses," *Cell* 163, no. 5 (2015), https://doi.org/10.1016/j.cell.2015.11.001.

9. Raul Y. Tito et al., "Insights from characterizing extinct human gut microbiomes," *PLoS ONE* 7, no. 12 (2012), https://doi.org/10.1371/journal.pone.0051146.

10. Raul Y. Tito et al., "Insights from characterizing."

11. Stephanie L. Schnorr et al., "Gut microbiome of the Hadza hunter-gatherers," *Nature Communications* 5, no. 1 (2014), https://doi.org/10.1038/ncomms4654.

12. Justin Sonnenburg, "Your Microbiome: What Is It, and How Can It Help or Hurt You?," YouTube, May 30, 2017, www.youtube.com/watch?v=EAvL0md46_M; Carlotta De Filippo et al., "Impact of diet in shaping gut microbiota revealed by a comparative study in children from Europe and rural Africa," *Proceedings of the National Academy of Sciences* 107, no. 33 (2010), https://doi.org/10.1073/pnas.1005963107.

13. Justin Sonnebury, "Your Microbiome"; Carlotta De Filippo et al., "Impact of Diet."

14. Carlos Augusto Monteiro et al., "The UN Decade of Nutrition, the NOVA food classification and the trouble with ultra-processing." *Public Health Nutrition* 21, no.1 (2017), https://doi.org/10.1017/s1368980017000234.

15. Alexandra Sifferlin, "Here's what eating nothing but McDonalds for 10 days does to your gut bacteria," *Time Magazine*, May 11, 2015.

16. Tim Spector, "What a hunter-gatherer diet does to the body in just three days," *CNN Health*, July 5, 2017, https://edition.cnn.com/2017/07/05/health/hunter-gatherer-diet-tanzania-the-conversation/index.html.

17. Michael W. Gray, Gertraud Burger, and B. Franz Lang, "The origin and early evolution of mitochondria," *Genome Biology* 2, no. 6 (2001), https://doi.org/10.1186/gb-2001-2-6-reviews1018.

18. C. G. Kurland and S. G. E. Andersson, "Origin and evolution of the mitochondrial proteome," *Microbiology and Molecular Biology Reviews* 64, no. 4 (2000), https://doi.org/10.1128/mmbr.64.4.786-820.2000.

19. Liping Zhao, "Genomics: the tale of our other genome," *Nature* 465, no.7300 (2010), https://doi.org/10.1038/465879a.

20. Walid Mottawea et al., "Altered intestinal microbiota–host mitochondria crosstalk in new onset Crohn's disease," *Nature Communications* 7 (2016), https://doi.org/10.1038/ncomms13419.

21. Dallas R. Donohoe et al., "The microbiome and butyrate regulate energy metabolism and autophagy in the mammalian colon," *Cell Metabolism* 13, no. 5 (2011), https://doi.org/10.1016/j.cmet.2011.02.018.

22. Z. Gao et al., "Butyrate improves insulin sensitivity and increases energy expenditure in mice," *Diabetes* 58, no. 7 (2009), https://doi.org/10.2337/db08-1637; Maria Pina Mollica et al., "Butyrate regulates liver mitochondrial function, efficiency, and dynamic, in insulin resistant obese mice," *Diabetes* 66, no. 5 (2017), https://doi.org/10.2337/db16-0924.

23. Gijs den Besten et al., "The role of short-chain fatty acids in the interplay between diet, gut microbiota, and host energy metabolism," *Journal of Lipid Research* 54, no. 9 (2013), https://doi.org/10.1194/jlr.r036012.

24. Siobhan F Clarke et al., "Exercise and associated dietary extremes impact on gut microbial diversity," *Gut* 63, no.12 (2014), https://doi.org/10.1136/gutjnl-2013-306541.

25. Joep Grootjans et al., "Human intestinal ischemia-reperfusion–induced inflammation characterized," *The American Journal of Pathology* 176, no. 5 (2010), https://doi.org/10.2353/ajpath.2010.091069; Mark A. Febbraio and Bente Klarlund Pedersen, "Muscle-derived interleukin-6: mechanisms for activation and possible biological roles," *The FASEB Journal* 16, no. 11 (2002), https://doi.org/10.1096/fj.01-0876rev.

26. Allison Clark and Núria Mach, "Exercise-induced stress behavior, gut-microbiota-brain axis and diet: a systematic review for athletes," *Journal of the International Society of Sports Nutrition* 13, no. 1 (2016), https://doi.org/10.1186/s12970-016-0155-6.

27. M. Y. Zeng, N. Inohara, and G. Nuñez, "Mechanisms of inflammation-driven bacterial dysbiosis in the gut," *Mucosal Immunology* 10, no. 1 (2017), https://doi.org/10.1038/mi.2016.75.

28. Masaki Igarashi and Leonard Guarente, "mTORC1 and SIRT1 cooperate to foster expansion of gut adult stem cells during calorie restriction," *Cell* 166, no. 2 (2016), https://doi.org/10.1016/j .cell.2016.05.044.

29. Elodie Lobet, Jean-Jacques Letesson, and Thierry Arnould, "Mitochondria: a target for bacteria," *Biochemical Pharmacology* 94, no. 3 (2015), https://doi.org/10.1016/j.bcp.2015.02.007.

30. Elodie Lobet, Jean-Jacques Letesson, and Thierry Arnould, "Mitochondria."

31. David B. Pyne et al., "Probiotics supplementation for athletes — clinical and physiological effects," *European Journal of Sport Science* 15, no. 1 (2015), https://doi.org/10.1080/17461391.20 14.97187.

32. Lauren Petersen (Associate Research Scientist, Athlete Microbiome Project, Jackson Laboratory, Sacramento, CA), in discussion with the author, March 8, 2018.

33. Orla O'Sullivan et al., "Exercise and the microbiota," *Gut Microbes* 6, no. 2 (2015), https://doi.org /10.1080/19490976.2015.1011875.

34. Timothy Wai and Thomas Langer, "Mitochondrial dynamics and metabolic regulation," *Trends in Endocrinology and Metabolism* 27, no. 2 (2016), https://doi.org/10.1016/j.tem.2015.12.001.

35. Núria Mach and Dolors Fuster-Botella, "Endurance exercise gut microbiota: a review," *Journal of Sport and Health Science* 6, no. 2 (2017), https://doi.org/10.1016/j.jshs.2016.05.001.

36. D. R. Green, L. Galluzzi, and G. Kroemer, "Mitochondria and the autophagy–inflammation–cell death axis in organismal aging," *Science* 333, no. 6046 (2011), https://doi.org/10.1126/ science.1201940.

37. Benjamin I. Rapoport, "Metabolic factors limiting performance in marathon runners. *PLoS Computational Biology* 6, no. 10 (2010), https://doi.org/10.1371/journal.pcbi.1000960.

38. Stephane Palazzetti et al., "Overloaded training increases exercise-induced oxidative stress and damage," *Canadian Journal of Applied Physiology* 28, no. 4 (2003), https://doi.org/10.1139 /h03-045.

39. Ergün Sahin et al., "Telomere dysfunction induces metabolic and mitochondrial compromise," *Nature* 470, no. 7355 (2011), https://doi.org/10.1038/nature10223.

40. Núria Mach et al., "Understanding the response to endurance exercise using a systems biology approach: combining blood metabolomics, transcriptomics and miRNomics in horses," *BMC Genomics* 18, no 1 (2017), https://doi.org/10.1186/s12864-017-3571-3.

41. A. Maleah Holland et al., "Influence of endurance exercise training on antioxidant enzymes, tight junction proteins, and inflammatory markers in the rat ileum," *BMC Res Notes* 8, no. 1 (2015), https://doi.org/10.1186/s13104-015-1500-6.

42. Kelsey Fisher-Wellman and Richard J Bloomer, "Acute exercise and oxidative stress: a 30 year history," *Dynnamic Medicine* 8, no. 1 (2009), https://doi.org/10.1186/1476-5918-8-1.

43. Ian Spreadbury, "Comparison with ancestral diets suggests dense acellular carbohydrates promote an inflammatory microbiota, and may be the primary dietary cause of leptin resistance and obesity," *Diabetes, Metabolic Syndrome and Obesity: Targets and Therapy* 5 (2012), https://doi .org/10.2147/dmso.s33473.

44. Elliott D. Crouser et al., "Endotoxin-induced mitochondrial damage correlates with impaired respiratory activity," *Critical Care Medicine* 30, no. 2 (2002), https://doi.org/10.1097 /00003246-200202000-00002.

45. Agnieszka Mika and Monika Fleshner, "Early-life exercise may promote lasting brain and metabolic health through gut bacterial metabolites," *Immunology and Cell Biology* 94, no. 2 (2016), https://doi.org/10.1038/icb.2015.113.

46. Charlie T. Seto et al., "Prolonged use of a proton pump inhibitor reduces microbial diversity: implications for Clostridium difficile susceptibility," *Microbiome 2, no. 1* (2014), https://doi.org /10.1186/2049-2618-2-42.

47. Robin M. Voigt et al., "Circadian disorganization alters intestinal microbiota," *PLoS ONE* 9, no. 5 (2014), https://doi.org/10.1371/journal.pone.0097500.

48. Harry J. Flint et al., "Polysaccharide utilization by gut bacteria: potential for new insights from genomic analysis," *Nature Reviews Microbiology* 6, no. 2 (2008), https://doi.org/10.1038/nrmicro1817.

49. Nicholas P. West et al., "Lactobacillus fermentum (PCC®) supplementation and gastrointestinal and respiratory-tract illness symptoms: a randomised control trial in athletes," *Nutrition Journal* 10, no. 1 (2011), https://doi.org/10.1186/1475-2891-10-30.

50. Justin Sonnenburg, "Your Microbiome"; Carlotta De Filippo et al., "Impact of diet."

51. Miguel Toribio-Mateas, "Harnessing the power of microbiome assessment tools as part of neuroprotective nutrition and lifestyle medicine interventions," *Microorganisms* 6, no. 35 (2018), https://doi.org/10.3390/microorganisms6020035.

## Chapter 3: Blood Sugars and Longevity

1. Carlos Augusto Monteiro et al., "Household availability of ultra-processed foods and obesity in nineteen European countries," *Public Health Nutrition* 21, no. 1 (2017), https://doi.org/10.1017/s1368980017001379.

2. Ramachandran S. Vasan et al., "Residual lifetime risk for developing hypertension in middle-aged women and men: the Framingham Heart Study," *JAMA* 287, no. 8 (2002), https://doi.org/10.1001/jama.287.8.1003; Earl S. Ford et al., "Prevalence of the metabolic syndrome among US adults: findings from the third National Health and Nutrition Examination Survey," *JAMA* 287, no. 3 (2002), https://doi.org/10.1001/jama.287.3.356.

3. Andy Menke et al., "Prevalence of and trends in diabetes among adults in the United States," *JAMA* 314, no. 10 (2015), https://doi.org/10.1001/jama.2015.10029.

4. David K. Foot et al., "Demographics and cardiology, 1950-2050," *Journal of the American College of Cardiology* 35, no. 5 (2000), https://doi.org/10.1016/s0735-1097(00)80055-8.

5. J. V. Bjornholt et al., "Fasting blood glucose: An underestimated risk factor for cardiovascular death," *Diabetes Care* 22, no. 1 (1999), https://doi.org/10.2337/diacare.22.1.45; E. Eschwege, B. Balkau, and A. Fontbonne, "The epidemiology of coronary heart disease in glucose intolerant and diabetic subjects," *Journal of Internal Medicine, Supplement* 736 (1994).

6. J. H. Fuller et al., "Mortality from coronary heart disease and stroke in relation to degree of glycaemia: the Whitehall study," *BMJ* 287, no. 6396 (1983), https://doi.org/10.1136/bmj.287.6396.867.

7. Elizabeth Barrett-Connor et al., "Is borderline fasting hyperglycemia a risk factor for cardiovascular death?," *Journal of Chronic Diseases* 37, no. 9-10 (1984), https://doi.org/10.1016/0021-9681(84)90046-8.

8. F. S. Facchini et al., "Insulin resistance as a predictor of age-related diseases," *Journal of Clinical Endocrinology and Metabolism* 86, no. 8 (2001), https://doi.org/10.1210/jc.86.8.3574; Gerald M. Reaven, "Role of insulin resistance in human disease," *Diabetes* 37, no. 12 (1988) https://doi.org/10.2337/diab.37.12.1595.

9. The DECODE Study Group, "Is the current definition for diabetes relevant to mortality risk from all causes and cardiovascular and noncardiovascular diseases?," *Diabetes Care* 26, no. 3 (2003), https://doi.org/10.2337/diacare.26.3.688.

10. Sang-Wook Yi et al., "Association between fasting glucose and all-cause mortality according to sex and age: a prospective cohort study," *Scientific Reports* 7, no. 1 (2017), https://doi.org/10.1038/s41598-017-08498-6.

11. Kevin D. Hall, "Did the food environment cause the obesity epidemic?," *Obesity* 26, no. 1, (2018) https://doi.org/10.1002/oby.22073.

12. Emma J. Stinson et al., "High fat and sugar consumption during ad libitum intake predicts weight gain," *Obesity* 26, no. 4 (2018), https://doi.org/10.1002/oby.22124.

13. W. B. Kannel and D. L. McGee, "Diabetes and cardiovascular risk factors: the Framingham study," *Diabetes Care* 2, no. 2 (1979), https://doi.org/10.2337/diacare.2.2.120; J. Lindsay, "Risk factors for Alzheimer's disease: a prospective analysis from the Canadian Study of Health and Aging," *American Journal of Epidemiology* 156, no. 5 (2002), https://doi.org/10.1093/aje/kwf074; R. Doll,

"The age distribution of cancer: implications for models of carcinogenesis," *Journal of the Royal Statistical Society. Series A (General)* 134, no. 4 (1971), https://doi.org/10.2307/2343684.

14. S. J. Olshansky, "Position statement on human aging," *Science of Aging Knowledge Environment* 2002, no. 24 (2002), https://doi.org/10.1126/sageke.2002.24.pe9.

15. Ronald C. W. Ma, "Genetics of cardiovascular and renal complications in diabetes," *Journal of Diabetes Investigation* 7, no. 2 (2015), https://doi.org/10.1111/jdi.12391; The Emerging Risk Factors Collaboration, "Diabetes mellitus, fasting blood glucose concentration, and risk of vascular disease: a collaborative meta-analysis of 102 prospective studies," *Lancet* 375, no. 9733 (2010) https://doi .org/10.1016/s0140-6736(10)60484-9; Saion Chatterjee et al., "Type 2 diabetes as a risk factor for dementia in women compared with men: a pooled analysis of 2.3 million people comprising more than 100,000 cases of dementia," *Diabetes Care* (2015), https://doi.org/10.2337/dc15-1588.

16. B. Vodenik, J. Rovira, and J. M. Campistol, "Mammalian target of rapamycin and diabetes: what does the current evidence tell us?," *Transplantation Proceedings* 41, no. 6 (2009) https://doi.org /10.1016/j.transproceed.2009.06.159.

17. Nir Barzilai et al., "Metformin as a tool to target aging," *Cell Metabolism* 23, no. 6 (2016), https:// doi.org/10.1016/j.cmet.2016.05.011.

18. Gloria Formoso et al., "Decreased in vivo oxidative stress and decreased platelet activation following metformin treatment in newly diagnosed type 2 diabetic subjects," *Diabetes/Metabolism Research and Reviews* 24, no. 3 (2008), https://doi.org/10.1002/dmrr.794; Yong-Syu Lee et al., "Combined metformin and resveratrol confers protection against UVC-induced DNA damage in A549 lung cancer cells via modulation of cell cycle checkpoints and DNA repair," *Oncology Reports* 35, no. 6 (2016) https://doi.org/10.3892/or.2016.4740.

19. Alejandro Martin-Montalvo et al., "Metformin improves healthspan and lifespan in mice," *Nature Communications* 4, no. 1 (2013), https://doi.org/10.1038/ncomms3192.

20. C. A. Bannister et al., "Can people with type 2 diabetes live longer than those without? A comparison of mortality in people initiated with metformin or sulphonylurea monotherapy and matched, non-diabetic controls," *Diabetes, Obesity and Metabolism* 16, no. 11 (2014), https://doi.org /10.1111/dom.12354.

21. Ralph DeFronzo et al., "Metformin-associated lactic acidosis: current perspectives on causes and risk," *Metabolism* 65, no. 2 (2016), https://doi.org/10.1016/j.metabol.2015.10.014.

22. D. Grahame Hardie, Fiona A. Ross, and Simon A. Hawley, "AMPK: a nutrient and energy sensor that maintains energy homeostasis," *Nature Reviews Molecular Cell Biology* 13, no. 4 (2012), https:// doi.org/10.1038/nrm3311; Maria M. Mihaylova and Reuben J. Shaw, "The AMPK signalling pathway coordinates cell growth, autophagy and metabolism," *Nature Cell Biology* 13, no. 9 (2011), https://doi.org/10.1038/ncb2329.

23. Catherine Rose Braunstein et al., "Effect of low-glycemic index/load diets on body weight: a systematic review and meta-analysis," *FASEB Supplement* 30, no. 1 (2016).

24. Christine Clar et al., "Low glycaemic index diets for the prevention of cardiovascular disease," *Cochrane Database of Systematic Reviews* 7, 2017, https://doi.org/10.1002/14651858.cd004467.pub3.

25. Alireza Milajerdi et al., "The effect of dietary glycemic index and glycemic load on inflammatory biomarkers: a systematic review and meta-analysis of randomized clinical trials," *The American Journal of Clinical Nutrition* 107, no. 4 (2018), https://doi.org/10.1093/ajcn/nqx042.

26. Huicui Meng et al., "Effect of macronutrients and fiber on postprandial glycemic responses and meal glycemic index and glycemic load value determinations," *The American Journal of Clinical Nutrition* 105, no. 4 (2017), https://doi.org/10.3945/ajcn.116.144162.

27. Andreea Zurbau et al., "Acute effect of equicaloric meals varying in glycemic index and glycemic load on arterial stiffness and glycemia in healthy adults: a randomized crossover trial," *European Journal of Clinical Nutrition* (2018), https://doi.org/10.1038/s41430-018-0182-2.

28. David Zeevi et al., "Personalized nutrition by prediction of glycemic responses," *Cell* 163, no. 5 (2015), https://doi.org/10.1016/j.cell.2015.11.001.

29. Gunjan Y. Gandhi et al., "Efficacy of continuous glucose monitoring in improving glycemic control and reducing hypoglycemia: a systematic review and meta-analysis of randomized trials," *Journal of Diabetes Science and Technology* 5, no. 4 (2011), https://doi.org/10.1177 /193229681100500419; L. B. E. A. Hoeks et al., "Real-time continuous glucose monitoring system for treatment of diabetes: a systematic review," *Diabetic Medicine* 28, no. 4 (2011), https:// doi.org/10.1111/j.1464-5491.2010.03177.x.

30. American Diabetes Association, "Diagnosis and classification of diabetes mellitus," *Diabetes Care* 34, Supplement 1 (2010), https://doi.org/10.2337/dc11-s062.

31. Ethan Bergman et al., "Position of the American Dietetic Association, Dietitians of Canada, and the American College of Sports Medicine: nutrition and athletic performance," *Journal of The American Dietetic Association* 100, no. 12 (2000), https://doi.org/10.1016/s0002-8223(00)00428-4.

32. Felicity Thomas et al., "Blood glucose levels of subelite athletes during 6 days of free living," *Journal of Diabetes Science and Technology* 10, no. 6 (2016), https://doi.org/10.1177/19322968 16648344.

33. Philip B. Maffetone and Paul B. Laursen, "Athletes: fit but unhealthy?," *Sports Medicine — Open* 2 (2016), https://dx.doi.org/10.1186%2Fs40798-016-0048-x.

34. S. R. Bloom et al., "Differences in the metabolic and hormonal response to exercise between racing cyclists and untrained individuals," *Journal of Physiology* 258, no. 1 (1976), https://doi.org /10.1113/jphysiol.1976.sp011403.

35. Nicole M. Ehrhardt et al., "The effect of real-time continuous glucose monitoring on glycemic control in patients with type 2 diabetes mellitus," *Journal of Diabetes Science and Technology* 5, no. 3 (2011), https://doi.org/10.1177/193229681100500320.

36. Jan-Willem Van Dijk et al., "Both resistance- and endurance-type exercise reduce the prevalence of hyperglycaemia in individuals with impaired glucose tolerance and in insulin-treated and non-insulin-treated type 2 diabetic patients," *Diabetologia* 55, no. 5 (2012), https://doi.org/10.1007/s00125-011-2380-5; Jan-Willem Van Dijk et al., "Exercise therapy in type 2 diabetes: is daily exercise required to optimize glycemic control?" *Diabetes Care* 35, no. 5 (2012), https://doi.org/10.2337/dc11-2112.

37. H. J. Yoo et al., "Use of real time continuous glucose monitoring system as a motivational device for poorly controlled type 2 diabetes," *Diabetes Research and Clinical Practice* 82, no. 1 (2008), https://doi.org/10.1016/j.diabres.2008.06.015.

38. G. W. Heath et al., "Effects of exercise and lack of exercise on glucose tolerance and insulin sensitivity," *Journal of Applied Physiology* 55, no. 2 (1983), https://doi.org/10.1152/jappl.1983.55.2.512; K. J. Mikines et al., "Effects of training and detraining on dose-response relationship between glucose and insulin secretion," *American Journal of Physiology-Endocrinology and Metabolism* 256, no. 5 (1989), https://doi.org/10.1152/ajpendo.1989.256.5.e588.

39. Jonathan P. Little et al., "Effects of high-intensity interval exercise versus continuous moderate-intensity exercise on postprandial glycemic control assessed by continuous glucose monitoring in obese adults," *Applied Physiology, Nutrition, and Metabolism* 39, no. 7 (2014), https://doi.org /10.1139/apnm-2013-0512.

40. Yasuo Sengoku et al., "Continuous glucose monitoring during a 100-km race: a case study in an elite ultramarathon runner," *International Journal of Sports Physiology and Performance* 10, no. 1 (2015), https://doi.org/10.1123/ijspp.2013-0493.

41. Yuichiro Nishida et al., "S(G), S(I), and EGP of exercise-trained middle-aged men estimated by a two-compartment labeled minimal model," *American Journal of Physiology-Endocrinology and Metabolism* 283, no. 4 (2002), https://doi.org/10.1152/ajpendo.00237.2001; M. Kjaer M et al., "Glucose turnover and hormonal changes during insulin-induced hypoglycemia in trained humans," *Journal of Applied Physiology* 57, no. 1 (1984), https://doi.org/10.1152/jappl.1984.57.1.21.

42. Felicity Thomas et al., "Blood glucose levels of subelite athletes during 6 days of free living," *Journal of Diabetes Science and Technology* 10, no. 6 (2016), https://doi.org/10.1177 /1932296816648344.

43. Markku Timonen et al., "Insulin resistance and depressive symptoms in young adult males: findings from Finnish military conscripts," *Psychosomatic Medicine* 69, no. 8 (2007), https://doi.org/10.1097/psy.0b013e318157ad2e.

44. Antti-Jussi Pyykkonen et al., "Depressive symptoms, antidepressant medication use, and insulin resistance: the PPP-Botnia Study," *Diabetes Care* 34, no. 12 (2011), https://doi.org/10.2337/dc11-0107.

45. J. C. Felger and F. E. Lotrich, "Inflammatory cytokines in depression: neurobiological mechanisms and therapeutic implications," *Neuroscience* 246 (2013), https://doi.org/10.1016/j.neuroscience.2013.04.060.

46. Emerging Risk Factors Collaboration, "Diabetes mellitus, fasting glucose, and risk of cause-specific death," *New England Journal of Medicine* 364, no. 9 (2011), https://doi.org/10.1056/nejmoa1008862.

47. Shane. M. Murphy, "Transitions in competitive sport: maximizing individual potential," in *Sport Psychology Interventions*, ed. Shane. M. Murphy (Champaign, IL: Human Kinetics, 1995), 331-46.

48. Jingzhen Yang et al., "Prevalence of and risk factors associated with symptoms of depression in competitive collegiate student athletes," *Clinical Journal of Sport Medicine* 17, no. 6 (2007), https://doi.org/10.1097/jsm.0b013e31815aed6b.

49. Satchin Panda, *The Circadian Code* (Vermillion, U.K.: Rodale, 2018).

50. Frank A. J. L. Scheer et al., "Adverse metabolic and cardiovascular consequences of circadian misalignment," *Proceedings of the National Academy of Sciences of the USA* 106, no. 11 (2009), https://doi.org/10.1073/pnas.0808180106.

51. Megumi Hatori et al., "Time-restricted feeding without reducing caloric intake prevents metabolic diseases in mice fed a high-fat diet," *Cell Metabolism* 15, no. 6 (2012), https://doi.org/10.1016/j.cmet.2012.04.019.

52. Elizabeth Sutton et al., "Early time-restricted feeding improves insulin sensitivity, blood pressure, and oxidative stress even without weight loss in men with prediabetes," *Cell Metabolism* 27, no. 6 (2018), https://doi.org/10.1016/j.cmet.2018.04.010.

53. Yun S. Lee et al., "Berberine, a natural plant product, activates AMP-activated protein kinase with beneficial metabolic effects in diabetic and insulin-resistant states," *Diabetes* 55, no. 8 (2006), https://doi.org/10.2337/db06-0006; Teayoun Kim et al., "Curcumin activates AMPK and suppresses gluconeogenic gene expression in hepatoma cells," *Biochemical and Biophysical Research Communications* 388, no. 2 (2009), https://doi.org/10.1016/j.bbrc.2009.08.018.

54. Saeid Golbidi, Mohammad Badran, and Ismail Laher, "Diabetes and alpha lipoic acid," *Frontiers in Pharmacology* 2, (2011), https://doi.org/10.3389/fphar.2011.00069.

55. Min-Seon Kim et al., "Anti-obesity effects of alpha-lipoic acid mediated by suppression of hypothalamic AMP-activated protein kinase," *Nature Medicine* 10, no. 7 (2004), https://doi.org/10.1038/nm1061.

56. Raul Zamora-Ros et al., "High concentrations of a urinary biomarker of polyphenol intake are associated with decreased mortality in older adults," *Journal of Nutrition* 143, no. 9 (2013), https://doi.org/10.3945/jn.113.177121.

57. Ying Huang et al., "The complexity of the Nrf2 pathway: beyond the antioxidant response," *The Journal of Nutritional Biochemistry* 26, no. 12 (2015), https://doi.org/10.1016/j.jnutbio.2015.08.001.

58. Kaitlyn. N. Lewis et al., "Nrf2, a guardian of healthspan and gatekeeper of species longevity," *Integrative and Comparative Biology* 50, no. 5 (2010), https://doi.org/10.1093/icb/icq034.

59. John D. Hayes and Michael McMahon, "Molecular basis for the contribution of the antioxidant responsive element to cancer chemoprevention," *Cancer Letters* 174, no. 2 (2001), https://doi.org/10.1016/s0304-3835(01)00695-4; Wulf Dröge and Hyman M. Schipper, "Oxidative stress and aberrant signaling in aging and cognitive decline," *Aging Cell* 6, no. 3 (2007), https://doi.org/10.1111/j.1474-9726.2007.00294.x.

60. Aaron J. Done, Michael J. Newell, and Tinna Traustadóttir, "Effect of exercise intensity on Nrf2 signalling in young men," *Free Radical Research* 51, no. 6 (2017), https://doi.org/10.1080/1071576 2.2017.1353689.

61. Kirk W. Beach, "A theoretical model to predict the behavior of glycosylated hemoglobin levels," *Journal of Theoretical Biology* 81, no. 3 (1979), https://doi.org/10.1016/0022-5193(79)90052-3.

62. Yasuhiro Tahara and Kenji Shima, "Kinetics of HbA1c, glycated albumin, and fructosamine and analysis of their weight functions against preceding plasma glucose level," *Diabetes Care* 18, no. 4 (1995), https://doi.org/10.2337/diacare.18.4.440.

## Chapter 4: Physique Nutrition

1. Alan A. Aragon et al., "International society of sports nutrition position stand: diets and body composition," *Journal of the International Society of Sports Nutrition* 14, no. 16 (2017), https://doi.org/10.1186/s12970-017-0174-y.

2. Centers for Disease Control and Prevention, "Hyperthermia and dehydration related deaths associated with intentional rapid weight loss in three collegiate wrestlers," *JAMA*, 279, no. 11 (1998), https://doi.org/10.1001/jama.279.11.824-jwr0318-3-1.

3. Robert O'Rourke, "Metabolic thrift and the genetic basis of human obesity," *Annals of Surgery* 259, no. 4 (2014), https://doi.org/10.1097/sla.0000000000000361.

4. Kevin D. Hall, "Did the food environment cause the obesity epidemic?" *Obesity* 26, no. 1, (2017), https://doi.org/10.1002/oby.22073.

5. Stephen A. McClave and Harvy L. Snider, "Dissecting the energy needs of the body," *Current Opinion in Clinical Nutrition and Metabolic Care* 4, no. 2 (2001), https://doi.org/10.1097/00075197 -200103000-00011.

6. Susan M. Kleiner, T. L. Bazzarre, and Mary Demarest Litchford, "Metabolic profiles, diet, and health practices of championship male and female bodybuilders," *Journal of the American Dietetic Association* 90, no. 7 (1990).

7. M. M. Manore and J. L. Thompson, "Energy requirements of the athlete: assessment and evidence of energy efficiency," in *Clinical Sports Nutrition*, 5th ed, eds. Louise Burke and Vicki Deakin (Sydney, Australia: McGraw-Hill, 2015), 114–39.

8. Barbara E. Ainsworth et al., "Compendium of physical activities," *Medicine and Science in Sports and Exercise* 43, no. 8 (2011), https://doi.org/10.1249/mss.0b013e31821ece12.

9. James A. Levine, "Nonexercise activity thermogenesis (NEAT): environment and biology," *American Journal of Physiology-Endocrinology and Metabolism* 285, no. 5 (2004), https://doi.org/10.1152 /ajpendo.00562.2003.

10. E. Jéquier, "Pathways to obesity," *International Journal of Obesity* 26, Supplement 2 (2002), https://doi.org/10.1038/sj.ijo.0802123.

11. Sadie B. Barr and Jonathan C. Wright, "Postprandial energy expenditure in whole-food and processed-food meals: implications for daily energy expenditure," *Food Nutrition Research* 54, no. 1 (2010), https://doi.org/10.3402/fnr.v54i0.5144.

12. S. Heymsfield et al., "Weight management using a meal replacement strategy: meta and pooling analysis from six studies," *International Journal of Obesity* 27, no. 5 (2003), https://doi.org/10.1038 /sj.ijo.0802258.

13. Eric Helms, "Nutrition for bodybuilders, hypertrophy and physique-focused athletes," *Dr. Bubbs Performance Podcast*, Podcast audio, February 15, 2018, https://drbubbs.com/season-2-podcast -episodes/2018/2/s2e7-nutrition-for-bodybuilders-hypertrophy-and-physique-focused-athletes -w-dr-eric-helms-phd.

14. Brad J. Schoenfeld, *Science and Development of Muscle Hypertrophy* (Champaign, IL: Human Kinetics, 2016).

15. Brad J. Schoenfeld, "Maximize hypertrophy training, fat loss myths and nutrition for building muscle," *Dr. Bubbs Performance Podcast*, Podcast audio, June 22, 2017, https://drbubbs.com

/podcastepisodes/2017/6/building-muscle-burning-fat-and-evidenced-based-nutrition-w-dr
-brad-schoenfeld.

16. Brad J. Schoenfeld et al., "Strength and hypertrophy adaptations between low- vs. high-load
resistance training: a systematic review and meta-analysis," *Journal of Strength and Conditioning
Research* 31, no. 12 (2017), https://doi.org/10.1519/jsc.0000000000002200.

17. Nicolas J. Pillon et al., "Crosstalk between skeletal muscle and immune cells: muscle-derived mediators and metabolic implications," *American Journal of Physiology-Endocrinology and Metabolism*
304, no. 5 (2013), https://doi.org/10.1152/ajpendo.00553.2012.

18. Brad J. Schoenfeld, Dan Ogborn, and James W. Krieger, "Dose-response relationship between weekly
resistance training volume and increases in muscle mass: a systematic review and meta-analysis,"
*Journal of Sports Sciences* 35, no. 11 (2017), https://doi.org/10.1080/02640414.2016.1210197.

19. Stefan M. Pasiakos and John W. Carbone, "Assessment of skeletal muscle proteolysis and the regulatory
response to nutrition and exercise," *IUBMB Life* 66, no. 7 (2014), https://doi.org/10.1002/iub.1291.

20. T. Van Wessel et al., "The muscle fiber type-fiber size paradox: hypertrophy or oxidative metabolism?" *European Journal of Applied Physiology* 110, no. 4 (2010), https://doi.org/10.1007/s00421
-010-1545-0.

21. Ina Garthe et al., "Effect of nutritional intervention on body composition and performance in elite
athletes," *European Journal of Sport Science* 13, no. 3 (2013), https://doi.org/10.1080/17461391.2011
.643923.

22. Gary Slater and Stuart M. Phillips, "Protein nutrition guidelines for strength sports: sprinting,
weightlifting, throwing events, and bodybuilding," *Journal of Sports Sciences* 29, Supplement 1
(2011), https://doi.org/10.1080/02640414.2011.574722.

23. Robert W. Morton et al., "A systematic review, meta-analysis and meta-regression of the effect
of protein supplementation on resistance training-induced gains in muscle mass and strength
in healthy adults," *British Journal of Sports Medicine* 5, no. 6 (2017), https://doi.org/10.1136
/bjsports-2017-097608.

24. Ralf Jäger et al., "International society of sports nutrition position stand: protein and exercise,"
*Journal of the International Society of Sports Nutrition* 14, no. 20 (2017), https://doi.org/10.1186
/s12970-017-0177-8.

25. Daniel A. Traylor, Stefan H. M. Gorissen, and Stuart M. Phillips, "Perspective: protein requirements and optimal intakes in aging: are we ready to recommend more than the recommended daily
allowance?," *Advances in Nutrition* 9, no. 3 (2018), https://doi.org/10.1093/advances/nmy003.

26. Adriano E. Lima-Silva et al., "Effects of a low- or high-carbohydrate diet on performance, energy
system contribution, and metabolic responses during supramaximal exercise," *Applied Physiology,
Nutrition, and Metabolism* 38, no. 9 (2013), https://doi.org/10.1139/apnm-2012-0467.

27. Joel B. Mitchell et al., "The effect of preexercise carbohydrate status on resistance exercise
performance," *International Journal of Sport Nutrition* 7, no. 3 (1997), https://doi.org/10.1123/ijsn
.7.3.185.

28. Eric R. Helms, Alan A. Aragon, and Peter J. Fitschen, "Evidence-based recommendations for natural bodybuilding contest preparation: nutrition and supplementation," *Journal of the International
Society of Sports Nutrition* 11, no. 1 (2014), https://doi.org/10.1186/1550-2783-11-20.

29. Stuart M. Phillips and Luc J. C. Van Loon, "Dietary protein for athletes: from requirements to
optimum adaptation," *Journal of Sports Sciences* 29, Supplement 1 (2011), https://doi.org/10.1080
/02640414.2011.619204.

30. A. J. Chappell, T. Simper, and M. E. Baker, "Nutritional strategies of high level natural bodybuilders during competition preparation," *Journal of the International Society of Sports Nutrition* 15, no. 4
(2018), https://doi.org/10.1186/s12970-018-0209-z.

31. J. Walberg et al., "Macronutrient content of a hypoenergy diet affects nitrogen retention and
muscle function in weight lifters," *International Journal of Sports Medicine* 9, no. 4 (1988), https://
doi.org/10.1055/s-2007-1025018.

32. Stefan M. Pasiakos et al., "Effects of high-protein diets on fat-free mass and muscle protein synthesis following weight loss: a randomized controlled trial," *The FASEB Journal* 27, no. 9 (2013), https://doi.org/10.1096/fj.13-230227.

33. Mary G. Murphy, "Dietary fatty acids and membrane protein function," *The Journal of Nutritional Biochemistry* 1, no. 2 (1990), https://doi.org/10.1016/0955-2863(90)90052-m.

34. Jacob M. Wilson et al., "The effects of 12 weeks of beta-hydroxy-beta-methylbutyrate free acid supplementation on muscle mass, strength, and power in resistance-trained individuals: a randomized, double-blind, placebo-controlled study," *European Journal of Applied Physiology* 114, no. 6 (2014), https://doi.org/10.1007/s00421-014-2854-5.

35. Richard B. Kreider et al., "International Society of Sports Nutrition position stand: safety and efficacy of creatine supplementation in exercise, sport, and medicine," *Journal of the International Society of Sports Nutrition* 14, no. 1 (2017), https://doi.org/10.1186/s12970-017-0173-z; Richard B. Kreider et al., "Effects of creatine supplementation on body composition, strength, and sprint performance," *Medicine and Science in Sports and Exercise* 30, no. 1 (1998), https://doi.org/10.1097/00005768-199801000-00011.

36. Ronald J. Maughan et al., "IOC consensus statement: dietary supplements and the high-performance athlete," *International Journal of Sport Nutrition and Exercise Metabolism* (2018), https://doi.org/10.1123/ijsnem.2018-0020.

37. Erica R. Goldstein et al., "International society of sports nutrition position stand: caffeine and performance," *Journal of the International Society of Sports Nutrition* 7, no. 1 (2010), https://doi.org/10.1186/1550-2783-7-5.

38. Ian C. Dunican et al., "Caffeine use in a Super Rugby game and its relationship to post-game sleep," *European Journal of Sport Science* 18, no. 4 (2018), https://doi.org/10.1080/17461391.2018.1433238.

39. Kevin D. Hall, Dale A. Schoeller, and Andrew W. Brown et al., "Reducing calories to lose weight," *JAMA* 319, no. 22 (2018), https://doi.org/10.1001/jama.2018.4257.

40. Antti A. Mero et al., "Moderate energy restriction with high protein diet results in healthier outcome in women," *Journal of the International Society of Sports Nutrition* 7, no. 1 (2010), https://doi.org/10.1186/1550-2783-7-4.

41. Ina Garthe et al., "Effect of two different weight-loss rates on body composition and strength and power-related performance in elite athletes," *International Journal of Sport Nutrition and Exercise Metabolism* 21, no. 2 (2011), https://doi.org/10.1123/ijsnem.21.2.97.

42. Eric Helms et al., "A systematic review of dietary protein during caloric restriction in resistance trained lean athletes: a case for higher intakes," *International Journal of Sport Nutrition and Exercise Metabolism* 24, no. 2 (2014), https://doi.org/10.1123/ijsnem.2013-0054.

43. Laura E. Newton et al., "Changes in psychological state and self-reported diet during various phases of training in competitive bodybuilders," *The Journal of Strength and Conditioning Research* 7, no. 3 (1993), https://doi.org/10.1519/00124278-199308000-00005.

44. Gail E. Butterfield, "Whole-body protein utilization in humans," *Medicine and Science in Sports and Exercise* 19 (1987), https://doi.org/10.1249/00005768-198710001-00010.

45. Paul Arciero et al., "Protein-pacing from food or supplementation improves physical performance in overweight men and women: the PRISE 2 study," *Nutrients* 8, no. 5 (2016), https://doi.org/10.3390/nu8050288.

46. Jose Antonio et al., "The effects of consuming a high protein diet (4.4 g/kg/d) on body composition in resistance-trained individuals," *Journal of the International Society of Sports Nutrition* 11, no. 1 (2014), https://doi.org/10.1186/1550-2783-11-19.

47. Jose Antonio et al., "A high protein diet has no harmful effects: a one-year crossover study in resistance-trained males," *Journal of Nutrition and Metabolism* 2016, 9104791 (2016), https://doi.org/10.1155/2016/9104792.

48. E. K. Hämäläinen et al., "Decrease of serum total and free testosterone during a low-fat high-fibre diet," *Journal of Steroid Biochemistry* 18, no. 3 (1983), https://doi.org/10.1016/0022-4731(83)90117-6.

49. Jarek Mäestu et al., "Anabolic and catabolic hormones and energy balance of the male bodybuilders during the preparation for the competition," *Journal of Strength and Conditioning Research* 24, no. 4 (2010), https://doi.org/10.1519/jsc.0b013e3181cb6fd3.

50. M. Veldhorst et al., "Protein-induced satiety: effects and mechanisms of different proteins," *Physiology and Behavior* 94, no. 2 (2008), https://doi.org/10.1016/j.physbeh.2008.01.003.

51. Ben Crighton, Graeme L. Close, and James P. Morton, "Alarming weight cutting behaviours in mixed martial arts: a cause for concern and a call for action," *British Journal of Sports Medicine* 50, no. 8 (2015), https://doi.org/10.1136/bjsports-2015-094732.

52. Luke Thomas, "ONE Championship's Yang Jian Bing dies from weight cutting complications," *MMA Fighting*, December 11, 2015, https://www.mmafighting.com/2015/12/11/9891100/one-championships-yang-jian-bing-dies-from-weight-cutting.

53. Marcus Smith et al., "The effects of restricted energy and fluid intake on simulated amateur boxing performance," *International Journal of Sport Nutrition and Exercise Metabolism* 11, no. 2 (2001), https://doi.org/10.1123/ijsnem.11.2.238.

54. James P. Morton et al., "Making the weight: a case study from professional boxing," *International Journal of Sport Nutrition and Exercise Metabolism* 20, no. 1 (2010), https://doi.org/10.1123/ijsnem.20.1.80.

55. James P. Morton et al., "Making the weight: a case study from professional boxing."

56. Joseph John Matthews and Ceri Nicholas, "Extreme rapid weight loss and rapid weight gain observed in UK mixed martial arts athletes preparing for competition," *International Journal of Sport Nutrition and Exercise Metabolism* 27, no. 2 (2017), https://doi.org/10.1123/ijsnem.2016-0174.

57. Joseph John Matthews and Ceri Nicholas, "Extreme rapid weight loss and rapid weight gain observed in UK mixed martial arts athletes preparing for competition."

58. Dale R. Wagner and Vivian H. Heyward, "Techniques of body composition assessment: a review of laboratory and field methods," *Research Quarterly for Exercise and Sport* 70, no. 2 (1999), https://doi.org/10.1080/02701367.1999.10608031.

59. Sanja Mazic et al., "Body composition assessment in athletes: a systematic review," *Medicinski Pregled* 67, no 7-8 (2014), https://doi.org/10.2298/mpns1408255m.

60. Julia L. Bone et al., "Manipulation of muscle creatine and glycogen changes DXA estimates of body composition," *Medicine and Science in Sports and Exercise* 49, no. 5 (2016), https://doi.org/10.1249/mss.0000000000001174.

61. Clodagh Toomey et al., "A review of body composition measurement in the assessment of health," *Topics in Clinical Nutrition* 30, no. 1 (2015), https://doi.org/10.1097/tin.0000000000000017; P. Cross et al., "Assessing various body composition measurements as an appropriate tool for estimating body fat in Division I female collegiate athletes," *Journal of Science and Medicine in Sport* 14, Supplement 1 (2011), https://doi.org/10.1016/j.jsams.2011.11.192.

62. Clodagh Toomey et al., "A review of body composition measurement in the assessment of health."

## Chapter 5: Endurance Nutrition

1. August Krogh and Johannes Lindhard, "The relative value of fat and carbohydrate as sources of muscular energy," *Biochemical Journal* 14, no. 3-4 (1920), https://doi.org/10.1042/bj0140290.

2. E. F. Coyle et al., "Carbohydrate feeding during prolonged strenuous exercise," *Journal of Applied Physiology* 55, no. 1 (1983), https://doi.org/10.1152/jappl.1983.55.1.230.

3. D. T. Thomas, K. A. Erdman, and L. M. Burke, "American College of Sports Medicine joint position statement: nutrition and athletic performance," *Medicine and Science in Sports and Exercise* 48, no. 3 (2016), https://doi.org/10.1249/MSS.0000000000000852.

4. G. L. Close et al., "New strategies in sport nutrition to increase exercise performance," *Free Radical Biology and Medicine* 98 (2016), https://doi.org/10.1016/j.freeradbiomed.2016.01.016.

5. N. Rodriguez et al., "American College of Sports Medicine position statement, nutrition and athletic performance," *Medicine and Science in Sports and Exercise* 41, no. 3 (2009), https://doi.org/10.1249/MSS.0b013e31890eb86.

6. John A. Hawley et al., "Carbohydrate-loading and exercise performance," *Sports Medicine* 24, no. 2 (1997), https://doi.org/10.2165/00007256-199724020-00001.

7. Trent Stellingwerff and Gregory R. Cox, "Systematic review: carbohydrate supplementation on exercise performance or capacity of varying durations," *Applied Physiology, Nutrition, and Metabolism* 39, no. 9 (2014), https://doi.org/10.1139/apnm-2014-0027.

8. Trent Stellingwerff et al., "Carbohydrate supplementation during prolonged cycling exercise spares muscle glycogen but does not affect intramyocellular lipid use," *Pflügers Archiv — European Journal of Physiology* 454, no. 4 (2007), https://doi.org/10.1007/s00424-007-0236-0; Javier T. Gonzalez et al., "Ingestion of glucose or sucrose prevents liver but not muscle glycogen depletion during prolonged endurance- type exercise in trained cyclists," *American Journal of Physiology-Endocrinology and Metabolism* 309, no. 12 (2015), https://doi.org/10.1152/ajpendo.00376.2015; Edward F. Coyle et al., "Muscle glycogen utilization during prolonged strenuous exercise when fed carbohydrate," *Journal of Applied Physiology* 61, no. 1 (1986), https://doi.org/10.1152/jappl.1986.61.1.165.

9. James M. Carter, Asker E. Jeukendrup, and David A. Jones, "The effect of carbohydrate mouth rinse on 1-h cycle time trial performance," *Medicine and Science in Sports and Exercise* 36 (2004), https://doi.org/10.1249/01.mss.0000147585.65709.6f.

10. Louise M. Burke and Ronald J. Maughan, "The Governor has a sweet tooth — mouth sensing of nutrients to enhance sports performance," *European Journal of Sport Science* 15, no. 1 (2015), https://doi.org/10.1080/17461391.2014.971880.

11. E. S. Chambers, M. W. Bridge, and D. A. Jones, "Carbohydrate sensing in the human mouth: effects on exercise performance and brain activity," *Journal of Physiology* 587, no. 8 (2009) https://doi.org/10.1113/jphysiol.2008.164285; Andreas M. Kasper et al., "Carbohydrate mouth rinse and caffeine improves high-intensity interval running capacity when carbohydrate restricted," *European Journal of Sport Science* 16, no. 5 (2015), https://doi.org/10.1080/17461391.2015.1041063.

12. Louise M. Burke et al., "Carbohydrates for training and competition," *Journal of Sports Sciences* 29, Supplement 1 (2011), https://doi.org/10.1080/02640414.2011.585473.

13. Kirsten F. Howlett et al., "The effect of exercise and insulin on AS160 phosphorylation and 14-3-3 binding capacity in human skeletal muscle," *American Journal of Physiology-Endocrinology and Metabolism* 294, no. 2 (2008), https://doi.org/10.1152/ajpendo.00542.2007.

14. Samuel G. Impey et al., "Fuel for the work required: a theoretical framework for carbohydrate periodization and the glycogen threshold hypothesis," *Sports Medicine* 48, no. 5 (2018), https://doi.org/10.1007/s40279-018-0867-7.

15. Wee Kian Yeo et al., "Skeletal muscle adaptation and performance responses to once versus twice every second day endurance training regimens," *Journal of Applied Physiology* 105, no. 5 (2008) https://doi.org/10.1152/japplphysiol.90882.2008; Andrew J. R. Cochran et al., "Manipulating carbohydrate availability between twice-daily sessions of high-intensity interval training over 2 weeks improves time-trial performance," *International Journal of Sport Nutrition and Exercise Metabolism* 25, no. 5 (2015), https://doi.org/10.1123/ijsnem.2014-0263.

16. Samuel G. Impey et al., "Leucine-enriched protein feeding does not impair exercise-induced free fatty acid availability and lipid oxidation: beneficial implications for training in carbohydrate-restricted states," *Amino Acids* 47, no. 2 (2015), https://doi.org/10.1007/s00726-014-1876-y.

17. Stephen C. Lane et al., "Effects of sleeping with reduced carbohydrate availability on acute training responses," *Journal of Applied Physiology* 119, no. 6 (2015), https://doi.org/10.1152/japplphysiol.00857.2014.

18. Carl J. Hulston et al., "Training with low muscle glycogen enhances fat metabolism in well-trained cyclists," *Medicine and Science in Sports and Exercise* 42, no. 11. 2010;42:2046–55. https://doi.org/10.1249/mss.0b013e3181dd5070.

19. Louise M. Burke et al., "Low carbohydrate, high fat diet impairs exercise economy and negates the performance benefit from intensified training in elite race walkers," *Journal of Physiology* 595, no. 9. (2017), https://doi.org/10.1113/jp273230.

20. Trent Stellingwerff et al., "Decreased PDH activation and glycogenolysis during exercise following fat adaptation with carbohydrate restoration," *American Journal of Physiology-Endocrinology and Metabolism* 290, no. 2 (2006), https://doi.org/10.1152/ajpendo.00268.2005.

21. Asker E. Jeukendrup, "Carbohydrate and exercise performance: the role of multiple transportable carbohydrates," *Current Opinion in Clinical Nutrition and Metabolic Care* 13, no. 4 (2010), https://doi.org/10.1097/mco.0b013e328339de9f; Asker E. Jeukendrup, "Carbohydrate feeding during exercise," *European Journal of Sport Science* 8, no. 2 (2008), https://doi.org/10.1080/1746139 0801918971.

22. James M. Carter et al., "The effect of glucose infusion on glucose kinetics during a 1-h time trial," *Medicine and Science in Sports and Exercise* 36, no. 9 (2004), https://doi.org/10.1249/01 .mss.0000139892.69410.d8.

23. Nicholas Gant, Cathy M. Stinear, and Winston D. Byblow, "Carbohydrate in the mouth immediately facilitates motor output," *Brain Research* 13, no. 4 (2010), https://doi.org/10.1016/j .brainres.2010.04.004.

24. Asker E. Jeukendrup, "Carbohydrate intake during exercise and performance," *Nutrition* 20, no. 7-8 (2004), https://doi.org/10.1016/j.nut.2004.04.017; Asker E. Jeukendrup and Edward S. Chambers, "Oral carbohydrate sensing and exercise performance," *Current Opinion in Clinical Nutrition and Metabolic Care* 13, no. 4 (2010), https://doi.org/10.1097/mco.0b013e328339de83.

25. Dana. M. Small et al., "The role of the human orbitofrontal cortex in taste and flavor processing," *Annals of the New York Academy of Sciences* 1121, no. 1 (2007), https://doi.org/10.1196/annals .1401.002.

26. M. L. Kringelbach, "Food for thought: hedonic experience beyond homeostasis in the human brain," *Neuroscience* 126, no. 4 (2004), https://doi.org/10.1016/j.neuroscience.2004.04.035; Edmund T. Rolls, "Sensory processing in the brain related to the control of food intake," *Proceedings of the Nutrition Society* 66, no. 1 (2007), https://doi.org/10.1017/s0029665107005332.

27. Roy L. P. G. Jentjens et al., "Oxidation of combined ingestion of glucose and fructose during exercise," *Journal of Applied Physiology* 96, no. 4 (2004), https://doi.org/10.1152/japplphysiol.00974 .2003.

28. Beate Pfeiffer et al., "CHO oxidation from a CHO gel compared with a drink during exercise," *Medicine and Science in Sports and Exercise* 42, no. 11 (2010), https://doi.org/10.1249/ mss.0b013e3181e0efe6; Beate Pfeiffer et al., "Oxidation of solid versus liquid CHO sources during exercise," *Medicine and Science in Sports and Exercise* 42, no. 11 (2010), https://doi.org/10.1249 /mss.0b013e3181e0efc9.

29. Asker E. Jeukendrup et al., "Exogenous carbohydrate oxidation during ultraendurance exercise," *Journal of Applied Physiology* 100, no. 4 (2006), https://doi.org/10.1152/japplphysiol.00981.2004.

30. John Eric W. Smith et al., "Evidence of a carbohydrate dose and prolonged exercise performance relationship," *Medicine and Science in Sports and Exercise* 42 (2010), https://doi.org/10.1249/01 .mss.0000385615.40977.c3.

31. Nicholas E. Kimber et al., "Energy balance during an ironman triathlon in male and female triathletes," *International Journal of Sport Nutrition and Exercise Metabolism* 12 (2002), https://doi .org/10.1123/ijsnem.12.1.47.

32. Tim Noakes, "The lore of running, hydration and increasing longevity," *Dr. Bubbs Performance Podcast*, Podcast audio, June 22, 2017, https://drbubbs.com/podcastepisodes/2017/10/episode -42-the-lore-of-running-hydration-increasing-longevity-w-prof-tim-noakes.

33. D. T. Thomas, K. A. Erdman, and L. M. Burke, "American College of Sports Medicine joint position statement: nutrition and athletic performance."

34. Philip B. Maffetone and Paul B. Laursen, "Athletes: Fit but Unhealthy?," *Sports Medicine — Open* 2 (2016), https://dx.doi.org/10.1186%2Fs40798-016-0048-x; Jeff S. Volek et al. "Metabolic characteristics of keto-adapted ultra-endurance runners," *Metabolism* 65, no. 3 (2016) https://doi .org/10.1016/j.metabol.2015.10.028.

35. Begoña Ruiz-Núñez et al., "Lifestyle and nutritional imbalances associated with western diseases: causes and consequences of chronic systemic low-grade inflammation in an evolutionary context," *Journal of Nutritional Biochemistry* 24, no. 7 (2013), https://doi.org/10.1016/j.jnutbio.2013.02.009.

36. Louise M. Burke et al., "Adaptations to short-term high-fat diet persist during exercise despite high carbohydrate availability," *Medicine and Science in Sports and Exercise* 34, no. 1 (2002), https://doi.org/10.1097/00005768-200201000-00014.

37. Lukas Cipryan et al., "Effects of a 4-week very low-carbohydrate diet on high-intensity interval training responses," *Journal of Sports Science and Medicine* 17, no. 2 (2018).

38. Ken J. Hetlelid et al., "Rethinking the role of fat oxidation: substrate utilisation during high-intensity interval training in well-trained and recreationally trained runners," *BMJ Open Sport and Exercise Medicine* 1, no. 1 (2015), https://doi.org/10.1136/bmjsem-2015-000047.

39. Fionn T. McSwiney et al., "Keto-adaptation enhances exercise performance and body composition responses to training in endurance athletes," *Metabolism* 83 (2018), https://doi.org/10.1016/j.metabol.2017.11.016.

40. Matthew S. Ganio et al., "Effect of caffeine on sport-specific endurance performance: a systematic review," *Journal of Strength and Conditioning Research* (2009), https://doi.org/10.1519/jsc.0b013e31818b979a.

41. Trent Stellingwerff, "Case-study: Body composition periodization in an Olympic-level female middle-distance runner over a 9-year career," *International Journal of Sport Nutrition and Exercise Metabolism* 28, no. 4 (2018), https://doi.org/10.1123/ijsnem.2017-0312.

42. Lawrence L. Spriet, "Exercise and sport performance with low doses of caffeine," *Sports Medicine* 44, Supplement 2 (2014), https://doi.org/10.1007/s40279-014-0257-8.

43. Knut Thomas Schneiker et al., "Effects of caffeine on prolonged intermittent-sprint ability in team-sport athletes," *Medicine and Science in Sports and Exercise* 38, no. 3 (2006), https://doi.org/10.1249/01.mss.0000188449.18968.62.

44. Nanci Guest et al., "Caffeine, CYP1A2 genotype, and endurance performance in athletes," *Medicine and Science in Sports and Exercise* 50, no. 8 (2018), https://doi.org/10.1249/mss.0000000000001596.

45. Andrew M. Jones, "Dietary nitrate supplementation and exercise performance," *Sports Medicine* 44, Supplement 1 (2014), https://doi.org/10.1007/s40279-014-0149-y.

46. Nathan S. Bryan, "Nitrite in nitric oxide biology: cause or consequence? A systems-based review," *Free Radical Biology and Medicine* 41, no. 5 (2006), https://doi.org/10.1016/j.freeradbiomed.2006.05.019.

47. Jon O. Lundberg et al., "Roles of dietary inorganic nitrate in cardiovascular health and disease," *Cardiovascular Research* 89, no. 3 (2010), https://doi.org/10.1093/cvr/cvq325; Andrew J. Webb et al., "Acute blood pressure lowering, vasoprotective, and antiplatelet properties of dietary nitrate via bioconversion to nitrite," *Hypertension* 51, no. 3 (2008), https://doi.org/10.1161/hypertensionaha.107.103523.

48. Louise M. Burke, "Practical considerations for bicarbonate loading and sports performance," *Nestlé Nutrition Institute Workshop Series* 75 (2013), https://doi.org/10.1159/000345814.

49. Amelia J. Carr et al., "Effect of sodium bicarbonate on (HCO3-), pH, and gastrointestinal symptoms," *International Journal of Sport Nutrition and Exercise Metabolism* 21, no. 3 (2011), https://doi.org/10.1123/ijsnem.21.3.189.

50. Daniel J. Owens et al., "Vitamin D supplementation does not improve human skeletal muscle contractile properties in insufficient young males," *European Journal of Applied Physiology* 114, no. 6 (2014), https://doi.org/10.1007/s00421-014-2865-2.

51. Pawel Bieganowski and Charles Brenner, "Discoveries of nicotinamide riboside as a nutrient and conserved NRK genes establish a Preiss–Handler independent route to NADþ in fungi and humans," *Cell* 117, no. 4 (2004), https://doi.org/10.1016/s0092-8674(04)00416-7; Carles Cantó, Keir J. Menzies, and Johan Auwerx, "NAD(þ) metabolism and the control of energy homeostasis:

a balancing act between mitochondria and the nucleus," *Cell Metabolism* 22, no. 1 (2015), https://doi.org/10.1016/j.cmet.2015.05.023.

52. G. Paulsen et al., "Vitamin C and E supplementation alters protein signalling after a strength training session, but not muscle growth during 10 weeks of training," *Journal of Physiology* 592, no. 24 (2014), https://doi.org/10.1113/jphysiol.2014.279950; Dale Morrison et al., "Vitamin C and E supplementation prevents some of the cellular adaptations to endurance-training in humans," *Free Radical Biology and Medicine* 89 (2015), https://doi.org/10.1016/j.freeradbiomed.2015.10.412.

53. Lasse Gliemann et al., "Resveratrol blunts the positive effects of exercise training on cardiovascular health in aged men," *The Journal of Physiology* 591, no. 20 (2013), https://doi.org/10.1113/jphysiol.2013.258061.

54. G. L. Close and M. J. Jackson, "Antioxidants and exercise: a tale of the complexities of relating signalling processes to physiological function?" *The Journal of Physiology* 592 (2014), https://doi.org/10.1113/jphysiol.2014.272294.

## Chapter 6: Team Sport Nutrition

1. Jens Bangsbo, Magni Mohr, and Peter Krustrup, "Physical and metabolic demands of training and match-play in the elite football player," *Journal of Sports Sciences* 24, no. 7 (2006), https://doi.org/10.1080/02640410500482529; Mark Russell, David Benton, and Michael Kingsley, "Carbohydrate ingestion before and during soccer match play and blood glucose and lactate concentrations," *Journal of Athletic Training* 49, no. 4 (2014), https://doi.org/10.4085/1062-6050-49.3.12; Tomas Stølen et al., "Physiology of soccer: an update," *Sports Medicine* 35, no. 6 (2005), https://doi.org/10.2165/00007256-200535060-00004; Clyde Williams and Ian Rollo, "Carbohydrate nutrition and team sport performance," *Sports Medicine* 45, Supplement 1 (2015), https://doi.org/10.1007/s40279-015-0399-3.

2. Arni Arnason et al., "Physical fitness, injuries, and team performance in soccer," *Medicine and Science in Sports and Exercise* 36, no. 2 (2004), https://doi.org/10.1249/01.mss.0000113478.92945.ca; Eduardo Iglesias-Gutiérrez et al., "Is there a relationship between the playing position of soccer players and their food and macronutrient intake?," *Applied Physiology, Nutrition, and Metabolism* 37, no. 2 (2012), https://doi.org/10.1139/h11-152.

3. Kathryn Beck et al., "Role of nutrition in performance enhancement and postexercise recovery," *Open Access Journal of Sports Medicine* 6 (2015), https://doi.org/10.2147/oajsm.s33605; D. Travis Thomas et al., "American College of Sports Medicine joint position statement, nutrition and athletic performance," *Medicine and Science in Sports and Exercise* 48, no. 3 (2016), https://doi.org/10.1249/MSS.0000000000000852.

4. Liam Anderson et al., "Energy intake and expenditure of professional soccer players of the English Premier League: evidence of carbohydrate periodization," *International Journal of Sport Nutrition and Exercise Metabolism*, 27 (2017), https://doi.org/10.1123/ijsnem.2016-0259.

5. Armand E. O. Bettonviel et al., "Nutritional status and daytime pattern of protein intake on match, post-match, rest and training days in senior professional and youth elite soccer players," *International Journal of Sport Nutrition and Exercise Metabolism* 26, no. 3 (2016), https://doi.org/10.1123/ijsnem.2015-0218.

6. T. P. Gunnarsson et al., "Effect of whey protein- and carbohydrate-enriched diet on glycogen resynthesis during the first 48 h after a soccer game," *Scandinavian Journal of Medicine and Science in Sports* 23 (2013), https://doi.org/10.1111/j.1600-0838.2011.01418.x.

7. Peter Krustrup et al., "Muscle and blood metabolites during a soccer game: implications for sprint performance," *Medicine and Science in Sports and Exercise* 38, no. 6 (2006), https://doi.org/10.1249/01.mss.0000222845.89262.cd.

8. Louise M. Burke et al., "Carbohydrates for training and competition," *Journal of Sports Sciences* 29, Supplement 1 (2011), https://doi.org/10.1080/02640414.2011.585473; Ajmol Ali and Clyde Williams, "Carbohydrate ingestion and soccer skill performance during prolonged intermittent exercise," *Journal of Sports Sciences* 27, no. 14 (2009), https://doi.org/10.1080/02640410903334772;

Ralph S. Welsh et al., "Carbohydrates and physical/mental performance during intermittent exercise to fatigue," *Medicine and Science in Sports and Exercise* 34, no. 4 (2002), https://doi.org/10.1097/00005768-200204000-00025.

9. Tae-Seok Jeong et al., "Quantification of the physiological loading of one week of 'pre-season' and one week of 'in-season' training in professional soccer players," *Journal of Sports Sciences* 29, no. 11 (2011), https://doi.org/10.1080/02640414.2011.583671; Mohamed Saifeddin Fessi et al., "Changes of the psychophysical state and feeling of wellness of professional soccer players during pre-season and in-season periods," *Research in Sports Medicine* 24, no. 4 (2016), https://doi.org/10.1080/15438627.2016.1222278.

10. Raquel Raizel et al., "Pre-season dietary intake of professional soccer players," *Nutrition and Health* 23, no. 4 (2017), https://doi.org/10.1177/0260106017737014.

11. Raquel Raizel et al., "Pre-season dietary intake of professional soccer players."

12. Raquel Raizel et al., "Pre-season dietary intake of professional soccer players."

13. Laura Sutton et al., "Body composition of English Premier League soccer players: influence of playing position, international status, and ethnicity," *Journal of Sports Sciences* 27, no. 10 (2009), https://doi.org/10.1080/02640410903030305; Christopher Carling and Emmanuel Orhant, "Variation in body composition in professional soccer players: interseasonal and intraseasonal changes and the effects of exposure time and player position," *Journal of Strength and Conditioning Research* 24, no. 5 (2010), https://doi.org/10.1519/jsc.0b013e3181cc6154.

14. Marc Briggs et al., "Assessment of energy intake and energy expenditure of male adolescent academy-level soccer players during a competitive week," *Nutrients* 7, no. 10 (2015), https://doi.org/10.3390/nu7105400.

15. James Cameron Morehen et al., "The assessment of total energy expenditure during a 14-day in-season period of professional rugby league players using the doubly labelled water method," *International Journal of Sport Nutrition and Exercise Metabolism* 26, no. 5 (2016), https://doi.org/10.1123/ijsnem.2015-0335.

16. Warren J. Bradley et al., "Energy intake and expenditure assessed 'in-season' in an elite European rugby union squad," *European Journal of Sport Science* 15, no. 6 (2015), https://doi.org/10.1080/17461391.2015.1042528.

17. Mark Russell et al., "Half-time strategies to enhance second-half performance in team-sports players: a review and recommendations," *Sports Medicine* 45, no. 3 (2015), https://doi.org/10.1007/s40279-014-0297-0.

18. Magni Mohr, Peter Krustrup, and Jens Bangsbo, "Fatigue in soccer: a brief review," *Journal of Sports Sciences* 23, no. 6 (2005), https://doi.org/10.1080/02640410400021286.

19. Mark Russell, David Benton, and Michael Kingsley, "Influence of carbohydrate supplementation on skill performance during a soccer match simulation," *Journal of Science and Medicine in Sport* 15, no. 4 (2012), https://doi.org/10.1016/j.jsams.2011.12.006.

20. Mark Russell, David Benton, and Michael Kingsley, "The effects of fatigue on soccer skills performed during a soccer match simulation," *International Journal of Sports Physiology and Performance* 6, no. 2 (2011), https://doi.org/10.1123/ijspp.6.2.221; Mark Russell, David Benton, and Michael Kingsley, "Reliability and construct validity of soccer skills tests that measure passing, shooting, and dribbling," *Journal of Sports Sciences* 28, no. 13 (2010), https://doi.org/10.1080/02640414.2010.511247; Mark Russell et al., "An exercise protocol that replicates soccer match-play," *International Journal of Sports Medicine* 32, no. 7 (2011), https://doi.org/10.1055/s-0031-1273742.

21. Emma J. Stevenson et al., "A comparison of isomaltulose versus maltodextrin ingestion during soccer-specific exercise," *European Journal of Applied Physiology* 117, no. 11 (2017), https://doi.org/10.1007/s00421-017-3750-6.

22. Andrew Foskett, Ajmol Ali, and Nicholas Gant, "Caffeine enhances cognitive function and skill performance during simulated soccer activity," *International Journal of Sport Nutrition and Exercise Metabolism* 19, no. 4 (2009), https://doi.org/10.1123/ijsnem.19.4.410.

23. Edward J. Ryan et al., "Caffeine gum and cycling performance: a timing study," *Journal of Strength and Conditioning Research* 27, no. 1 (2013), https://doi.org/10.1519/jsc.0b013e3182541d03.

24. Anthony J. Sargeant, "Effect of muscle temperature on leg extension force and short-term power output in humans," *European Journal of Applied Physiology and Occupational Physiology* 56, no. 6 (1987), https://doi.org/10.1007/bf00424812.

25. Liam P. Kilduff et al., "The influence of passive heat maintenance on lower body power output and repeated sprint performance in professional rugby league players," *Journal of Science and Medicine in Sport* 16, no. 5 (2013), https://doi.org/10.1016/j.jsams.2012.11.889.

26. Mayur Krachna Ranchordas, Joel T. Dawson, and Mark Russell, "Practical nutritional recovery strategies for elite soccer players when limited time separates repeated matches," *Journal of the International Society of Sports Nutrition* 14, no. 1 (2017), https://doi.org/10.1186/s12970-017-0193-8.

27. Louise M. Burke, Anne B. Loucks, and Nick Broad, "Energy and carbohydrate for training and recovery," *Journal of Sports Sciences* 24, no.7 (2006), https://doi.org/10.1080/02640410500482602.

28. Pablo García-Rovés et al., "Nutrient intake and food habits of soccer players: analyzing the correlates of eating patterns," *Nutrients* 6, no. 7 (2014), https://doi.org/10.3390/nu6072697.

29. Ronald J. Maughan et al., "Fluid and electrolyte intake and loss in elite soccer players during training," *International Journal of Sport Nutrition and Exercise Metabolism* 14, no. 3 (2004), https://doi.org/10.1123/ijsnem.14.3.333.

30. Kelly B. Jouris, Edward P. Weiss, and Jennifer L. McDaniel, "The effect of omega-3 fatty acid supplementation on the inflammatory response to eccentric strength exercise," *Journal of Sports Science and Medicine* 10, no. 3 (2011).

31. Timothy D. Mickleborough, "Omega-3 polyunsaturated fatty acids in physical performance optimization," *International Journal of Sport Nutrition and Exercise Metabolism* 23, no. 1 (2013), https://doi.org/10.1123/ijsnem.23.1.83.

32. A. P. Simopoulos, "Evolutionary aspects of diet and essential fatty acids," in *Fatty Acids and Lipids — New Findings*, Volume 88, eds. T. Hamazaki and H. Okuyama (Basel, Switzerland: Karger, 2001), 18–27.

33. Margot Mountjoy et al., "The IOC consensus statement: beyond the female athlete triad — relative energy deficiency in sport (RED-S)," *British Journal of Sports Medicine* 48, no. 7 (2014), https://doi.org/10.1136/bjsports-2014-093502.

34. Ben House, "The low testosterone epidemic, root causes of 'low T' and evidence-based solutions," *Dr. Bubbs Performance Podcast*, Podcast audio, March 17, 2017, https://drbubbs.com/podcastepisodes/2017/3/episode-12-the-low-testosterone-epidemic-root-causes-of-low-t-evidence-based-solutions-dr-ben-house.

35. Susan Kleiner, "Weight Loss For Women, Female Athletes & Body Composition," *Dr. Bubbs Performance Podcast*, Podcast audio, December 14th, 2017, https://drbubbs.com/podcastepisodes/2017/12/weight-loss-for-women-female-athletes-body-composition-w-dr-susan-kleiner.

36. G. L. Close et al., "New strategies in sport nutrition to increase exercise performance," *Free Radical Biology and Medicine* 98 (2016), https://doi.org/10.1016/j.freeradbiomed.2016.01.016.

37. G. L. Close et al., "Assessment of vitamin D concentration in non-supplemented professional athletes and healthy adults during the winter months in the UK: implications for skeletal muscle function," *Journal of Sports Sciences* 31, no. 4 (2013), https://doi.org/10.1080/02640414.2012.733822.

38. Daniel J. Owens et al., "Vitamin D supplementation does not improve human skeletal muscle contractile properties in insufficient young males," *European Journal of Applied Physiology* 114, no. 6 (2014), https://doi.org/10.1007/s00421-014-2865-2.

39. Philippe Autier, "Vitamin D status as a synthetic biomarker of health status," *Endocrine* 51, no. 2 (2015), https://doi.org/10.1007/s12020-015-0837-x.

40. Institute of Medicine, Food and Nutrition Board, *Dietary Reference Intakes for Vitamin A, Vitamin K, Arsenic, Boron, Chromium, Copper, Iodine, Iron, Manganese, Molybdenum, Nickel, Silicon,*

*Vanadium, and Zinc: a Report of the Panel on Micronutrients,* (Washington, DC: National Academy Press, 2001).

41. Institute of Medicine, Food and Nutrition Board, *Dietary Reference Intakes.*

42. Institute of Medicine, Food and Nutrition Board, *Dietary Reference Intakes.*

43. Peter Peeling et al., "Athletic induced iron deficiency: new insights into the role of inflammation, cytokines and hormones," *European Journal of Applied Physiology* 103, no. 4 (2008), https://doi.org/10.1007/s00421-008-0726-6.

44. Peter Peeling et al., "Iron status and the acute post-exercise hepcidin response in athletes," *PloS ONE* 9, no. 3 (2014), https://doi.org/10.1371/journal.pone.0093002.

## Chapter 7: Periodized Recovery

1. Romain Meeusen et al., "Prevention, diagnosis, and treatment of the overtraining syndrome: joint consensus statement of the European College of Sport Science and the American College of Sports Medicine," *Medicine and Science in Sports and Exercise* 45, no. 1 (2013), https://doi.org/10.1249/mss.0b013e318279a10a; Robert J. Aughey, "Applications of GPS technologies to field sports," *International Journal of Sports Physiology and Performance* 6, no. 3 (2011), https://doi.org/10.1123/ijspp.6.3.295; Ric Lovell and Grant Abt, "Individualisation of time-motion analysis: a case-cohort example," *International Journal of Sports Physiology and Performance* 8, no. 4 (2013), https://doi.org/10.1123/ijspp.8.4.456; Craig Twist and Jamie Highton, "Monitoring fatigue and recovery in rugby league players," *International Journal of Sports Physiology and Performance* 8, no. 5 (2013), https://doi.org/10.1123/ijspp.8.5.467.

2. Philippe Hellard et al., "Training-related risk of common illnesses in elite swimmers over a 4-yr period," *Medicine and Science in Sports and Exercise* 47, no. 4 (2015), https://doi.org/10.1249/mss.0000000000000461.

3. John S. Raglin and Gregory S. Wilson, "Overtraining in athletes," in *Emotions in Sports*, ed. Yuri L. Hanin (Champaign, IL: Human Kinetics; 2000), 191–207; Michael Lambert and Iñigo Mujika, "Physiology of exercise training," in *Recovery for Performance in Sport*, eds. Christophe Hausswirth and Iñigo Mujika (Champaign, IL: Human Kinetics, 2013), 3–8.

4. Richard B. Kreider, Andrew C. Fry, and Mary L. O'Toole, eds., *Overtraining In Sport: Terms, Definitions, and Prevalence* (Champaign, IL: Human Kinetics, 1998).

5. Tudor O. Bompa and Carlo A. Buzzichelli, eds., *Periodization Training: Theory and Methodology*, 4th ed. (Champaign, IL: Human Kinetics, 1999).

6. Kent Sahlin, "Metabolic factors in fatigue," *Sports Medicine* 13, no. 2 (1992), https://doi.org/10.2165/00007256-199213020-00005.

7. Kristie-Lee Taylor et al., "Fatigue monitoring in high performance sport: a survey of current trends," *Journal of Australian Strength and Conditioning* 20, no. 1 (2012).

8. Romain Meeusen et al., "Prevention, diagnosis, and treatment of the overtraining syndrome: joint consensus statement of the European College of Sport Science and the American College of Sports Medicine."

9. Jonathan M. Peake et al., "Muscle damage and inflammation during recovery from exercise," *Journal of Applied Physiology* 122, no. 3 (1985), https://doi.org/10.1152/japplphysiol.00971.2016.

10. Romain Meeusen et al., "Hormonal responses in athletes: the use of a two bout exercise protocol to detect subtle differences in (over)training status," *European Journal of Applied Physiology* 91, no. 2-3 (2004), https://doi.org/10.1007/s00421-003-0940-1.

11. Martine Duclos, "A critical assessment of hormonal methods used in monitoring training status in athletes," *International SportMed Journal* 9, no. 2 (2008).

12. Axel Urhausen, Holger Gabriel, and Wilfried Kindermann, "Blood hormones as markers of training stress and overtraining," *Sports Medicine* 20, no. 4 (1995), https://doi.org/10.2165/00007256-199520040-00004; Manfred Lehman, Carl Foster, and Joseph Keul, "Overtraining in endurance athletes: a brief review," *Medicine and Science in Sports and Exercise* 25, no. 7 (1993), https://doi.org/10.1249/00005768-199307000-00015.

13. Romain Meeusen et al., "Prevention, diagnosis and treatment of the overtraining syndrome: ECSS position statement 'task force,'" *European Journal of Sport Science* 6, no. 1 (2006), https://doi.org/10.1080/17461390600617717.

14. Martine Duclos et al., "Trained versus untrained men: different immediate post-exercise responses of pituitary–adrenal axis," *European Journal of Applied Physiology* 75, no. 4 (1997), https://doi.org/10.1007/s004210050170; Caroline Gouarné et al., "Overnight urinary cortisol and cortisone add new insights into adaptation to training," *Medicine and Science in Sports and Exercise* 37, no. 7 (2005), https://doi.org/10.1249/01.mss.0000170099.10038.3b.

15. Romain Meeusen et al., "Prevention, diagnosis, and treatment of the overtraining syndrome."

16. Romain Meeusen et al., "Prevention, diagnosis, and treatment of the overtraining syndrome."

17. Axel Urhausen, Holger H. W. Gabriel, and Wilfried Kindermann, "Impaired pituitary hormonal response to exhaustive exercise in overtrained endurance athletes," *Medicine and Science in Sports and Exercise* 30, no. 3 (1998), https://doi.org/10.1097/00005768-199803000-00011.

18. Stuart M. Phillips and Luc J. C. Van Loon, "Dietary protein for athletes: from requirements to optimum adaptation," *Journal of Sports Sciences* 29, Supplement 1 (2011), https://doi.org/10.1080/02640414.2011.619204; Louise M. Burke et al., "Carbohydrates for training and competition," *Journal of Sports Sciences* 29, Supplement 1 (2011), https://doi.org/10.1080/02640414.2011.585473.

19. Cassandra M. McIver, Thomas P. Wycherley, and Peter M. Clifton, "MTOR signaling and ubiquitin-proteosome gene expression in the preservation of fat free mass following high protein, calorie restricted weight loss," *Nutrition and Metabolism* 9, no. 1 (2012), https://doi.org/10.1186/1743-7075-9-83; Tyler A. Churchward-Venne et al., "Role of protein and amino acids in promoting lean mass accretion with resistance exercise and attenuating lean mass loss during energy deficit in humans," *Amino Acids* 45, no. 2 (2013), https://doi.org/10.1007/s00726-013-1506-0.

20. Ina Garthe et al., "Effect of nutritional intervention on body composition and performance in elite athletes," *European Journal of Sport Science* 13, no. 3 (2013), https://doi.org/10.1080/17461391.2011.643923.

21. D. T. Thomas, K. A. Erdman, and L. M. Burke, "American College of Sports Medicine joint position statement. Nutrition and athletic performance," *Medicine and Science in Sports and Exercise* 48, no. 3 (2016), https://doi.org/10.1249/MSS.0000000000000852; J. S. Volek, "Nutritional aspects of women strength athletes," *British Journal of Sports Medicine* 40, no. 9 (2006), https://doi.org/10.1136/bjsm.2004.016709.

22. Iñigo Mujika et al., "An integrated, multifactorial approach to periodization for optimal performance in individual and team sports," *International Journal of Sports Physiology and Performance* 13, no. 5 (2018), https://doi.org/10.1123/ijspp.2018-0093.

23. Jennifer Sygo et al., "Prevalence of indicators of low energy availability in elite female sprinters," *International Journal of Sport Nutrition and Exercise Metabolism* 28, no. 5 (2018), https://doi.org/10.1123/ijsnem.2017-0397.

24. Jennifer Sygo et al., "Prevalence of indicators of low energy availability in elite female sprinters."

25. Jonathan Bloomfield, Remco Polman, and Peter O'Donoghue, "Physical demands of different positions in FA Premier League soccer," *Journal of Sports Science and Medicine* 6, no. 1 (2007); Christopher Carling, Franck Le Gall, and Gregory Dupont, "Analysis of repeated high-intensity running performance in professional soccer," *Journal of Sports Sciences* 30, no. 4 (2012), https://doi.org/10.1080/02640414.2011.652655.

26. Stuart M. Phillips and Luc J. C. Van Loon, "Dietary protein for athletes."

27. Jonathan M. Oliver et al., "Macronutrient intake in Collegiate powerlifters participating in off season training," *Journal of the International Society of Sports Nutrition* 7, Supplement 1 (2010), https://doi.org/10.1186/1550-2783-7-s1-p8.

28. Chad Kerksick et al., "International society of sports nutrition position stand: nutrient timing," *Journal of the International Society of Sports Nutrition* 14, no. 1 (2017), https://doi.org/10.1186/1550-2783-5-18.

29. Anthony A. Duplanty et al., "Effect of acute alcohol ingestion on resistance exercise induced mTORC1 signaling in human muscle," *Journal of Strength and Conditioning Research* 31, no. 1 (2017), https://doi.org/10.1519/jsc.0000000000001468.

30. Louise M. Burke et al., "Carbohydrates for training and competition."

31. Francis E. Holway and Lawrence L. Spriet, "Sport-specific nutrition: practical strategies for team sports," *Journal of Sports Sciences* 29, Supplement 1 (2011), https://doi.org/10.1080/02640414. 2011.605459; P. D. Balsom et al., "Carbohydrate intake and multiple sprint sports: with special reference to football (soccer)," *International Journal of Sports Medicine* 20, no. 1 (1999), https://doi .org/10.1055/s-2007-971091.

32. T. Gunnarsson et al., "Effect of whey protein- and carbohydrate-enriched diet on glycogen resynthesis during the first 48 h after a soccer game," *Scandinavian Journal of Medicine and Science in Sports* 23, no. 4 (2011), https://doi.org/10.1111/j.1600-0838.2011.01418.x; Peter Krustrup et al., "Maximal voluntary contraction force, SR function and glycogen resynthesis during the first 72 h after a high-level competitive soccer game," *European Journal of Applied Physiology* 111, no. 12 (2011), https://doi.org/10.1007/s00421-011-1919-y.

33. Lisa E. Heaton et al., "Selected in-season nutritional strategies to enhance recovery for team sport athletes: a practical overview," *Sports Medicine* 47, no. 11 (2017), https://doi.org/10.1007 /s40279-017-0759-2.

34. Thomas Reilly et al., "Nutrition for travel," *Journal of Sports Sciences* 25, Supplement 1 (2007), https://doi.org/10.1080/02640410701607445; Shona L. Halson, "Sleep in elite athletes and nutritional interventions to enhance sleep," *Sports Medicine* 44, Supplement 1 (2014), https://doi .org/10.1007/s40279-014-0147-0.

35. Chris McGlory et al., "Temporal changes in human skeletal muscle and blood lipid composition with fish oil supplementation," *Prostaglandins Leukot Essent Fatty Acids* 90, no. 6 (2014), https://doi. org/10.1016/j.plefa.2014.03.001.

36. Kelly B. Jouris, Jennifer L. McDaniel, and Edward P. Weiss, "The effect of omega-3 fatty acid supplementation on the inflammatory response to eccentric strength exercise," *Journal of Sports Science and Medicine* 10, no. 3 (2011); Bakhtiar Tartibian, Behzad Hajizadeh Maleki, and Asghar Abbasi, "The effects of omega-3 supplementation on pulmonary function of young wrestlers during intensive training," *Journal of Science and Medicine in Sport* 13, no. 2 (2010), https://doi .org/10.1016/j.jsams.2008.12.634.

37. Susan M. Ring, Erin A. Dannecker, and Catherine A. Peterson, "Vitamin D status is not associated with outcomes of experimentally-induced muscle weakness and pain in young, healthy volunteers," *Journal of Nutrition and Metabolism* 2010 (2010), https://doi.org/10.1155/2010/674240.

38. Tyler Barker, "Supplemental vitamin D enhances the recovery in peak isometric force shortly after intense exercise," *Nutrition and Metabolism* 10, no. 1 (2013), https://doi.org/10.1186 /1743-7075-10-69.

39. Daniel J. Owens et al., "A systems based investigation into vitamin D and skeletal muscle repair, regeneration and hypertrophy," *American Journal of Physiology-Endocrinology and Metabolism* 309, no. 12 (2015), https://doi.org/10.1152/ajpendo.00375.2015.

40. Jaouad Bouayed and Torsten Bohn, "Exogenous antioxidants: double-edged swords in cellular redox state: health beneficial effects at physiologic doses versus deleterious effects at high doses," *Oxidative Medicine and Cellular Longevity* 3, no. 4 (2010), https://doi.org/10.4161/oxim.3.4.12858.

41. G. L. Close et al., "New strategies in sport nutrition to increase exercise performance," *Free Radical Biology and Medicine* 98 (2016), https://doi.org/10.1016/j.freeradbiomed.2016.01.016; Robert T. Mankowski et al., "Dietary antioxidants as modifiers of physiologic adaptations to exercise," *Medicine and Science in Sports and Exercise* 47, no. 9 (2015), https://doi.org/10.1249/mss.0000000000000620.

42. Dale Morrison et al., "Vitamin C and E supplementation prevents some of the cellular adaptations to endurance-training," *Free Radical Biology and Medicine* 89 (2015), https://doi.org/10.1016/j .freeradbiomed.2015.10.412.

43. Andrea J. Braakhuis and Will G. Hopkins, "Impact of dietary antioxidants on sport performance: a review," *Sports Medicine* 45, no. 7 (2015), https://doi.org/10.1007/s40279-015-0323-x; Andrea J. Braakhuis, "Effect of vitamin C supplements on physical performance," *Current Sports Medicine Reports* 11, no. 4 (2012), https://doi.org/10.1249/jsr.0b013e31825e19cd.

44. William Clements, Sang-Rok Lee, and Richard Bloomer, "Nitrate ingestion: a review of the health and physical performance effects," *Nutrients* 6, no. 11 (2014), https://doi.org/10.3390/nu6115224.

45. Phillip Bell et al., "The effects of Montmorency tart cherry concentrate supplementation on recovery following prolonged, intermittent exercise," *Nutrients* 8, no. 7 (2016), https://doi.org/10.3390/nu8070441; Kyle Levers et al., "Effects of powdered Montmorency tart cherry supplementation on acute endurance exercise performance in aerobically trained individuals," *Journal of the International Society of Sports Nutrition* 13, no. 1 (2016), https://doi.org/10.1186/s12970-016-0133-z.

46. Achraf Ammar et al., "Pomegranate supplementation accelerates recovery of muscle damage and soreness and inflammatory markers after a weightlifting training session," *PloS ONE* 11, no. 10 (2016), https://doi.org/10.1371/journal.pone.0160305; Justin R. Trombold et al., "The effect of pomegranate juice supplementation on strength and soreness after eccentric exercise," *Journal of Strength and Conditioning Research* 27, no. 7 (2011), https://doi.org/10.1519/jsc.0b013e318220d992.

47. Alexander T. Hutchison et al., "Black currant nectar reduces muscle damage and inflammation following a bout of high-intensity eccentric contractions," *Journal of Dietary Supplements* 13, no. 1 (2016), https://doi.org/10.3109/19390211.2014.952864.

48. Eric S. Rawson and Adam. M. Persky, "Mechanisms of muscular adaptations to creatine supplementation," *International Sport Med Journal* 8, no. 2 (2007); Matthew B. Cooke et al., "Creatine supplementation enhances muscle force recovery after eccentrically-induced muscle damage in healthy individuals," *Journal of the International Society of Sports Nutrition* 6, no. 1 (2009), https://doi.org/10.1186/1550-2783-6-13.

49. Kelly F. Veggi et al., "Oral creatine supplementation augments the repeated bout effect," *International Journal of Sport Nutrition and Exercise Metabolism* 23, no. 4 (2013), https://doi.org/10.1123/ijsnem.23.4.378.

50. R. A. Bassit, R. Curi, and L. F. B. P. Costa Rosa, "Creatine supplementation reduces plasma levels of pro-inflammatory cytokines and PGE2 after a half-ironman competition," *Amino Acids* 35, no. 2 (2007), https://doi.org/10.1007/s00726-007-0582-4.

51. R. V. T. Santos et al., "The effect of creatine supplementation upon inflammatory and muscle soreness markers after a 30 km race," *Life Sciences* 75, no. 16 (2004), https://doi.org/10.1016/j.lfs.2003.11.036.

52. G. Yuan, M. L. Wahlqvist, G. He, et al., "Natural products and anti-inflammatory activity," *Asia Pacific Journal of Clinical Nutrition* 15, no. 2 (2006).

53. Brian K. McFarlin et al., "Reduced inflammatory and muscle damage biomarkers following oral supplementation with bioavailable curcumin," *BBA Clinical* 5 (2016), https://doi.org/10.1016/j.bbacli.2016.02.003.

54. Lesley M. Nicol et al., "Curcumin supplementation likely attenuates delayed onset muscle soreness (DOMS)," *European Journal of Applied Physiology* 115, no. 8 (2015), https://doi.org/10.1007/s00421-015-3152-6.

55. Joseph N. Sciberras et al., "The effect of turmeric (curcumin) supplementation on cytokine and inflammatory marker responses following 2 hours of endurance cycling," *Journal of the International Society of Sports Nutrition* 12, no. 1 (2015), https://doi.org/10.1186/s12970-014-0066-3.

56. Jennifer Z. Paxton, Liam M. Grover, and Keith Baar, "Engineering an in vitro model of a functional ligament from bone to bone," *Tissue Engineering Part A* 16, no. 11 (2010), https://doi.org/10.1089/ten.tea.2010.0039.

57. Gregory Shaw et al., "Vitamin C-enriched gelatin supplementation before intermittent activity augments collagen synthesis," *American Journal of Clinical Nutrition* 105, no. 1 (2016), https://doi .org/10.3945/ajcn.116.138594.

58. Kristine L. Clark et al., "24-week study on the use of collagen hydrolysate as a dietary supplement in athletes with activity-related joint pain," *Current Medical Research Opinion* 24, no. 5 (2008), https://doi.org/10.1185/030079908x291967.

59. T. E. McAlindon et al., "Change in knee osteoarthritis cartilage detected by delayed gadolinium enhanced magnetic resonance imaging following treatment with collagen hydrolysate: a pilot randomized controlled trial," *Osteoarthritis Cartilage* 19, no. 4 (2011), https://doi.org/10.1016/j .joca.2011.01.001.

## Chapter 8: Athlete Immunity

1. Michael Gleeson, "Immunological aspects of sport nutrition," *Immunology and Cell Biology* 94, no. 2 (2016), https://doi.org/10.1038/icb.2015.109.

2. Michael Gleeson, Nicolette Bishop, and Neil Walsh, *Exercise Immunology* (London, U.K.: Routledge, 2013).

3. David C. Nieman, "Exercise, upper respiratory tract infection, and the immune system," *Medicine and Science in Sports and Exercise* 26, no. 2 (1994), https://doi.org/10.1249/00005768 -199402000-00002.

4. David C. Nieman et al., "Infectious episodes in runners before and after the Los Angeles Marathon," *Journal of Sports Medicine and Physical Fitness* 30, no. 3 (1990).

5. E. M. Peters and E. D. Bateman, "Ultramarathon running and upper respiratory tract infections. An epidemiological survey," *South African Medical Journal* 64, no. 15 (1983).

6. Martin Schwellnus et al., "How much is too much? (Part 2) International Olympic Committee consensus statement on load in sport and risk of illness," *British Journal of Sports Medicine* 50, no. 17 (2016), https://doi.org/10.1136/bjsports-2016-096572.

7. Sandra Mårtensson, Kristina Nordebo, and Christer Malm, "High training volumes are associated with a low number of self-reported sick days in elite endurance athletes," *Journal of Sports Science and Medicine* 13, no. 4 (2014).

8. David C. Nieman, "Is infection risk linked to exercise workload?," *Medicine and Science in Sports and Exercise* 32, no. 7 (2000), https://doi.org/10.1097/00005768-200007001-00005.

9. C. Malm, "Susceptibility to infections in elite athletes: the S-curve," *Scandinavian Journal of Medicine and Science in Sports* 16, no. 1 (2006), https://doi.org/10.1111/j.1600-0838.2005.00499.x.

10. Juan-Manuel Alonso et al., "Occurrence of injuries and illnesses during the 2009 IAAF World Athletics Championships," *British Journal of Sports Medicine* 44, no. 15 (2010), https://doi.org /10.1136/bjsm.2010.078030.

11. T. G. Weidner, "Literature review: upper respiratory illness and sport and exercise," *International Journal of Sports Medicine* 15, no. 1 (1994), https://doi.org/10.1055/s-2007-1021011; Luke Spence et al., "Incidence, etiology, and symptomatology of upper respiratory illness in elite athletes," *Medicine and Science in Sports and Exercise* 39, no. 4 (2007), https://doi.org/10.1249/mss .0b013e31802e851a.

12. L. J. Taylor, "An evaluation of handwashing techniques," *Nursing Times*, January 1978.

13. N. P. Walsh et al., "Position statement. Part one: immune function and exercise," *Exercise Immunology Review* 17 (2011).

14. N.P. Walsh et al., "Position statement. Part two: maintaining immune health," *Exercise Immunology Review* 17, (2011).

15. Michael Gleeson, "Immunological aspects of sport nutrition," *Immunology and Cell Biology* 94, no. 2 (2015), https://doi.org/10.1038/icb.2015.109.

16. Kenneth Ostrowski et al., "Pro- and anti-inflammatory cytokine balance in strenuous exercise in humans," *The Journal of Physiology* 515, no. 1 (1999), https://doi.org/10.1111/j.1469-7793.1999.287ad.x.

17. Helen G. Hanstock et al., "Tear fluid sIgA as a non-invasive biomarker of mucosal immunity and common cold risk," *Medicine and Science in Sports and Exercise* 48, no. 3 (2016), https://doi.org/10.1249/mss.0000000000000801.

18. N. P. Walsh et al., "Position statement. Part one: immune function and exercise."

19. J. M. Peake, "Exercise-induced alterations in neutrophil degranulation and respiratory burst activity: possible mechanisms of action," *Exercise Immunology Review* 8 (2002); Peter Peeling et al., "Cumulative effects of consecutive running sessions on hemolysis, inflammation and hepcidin activity," *European Journal of Applied Physiology* 106, no. 1 (2009), https://doi.org/10.1007/s00421-009-0988-7.

20. J. M. Peake, "Exercise-induced alterations in neutrophil degranulation and respiratory burst activity: possible mechanisms of action."

21. J. M. Peake, "Exercise-induced alterations in neutrophil degranulation and respiratory burst activity: possible mechanisms of action."

22. Ola Ronsen et al., "Recovery time affects immunoendocrine responses to a second bout of endurance exercise," *American Journal of Physiology-Cell Physiology* 283, no. 6 (2002), https://doi.org/10.1152/ajpcell.00242.2002.

23. A. Bøyum et al., "Chemiluminescence response of granulocytes from elite athletes during recovery from one or two intense bouts of exercise," *European Journal of Applied Physiology* 88, no. 1-2 (2002), https://doi.org/10.1007/s00421-002-0705-2.

24. Vernon Neville, Michael Gleeson, and Jonathan P. Folland, "Salivary IgA as a risk factor for upper respiratory infections in elite professional athletes," *Medicine and Science in Sports and Exercise* 40, no. 7 (2008), https://doi.org/10.1249/mss.0b013e31816be9c3.

25. Gerald D. Tharp and Marc W. Barnes, "Reduction of saliva immunoglobulin levels by swim training," *European Journal of Applied Physiology and Occupational Physiology* 60, no. 1 (1990), https://doi.org/10.1007/bf00572187.

26. Mariane M. Fahlman and Hermann-J. Engels, "Mucosal IgA and URTI in American college football players: a year longitudinal study," *Medicine and Science in Sports and Exercise* 37, no. 3 (2005), https://doi.org/10.1249/01.mss.0000155432.67020.88.

27. Vernon Neville, Michael Gleeson, and Jonathan P. Folland, "Salivary IgA as a risk factor for upper respiratory infections in elite professional athletes."

28. Gerald D. Tharp and Marc W. Barnes, "Reduction of saliva immunoglobulin levels by swim training."

29. Sheldon Cohen et al., "Sleep habits and susceptibility to the common cold," *Archives of Internal Medicine* 169, no. 1 (2009), https://doi.org/10.1001/archinternmed.2008.505; Aric A. Prather et al., "Behaviorally assessed sleep and susceptibility to the common cold," *Sleep* 38, no. 9 (2015), https://doi.org/10.5665/sleep.4968.

30. Michael R. Irwin, "Why sleep is important for health: a psychoneuroimmunology perspective," *Annual Review of Psychology* 66, no. 1 (2015), https://doi.org/10.1146/annurev-psych-010213-115205.

31. Marc Cuesta et al., "Simulated night shift disrupts circadian rhythms of immune functions in humans," *The Journal of Immunology* 196, no. 6 (2016), https://doi.org/10.4049/jimmunol.1502422.

32. Aric A. Prather et al., "Sleep and antibody response to hepatitis B vaccination," *Sleep* 35, no. 8 (2012), https://doi.org/10.5665/sleep.1990.

33. Sheldon Cohen, David A. J. Tyrrell, and Andrew P. Smith, "Psychological stress and susceptibility to the common cold," *New England Journal of Medicine* 325, no. 9 (1991), https://doi.org/10.1056/nejm199108293250903.

34. Vicki Stover Hertzberg et al., "Behaviors, movements, and transmission of droplet-mediated respiratory diseases during transcontinental airline flights," *Proceedings of the National Academy of Sciences* 115, no. 14 (2018), https://doi.org/10.1073/pnas.1711611115.

35. Robert L. Sack, "Jet lag," *The New England Journal of Medicine* 362, no. 5 (2010), https://doi.org/10.1056/NEJMcp0909838.

36. Cheng Shiun He et al., "Is there an optimal vitamin D status for immunity in athletes and military personnel?" *Exercise Immunology Review* 22 (2016).

37. N. P. Walsh et al., "Position statement. Part two: maintaining immune health."

38. Jonathan M. Peake et al., "Recovery of the immune system after exercise," *Journal of Applied Physiology* 122, no. 5 (2017), https://doi.org/10.1152/japplphysiol.00622.2016.

39. Graeme L. Lancaster et al., "Effect of pre-exercise carbohydrate ingestion on plasma cytokine, stress hormone, and neutrophil degranulation responses to continuous, high-intensity exercise," *International Journal of Sport Nutrition and Exercise Metabolism* 13, no. 4 (2003), https://doi.org /10.1123/ijsnem.13.4.436 .

40. Nicolette E. Bishop et al., "Pre-exercise carbohydrate status and immune responses to prolonged cycling: II. Effect on plasma cytokine concentration," *International Journal of Sport Nutrition and Exercise Metabolism* 11 (2001), https://doi.org/10.1123/ijsnem.11.4.503; Michael Gleeson et al., "Effect of low- and high-carbohydrate diets on the plasma glutamine and circulating leukocyte responses to exercise," *International Journal of Sport Nutrition* 8, no. 1 (1998), https:// doi.org/10.1123/ijsn.8.1.49; J. B. Mitchell et al., "Influence of carbohydrate status on immune responses before and after endurance exercise," *Journal of Applied Physiology* 84, no. 6 (1998), https://doi.org/10.1152/jappl.1998.84.6.1917.

41. John A. Hawley and Louise M. Burke, "Carbohydrate availability and training adaptation: effects on cell metabolism," *Exercise and Sport Sciences Reviews* 38, no. 4 (2010), https://doi.org/10.1097 /jes.0b013e3181f44dd9.

42. Oliver C. Witard et al., "High dietary protein restores overreaching induced impairments in leu-kocyte trafficking and reduces the incidence of upper respiratory tract infection in elite cyclists," *Brain, Behavior, and Immunity* 39 (2014), https://doi.org/10.1016/j.bbi.2013.10.002.

43. N. P. Walsh et al., "Position statement. Part two: maintaining immune health."

44. Thomas B. Tomasi et al., "Immune parameters in athletes before and after strenuous exercise"; Neil P. Walsh et al., "Salivary IgA response to prolonged exercise in a cold environment in trained cyclists"; A. K. Blannin et al., "Effects of submaximal cycling and long endurance training on neutrophil phagocytic activity in middle aged men."

45. Sarah King et al., "Effectiveness of probiotics on the duration of illness in healthy children and adults who develop common acute respiratory infectious conditions: a systematic review and meta-analysis," *British Journal of Nutrition* 112, no. 1 (2014), https://doi.org/10.1017/s0007114514000075.

46. Qiukui Hao, Bi Rong Dong, and Taixiang Wu, "Probiotics for preventing acute upper respiratory tract infections," *Cochrane Database of Systematic Reviews*, no. 2 (2015), https://doi. org/10.1002/14651858.cd006895.pub3.

47. Nicholas P. West et al., "Probiotic supplementation for respiratory and gastrointestinal illness symptoms in healthy physically active individuals," *Clinical Nutrition* 33, no. 4 (2014), https://doi .org/10.1016/j.clnu.2013.10.002.

48. Michael Gleeson et al., "Daily probiotic's (Lactobacillus casei Shirota) reduction of infection incidence in athletes," *International Journal of Sport Nutrition and Exercise Metabolism* 21, no. 1 (2011), https://doi.org/10.1123/ijsnem.21.1.55.

49. Lee A. Zella et al., "Vitamin D-binding protein influences total circulating levels of 1,25-dihydroxyvitamin D3 but does not directly modulate the bioactive levels of the hormone in vivo," *Endocrinology* 149, no. 7 (2008), https://doi.org/10.1210/en.2008-0042.

50. Daniel D. Bikle, "Vitamin D and immune function: understanding common pathways," *Current Osteoporosis Reports* 7, no. 2 (2009), https://doi.org/10.1007/s11914-009-0011-6; Tanya M. Halli-day et al., "Vitamin D status relative to diet, lifestyle, injury, and illness in college athletes," *Medicine and Science in Sports and Exercise* 43, no. 2 (2011), https://doi.org/10.1249/mss.0b013e3181eb9d4d.

51. Cheng Shiun He et al., "Influence of vitamin D status on respiratory infection incidence and immune function during 4 months of winter training in endurance sport athletes," *Exercise Immunology Review* 19 (2013).

52. Harri Hemilä, "Zinc lozenges may shorten the duration of colds: a systematic review," *Open Respiratory Medicine Journal* 5, no. 1 (2011), https://doi.org/10.2174/1874306401105010051.

53. Xiaoshuang Dai et al., "Consuming *Lentinula edodes* (shiitake) mushrooms daily improves human immunity: a randomized dietary intervention in healthy young adults," *Journal of the American College of Nutrition* 34, no. 6 (2015), https://doi.org/10.1080/07315724.2014.950391.

54. Alan L. Buchman, "Glutamine: commercially essential or conditionally essential? A critical appraisal of human data," *American Journal of Clinical Nutrition* 74, no. 1 (2001), https://doi.org/10.1093/ajcn/74.1.25.

## Chapter 9: Athlete Monitoring and Recovery Strategies

1. Manfred Lehmann et al., eds., *Overload, Performance Incompetence, and Regeneration in Sport* (New York: Springer, 1999); Sean O. Richardson, Mark Andersen, and Tony Morris, *Overtraining Athletes: Personal Journeys in Sport* (Champaign, IL: Human Kinetics, 2008).

2. Romain Meeusen et al., "Prevention, diagnosis and treatment of the overtraining syndrome" *European Journal Sport Science* 6, no. 1 (2006), https://doi.org/10.1080/17461390600617717.

3. Rod W. Fry, Alan R. Morton, and David Keast, "Overtraining in athletes: an update," *Sports Medicine* 12, no. 1 (1991), https://doi.org/10.2165/00007256-199112010-00004.

4. Anthony Turner and Paul Comfort, eds., *Advanced Strength and Conditioning — An Evidence-Based Approach* (London, U.K.: Routledge, 2018).

5. Thierry Busso, "Variable dose response relationship between exercise training and performance," *Medicine and Science in Sports and Exercise* 35, no. 7 (2003), https://doi.org/10.1249/01.mss.0000074465.13621.37.

6. Nijem Ramsey (Head Strength and Conditioning Coach for NBA Sacramento Kings), in discussion with the author, June 18, 2018.

7. Kent Sahlin, "Metabolic factors in fatigue," *Sports Medicine* 13, no. 2 (1992), https://doi.org/10.2165/00007256-199213020-00005.

8. Tim J. Gabbett, "Influence of training and match intensity on injuries in rugby league," *Journal of Sports Sciences* 22, no. 5 (2004), https://doi.org/10.1080/02640410310001641638.

9. Tim J. Gabbet, "Reductions in pre-season training loads reduce training injury rates in rugby league players," *British Journal of Sports Medicine* 38, no. 6 (2004), https://doi.org/10.1136/bjsm.2003.008391.

10. Billy T. Hulin et al., "The acute:chronic workload ratio predicts injury: High chronic workload may decrease injury risk in elite rugby players," *British Journal of Sports Medicine* 50, no. 4 (2016), https://doi.org/10.1136/bjsports-2015-094817.

11. Shane Malone et al., "Aerobic fitness and playing experience protect against spike in workload: the role of the acute:chronic workload ratio on injury risk in elite Gaelic football," *International Journal of Sports Physiology and Performance* 12, no. 3 (2016), http://dx.doi.org/10.1123/ijspp.2016-0090.

12. Billy T. Hulin et al., "Spikes in acute workload are associated with increased injury risk in elite cricket fast bowlers," *British Journal of Sports Medicine* 48, no. 8 (2013), https://doi.org/10.1136/bjsports-2013-092524.

13. Billy T. Hulin et al., "Low chronic workload and the acute:chronic workload ratio are more predictive of injury than between match recovery time:a two season prospective cohort study in elite rugby league players," *British Journal of Sports Medicine* 50, no. 16 (2016), https://doi.org/10.1136/bjsports-2015-095364; Nicholas B. Murray et al., "Calculating acute:chronic workload ratios using exponentially weighted moving averages provides a more sensitive indicator of injury likelihood than rolling averages," *British Journal of Sports Medicine* 51, no. 9 (2016), https://doi.org/10.1136/bjsports-2016-097152.

14. Shane Malone et al., "High chronic training loads and exposure to bouts of maximal velocity running reduce injury risk in Gaelic football," *Journal of Science and Medicine in Sport* 20, no. 3 (2017), https://doi.org/10.1016/j.jsams.2016.08.005.

15. Axel Urhausen and Wilfried Kindermann, "Diagnosis of overtraining: what tools do we have?," *Sports Medicine* 32, no. 2 (2002), https://doi.org/10.2165/00007256-200232020-00002.

16. Brent S. Rushall, "A tool for measuring stress tolerance in elite athletes," *Journal of Applied Sport Psychology* 2, no. 1 (1990), https://doi.org/10.1080/10413209008406420.

17. John S. Raglin, "Psychological factors in sport performance: the mental health model revisited," *Sports Medicine* 31, no. 12 (2001), https://doi.org/10.2165/00007256-200131120-00004.

18. Paul B. Gastin, Denny Meyer, and Dean Robinson, "Perceptions of wellness to monitor adaptive responses to training and competitions in elite Australian football," *Journal of Strength and Conditioning Research* 27, no. 9 (2013), https://doi.org/10.1519/jsc.0b013e31827fd600.

19. Kristie-Lee Taylor et al., "Fatigue monitoring in high performance sport: a survey of current trends," *Journal of Australian Strength and Conditioning* 20, no. 1 (2012).

20. Anna E. Saw, Luana C. Main, and Paul B. Gastin, "Monitoring the athlete training response: subjective self-reported measure trump commonly used objective measures: a systematic review," *British Journal of Sports Medicine* 50, no. 5 (2016), https://doi.org/10.1136/bjsports-2015-094758.

21. Maamer Slimani et al., "Rating of perceived exertion for quantification of training and combat loads during combat sport-specific activities: a short review," *Journal of Strength and Conditioning Research* 31, no. 10 (2017), https://doi.org/10.1519/jsc.0000000000002047.

22. James Faulkner, Gaynor Parfitt, and Roger Eston, "The rating of perceived exertion during competitive running scales with time," *Psychophysiology* 45, no. 6 (2008), https://doi.org/10.1111/j.1469-8986.2008.00712.x.

23. Franco M. Impellizzeri et al., "Use of RPE-Based Training Load in Soccer." *Medicine and Science in Sports and Exercise* 36, no. 6 (2004), https://doi.org/10.1249/01.mss.0000128199.23901.2f.

24. Marco C. Uchida et al., "Does the timing of measurement alter session-RPE in boxers?," *Journal of Sports Science and Medicine* 13, no. 1 (2014).

25. Anthony Turner and Paul Comfort, eds., *Advanced Strength and Conditioning.*

26. Fred Schafer and J. P. Ginsberg, "An overview of heart rate variability metrics and norms," *Frontiers in Public Health* 5, no. 285 (2017), https://doi.org/10.3389/fpubh.2017.00258.

27. Daniela Grimaldi et al., "Adverse impact of sleep restriction and circadian misalignment on autonomic function in healthy young adults," *Hypertension* 68, no. 1 (2016), https://doi.org/10.1161/hypertensionaha.115.06847.

28. Michelle M. Meyer et al., "Association of glucose homeostasis measures with heart rate variability among Hispanic/Latino adults without diabetes: the Hispanic Community Health Study/Study of Latinos (HCHS/SOL)," *Cardiovascular Diabetology* 15, no. 1 (2016), https://doi.org/10.1186/s12933-016-0364-y.

29. Andrew H. Kemp et al., "Impact of depression and antidepressant treatment on heart rate variability: a review and meta-analysis," *Biological Psychiatry* 67, no. 11 (2010), https://doi.org/10.1016/j.biopsych.2009.12.012.

30. Stavros Kavouras, "Hydration and heat acclimatization in athletes," *Dr. Bubbs Performance Podcast*, Podcast audio, February 1, 2018, https://drbubbs.com/season-2-podcast-episodes/2018/2/s2-episode-5-hydration-heat-acclimatization-in-athletes-stavros-kavouras.

31. Mauricio Castro-Sepulveda et al., "Hydration status after exercise affect resting metabolic rate and heart rate variability," *Nutricion Hospitalaria* 31, no. 3 (2014), https://doi.org/10.3305/nh.2015.31.3.8523.

32. Usman Zulfiqar et al., "Relation of high heart rate variability to healthy longevity," *American Journal of Cardiology* 105, no. 8 (2010), https://doi.org/10.1016/j.amjcard.2009.12.022.

33. Paul Poirier et al., "Exercise, heart rate variability, and longevity: the cocoon mystery?," *Circulation* 129, no. 21 (2014), https://doi.org/10.1161/circulationaha.114.009778.

34. Julian Koenig et al., "Impact of caffeine on heart rate variability: a systematic review," *Journal of Caffeine Research* 3, no. 1 (2013), https://doi.org/10.1089/jcr.2013.0009.

35. Andrew A. Flatt, Michael R. Esco, and Fabio Y. Nakamura, "Individual heart rate variability responses to pre-season training in high level female soccer players," *Journal Strength Conditioning Research* 31, no. 2 (2017).

36. Danilo F. da Silva et al., "Endurance running training individually-guided by HRV in untrained women," *Journal of Strength and Conditioning Research* (2017), https://doi.org/10.1519/jsc .0000000000002001.

37. Daniel J. Plews et al., "Evaluating training adaptation with heart-rate measures: a methodological comparison," *International Journal of Sports Physiology and Performance* 8, no. 6 (2013), https://doi .org/10.1123/ijspp.8.6.688.

38. Jonathan Leeder et al., "Cold water immersion and recovery from strenuous exercise; a meta-analysis," *British Journal of Sports Medicine* 46, no. 4 (2012), https://doi.org/10.1136/bjsports-2011-090061.

39. Jonathan M. Peake et al., "The effects of cold water immersion and active recovery on inflammation and cell stress responses in human skeletal muscle after resistance exercise," *Journal of Physiology* 595, no. 3 (2017), https://doi.org/10.1113/jp272881.

40. Mohammed Ihsan, Greig Watson, and Chris R. Abbiss, "What are the physiological mechanisms for post-exercise cold water immersion in the recovery form prolonged endurance and intermittent exercise?," *Sports Medicine* 46, no. 8 (2016), https://doi.org/10.1007/s40279-016-0483-3.

41. Chris Bleakely et al., "Cold-water immersion (cryotherapy) for preventing and treating muscle soreness after exercise," *Cochrane Database of Systematic Reviews*, no. 2 (2012), https://doi.org /10.1002/14651858.CD008262.pub2.

42. Nathan G. Versey, Shona L. Halson, and Brian T. Dawson, "Water immersion recovery for athletes: effect on exercise performance and practical recommendations," *Sports Medicine* 43, no. 11 (2013), https://doi.org/10.1007/s40279-013-0063-8.

43. Joanna Vaile et al., "Effect of hydrotherapy on recovery from fatigue," *International Journal of Sports Medicine* 29, no. 7 (2008), https://doi.org/10.1055/s-2007-989267.

44. Joanna Vaile et al., "Effect of hydrotherapy on signs and symptoms of delayed onset muscle soreness," *European Journal of Applied Physiology* 103, no. 1 (2008), https://doi.org/10.1007/s00421-007-0653-y.

45. Shona L. Halson, "Controversies in Recovery," (presentation, University of Notre Dame and Australian Catholic University Human Performance Summit: The 24 Hour Athlete, South Bend, Indiana, USA, June 2018).

46. Christophe Hausswirth et al., "Effects of whole body cryotherapy vs. far-infrared vs. passive modalities on recovery from exercise-induced muscle damage in highly-trained runners," *PLoS ONE* 6, no. 12 (2011), https://doi.org/10.1371/journal.pone.0027749; B. Fonda and N. Sarabon, "Effects of whole-body cryotherapy on recovery after hamstring damaging exercise: a crossover study," *Scandinavian Journal of Medicine and Science in Sports* 23, no. 5 (2013), https://doi.org/10.1111/sms.12074.

47. J. Costello et al., "Effects of whole-body cryotherapy and cold-water immersion on knee skin temperature," *International Journal of Sports Medicine* 35, no. 1 (2014), https://doi.org/10.1055 /s-0033-1343410.

48. Abd-Elbasset Abaïdia et al., "Recovery from exercise-induced muscle damage: cold water immersion versus whole body cryotherapy," *International Journal of Sports Physiology and Performance* 12, no. 3 (2017), https://doi.org/10.1123/ijspp.2016-0186.

49. Laura J. Wilson et al., "Recovery following a marathon: a comparison of cold water immersion, whole body cryotherapy and a placebo control," *European Journal of Applied Physiology* 118, no. 1 (2018), https://doi.org/10.1007/s00421-017-3757-z.

50. Jessica A. Hill et al., "Compression garments and recovery from exercise-induced muscle damage: a meta-analysis," *British Journal of Sports Medicine* 48, no. 18 (2014), https://doi.org/10.1136 /bjsports-2013-092456.

51. Jessica A. Hill et al., "Influence of compression garments on recovery after marathon running," *Journal of Strength and Conditioning Research* 28, no. 8 (2014), https://doi.org/10.1519/jsc .0000000000000469.

52. Jessica A. Hill et al., "Effects of compression garment pressure on recovery from strenuous exercise," *International Journal of Sports Physiology and Performance* 12, no. 8 (2017), https://doi .org/10.1123/ijspp.2016-0380.

53. Llion A. Roberts et al., "Post-exercise cold water immersion attenuates acute anabolic signaling and long-term adaptations in muscle to strength training," *Journal of Physiology* 593, no. 18 (2015), https://doi.org/10.1113/jp270570.

54. Shona L. Halson et al., "Does hydrotherapy help or hinder adaptation to training in competitive cyclists?," *Medicine and Science in Sports and Exercise* 46, no. 8 (2014), https://doi.org/10.1249 /mss.0000000000000268.

55. C. H. Joo et al., "Passive and post-exercise cold-water immersion augments PGC-1a and VEGF expression in human skeletal muscle," *European Journal of Applied Physiology* 116, no. 11-12 (2016), https://doi.org/10.1007/s00421-016-3480-1.

## Chapter 10: Brain Health and Concussions

1. John Kein, "Mark Rypien opens up on mental health issues, attempted suicide," *ABC News*, March 30, 2018, https://abcnews.go.com/Sports/mark-rypien-opens-mental-health-issues-attempted-suicide /story?id=54132326.

2. Nick Boynton, "Everything is not O.K.," *The Players' Tribune*, June 13, 2018, www.theplayers tribune.com/en-us/articles/nick-boynton-everythings-not-ok.

3. Jeanne Marie Laskas, "Bennet Omalu, concussions and the NFL: how one doctor changed football forever," *GQ*, September 2009, www.gq.com/story/nfl-players-brain-dementia-study-memory -concussions.

4. Bennet I. Omalu, "Chronic traumatic encephalopathy, suicides and parasuicides in professional American athletes: the role of the forensic pathologist," *American Journal of Forensic Medicine and Pathology* 31, no. 3 (2010), https://doi.org/10.1097/PAF.0b013e3181ca7f35.

5. G. C. Kennedy, "The role of depot fat in the hypothalamic control of food intake in the rat," *Proceedings of the Royal Society of London B: Biological Sciences* 140, no. 901 (1953), https://doi.org /10.1098/rspb.1953.0009.

6. Stephan Guyenet, *The Hungry Brain* (New York: Flatiron Books, 2017).

7. Kevin W. McConeghy et al., "A review of neuroprotection pharmacology and therapies in patients with acute traumatic brain injury," *CNS Drugs* 26, no. 7 (2012), https://doi.org/10.2165 /11634020-000000000-00000.

8. Zachary M. Weil, Kristopher R. Gaier, and Kate Karelina, "Injury timing alters metabolic, inflammatory and functional outcomes following repeated mild traumatic brain injury," *Neurobiology of Disease* 70 (2014), https://doi.org/10.1016/j.nbd.2014.06.016.

9. Michael McCrea and Kevin Guskiewicz, "Evidence-based management of sport-related concussion," *Progress in Neurological Surgery* 28 (2014), https://doi.org/10.1159/000358769.

10. Lyndsey E. Collins-Praino et al., "The effect of an acute systemic inflammatory insult on the chronic effects of a single mild traumatic brain injury," *Behavioural Brain Research* 336 (2018), https://doi.org/10.1016/j.bbr.2017.08.035.

11. Shao-Hua Su et al., "Elevated C-reactive protein levels may be a predictor of persistent unfavourable symptoms in patients with mild traumatic brain injury: a preliminary study," *Brain, Behavior, and Immunity* 38 (2014), https://doi.org/10.1016/j.bbi.2014.01.009.

12. Paul McRory et al., "Consensus statement on concussion in sport — the 5th international conference on concussion in sport held in Berlin, October 2016," *British Journal of Sports Medicine* 51, no. 11 (2017), https://doi.org/10.1136/bjsports-2017-097699.

13. Abhimanyu Sud, "The opioid epidemic, meditation & managing chronic pain," *Dr. Bubbs Performance Podcast,* Podcast audio, April 14, 2018, https://drbubbs.com/season-2-podcast-episodes/2018/4/s2 -episode-14-the-opioid-epidemic-meditation-managing-chronic-pain-w-dr-abhimanyu-sud-md.

14. Abhimanyu Sud, "The opioid epidemic, meditation & managing chronic pain."

15. Abhimanyu Sud, "The opioid epidemic, meditation & managing chronic pain."

16. Abhimanyu Sud, "The opioid epidemic, meditation & managing chronic pain."

17. Sara W. Lazar et al., "Meditation experience is associated with increased cortical thickness," *Neuroreport* 16, no. 17 (2005), https://doi.org/10.1097/01.wnr.0000186598.66243.19.

18. Hiroki Nakata, Kiwako Sakamoto, and Ryusuke Kakigi, "Meditation reduces pain-related neural activity in the anterior cingulate cortex, insula, secondary. somatosensory cortex, and thalamus," *Frontiers in Psychology* 5 (2014), https://doi.org/10.3389/fpsyg.2014.01489.

19. Maximilian Wiesmann, Amanda J Kiliaan, and Jurgen A. H. R. Claassen, "Vascular aspects of cognitive impairment and dementia," *Journal of Cerebral Blood Flow and Metabolism* 33, no. 11 (2013), https://doi.org/10.1038/jcbfm.2013.159.

20. Mary N. Haan et al., "Prevalence of dementia in older Latinos: the influence of type 2 diabetes mellitus, stroke and genetic factors," *Journal of the American Geriatrics Society* 51, no. 2 (2003), https://doi.org/10.1046/j.1532-5415.2003.51054.x.

21. Christiane Reitz, Carol Brayne, and Richard Mayeux, "Epidemiology of Alzheimer disease," *Nature Reviews Neurology* 7, no. 3 (2011), https://doi.org/10.1038/nrneurol.2011.2; Elham Saedi et al., "Diabetes mellitus and cognitive impairments," *World Journal of Diabetes* 7, no. 17 (2016), https://doi.org/10.4239/wjd.v7.i17.412.

22. Sarah T. Pendlebury and Peter M. Rothwell, "Prevalence, incidence, and factors associated with pre-stroke and post-stroke dementia: a systematic review and meta-analysis," *The Lancet Neurology* 8, no. 11 (2009), https://doi.org/10.1016/s1474-4422(09)70236-4.

23. Wendy A. Davis et al., "Dementia onset, incidence and risk in type 2 diabetes: a matched cohort study with the Fremantle Diabetes Study Phase I," *Diabetologia*, 60, no. 1 (2016), https://doi.org/10.1007/s00125-016-4127-9.

24. Juliette Janson et al., "Increased risk of type 2 diabetes in Alzheimer disease," *Diabetes* 53, no. 2 (2004), https://doi.org/10.2337/diabetes.53.2.474.

25. Lindsey A. Farrer et al., "Effects of age, sex, and ethnicity on the association between apolipoprotein E genotype and Alzheimer disease. A meta-analysis," *JAMA* 278, no. 16 (1997), https://doi.org/10.1001/jama.1997.03550160069041; E. H. Corder et al., "Gene dose of apolipoprotein E type 4 allele and the risk of Alzheimer's disease in late onset families," *Science* 261, no. 5123 (1993), https://doi.org/10.1126/science.8346443.

26. Heidi Terrio et al., "Traumatic brain injury screening: preliminary findings in a US Army Brigade Combat Team," *Journal of Head Trauma Rehabilitation* 24, no. 1 (2014), https://doi.org/10.1097/htr.0b013e31819581d8.

27. Nazanin Bahraini et al., "Traumatic brain injury and posttraumatic stress disorder," *The Psychiatric Clinics of North America* 37, no. 1 (2014), https://doi.org/10.1016/j.psc.2013.11.002.

28. Julia Halford et al., "New astroglial injury-defined biomarkers for neurotrauma assessment," *Journal of Cerebral Blood Flow and Metabolism* 37, no. 10 (2017), https://doi.org/10.1177/0271678x17724681.

29. Leslie C. Aiello and Peter Wheeler, "The expensive-tissue hypothesis: the brain and the digestive system in human and primate evolution," *Current Anthropology* 36, no. 2 (1995), https://doi.org/10.1086/204350.

30. Mark Grabowski, "Bigger brains led to bigger bodies?: The correlated evolution of human brain and body size," *Current Anthropology* 57, no. 2 (2016), https://doi.org/10.1086/685655.

31. Dorothée G. Drucker et al., "Isotopic analyses suggest mammoth and plant in the diet of the oldest anatomically modern humans from far southeast Europe," *Scientific Reports* 7, no. 1 (2017), https://doi.org/10.1038/s41598-017-07065-3.

32. Christopher Stringer, "Why have our brains started to shrink?," *Scientific American*, November 2014, https://www.scientificamerican.com/article/why-have-our-brains-started-to-shrink.

33. J. L. Mathias and P. K. Alvaro, "Prevalence of sleep disturbances, disorders, and problems following traumatic brain injury: a meta-analysis," *Sleep Medicine* 13, no. 7 (2012), https://doi.org/10.1016/j.sleep.2012.04.006.

34. Julia Kempf et al., "Sleep-wake disturbances 3 years after traumatic brain injury," *Journal of Neurology, Neurosurgery and Psychiatry* 81, no. 12 (2010), https://doi.org/10.1136/jnnp.2009.201913.

35. Durgul Ozdemir et al., "Protective effect of melatonin against head trauma-induced hippocampal damage and spatial memory deficits in immature rats," *Neuroscience Letters* 385, no. 3 (2005), https://doi.org/10.1016/j.neulet.2005.05.055; Fatemeh Dehghan et al., "Effect of melatonin on intracranial pressure and brain edema following traumatic brain injury: role of oxidative stresses," *Archives of Medical Research* 44, no. 4 (2013), https://doi.org/10.1016/j.arcmed.2013.04.002.

36. Richelle Mychasiuk et al., "Dietary intake alters behavioral recovery and gene expression profiles in the brain of juvenile rats that have experienced a concussion," *Frontiers in Behavioral Neuroscience* 9 (2015), https://doi.org/10.3389/fnbeh.2015.00017.

37. Yuan Liu et al., "Short-term caloric restriction exerts neuroprotective effects following mild traumatic brain injury by promoting autophagy and inhibiting astrocyte activation," *Behavioural Brain Research* 331 (2017), https://doi.org/10.1016/j.bbr.2017.04.024.

38. J. Pérez-Jiménez et al., "Identification of the 100 richest dietary sources of polyphenols: an application of the Phenol-Explorer database," *European Journal of Clinical Nutrition* 64, Supplement 3 (2010), https://doi.org/10.1038/ejcn.2010.221.

39. Richard L. Veech, Britton Chance, and Yoshihiro Kashiwaya et al., "Ketone bodies, potential therapeutic uses," *International Union of Biochemistry and Molecular Biology: Life* 51, no. 4 (2001), https://doi.org/10.1080/152165401753311780.

40. Denize R. Ziegler et al., "Ketogenic diet increases glutathione peroxidase activity in rat hippocampus," *Neurochemical Research* 28, no. 12 (2003).

41. Yun-Hee Youm et al., "The ketone metabolite β-hydroxybutyrate blocks NLRP3 inflammasome-mediated inflammatory disease," *Nature Medicine* 21, no. 3 (2015), https://doi.org/10.1038/nm.3804; Marwan Maalouf, Jong M. Rho, and Mark P. Mattso, "The neuroprotective properties of calorie restriction, the ketogenic diet, and ketone bodies," *Brain Research Reviews* 59, no. 2 (2009), https://doi.org/10.1016/j.brainresrev.2008.09.002.

42. Kimberley R. Byrnes et al., "FDG-PET imaging in mild traumatic brain injury: a critical review," *Frontiers in Neuroenergetics* 5 (2013), https://doi.org/10.3389/fnene.2013.00013.

43. George F. Cahill Jr. and Richard L. Veech, "Ketoacids? Good medicine?" *Transactions of the American Clinical and Climatological Association* 114 (2003).

44. Daniella Tassoni et al., "The role of eicosanoids in the brain," *Asia Pacific Journal of Clinical Nutrition* 17, Supplement 1 (2008).

45. James D. Mills et al., "Omega-3 fatty acid supplementation and reduction of traumatic axonal injury in a rodent head injury model," *Journal of Neurosurgery* 114, no. 1 (2011), https://doi.org/10.3171/2010.5.jns08914.

46. Ernst J. Schaefer et al., "Plasma phosphatidylcholine docosahexaenoic acid content and risk of dementia and Alzheimer disease: the Framingham Heart Study," *Archives of Neurology* 63, no. 11 (2006), https://doi.org/10.1001/archneur.63.11.1545.

47. Parvathy R. Kumar et al., "Omega-3 fatty acids could alleviate the risks of traumatic brain injury – a mini review," *Journal of Traditional and Complementary Medicine* 4, no. 2 (2014), https://doi.org/10.4103/2225-4110.130374.

48. Jonathan M. Oliver et al., "Effect of docosahexaenoic acid on a biomarker of head trauma in American football," *Medicine and Science in Sports and Exercise* 48, no. 6 (2016), https://doi.org/10.1249/mss.0000000000000875.

49. Michael D. Lewis, "Concussions, traumatic brain injury, and the innovative use of omega-3s," *Journal of the American College of Nutrition* 35, no. 5 (2016), https://doi.org/10.1080/07315724.2016.1150796.

50. Philip John Ainsley Dean et al., "Potential for use of creatine supplementation following mild traumatic brain injury," *Concussion* 2, no. 2 (2017), https://doi.org/10.2217/cnc-2016-0016.

51. Bruno Gualano et al., "Creatine supplementation in the aging population: effects on skeletal muscle, bone and brain," *Amino Acids* 48, no. 8 (2016), https://doi.org/10.1007/s00726-016-2239-7.

52. Aiguo Wu, Zhe Ying, and Fernando Gomez-Pinilla, "Omega-3 fatty acids supplementation restores mechanisms that maintain brain homeostasis in traumatic brain injury," *Journal of Neurotrauma* 24, no. 10 (2007), https://doi.org/10.1089/neu.2007.0313.

53. Katherine H. M. Cox, Andrew Pipingas, and Andrew B. Scholey, "Investigation of the effects of solid lipid curcumin on cognition and mood in a healthy older population," *Journal of Psychopharmacology* 29, https://doi.org/10.1177/0269881114552744.

54. Kara N. Corps, Theodore L. Roth, and Dorian B. McGavern, "Inflammation and neuroprotection in traumatic brain injury," *JAMA Neurology* 72, no. 3 (2015), https://doi.org/10.1001/jamaneurol.2014.3558.

55. Qiuhua Shen et al., "Systematic review of traumatic brain injury and the impact of antioxidant therapy on clinical outcomes," *Worldviews on Evidence-Based Nursing* 13, no. 5 (2016), https://doi.org/10.1111/wvn.12167.

## Chapter 11: Emotions and Mindset

1. Aditi Narurkar et al., "When physicians counsel about stress: results of a national study," *JAMA Internal Medicine* 173, no. 1 (2013), https://doi.org/10.1001/2013.jamainternmed.480.

2. Armita Golkar et al., "The influence of work-related chronic stress on the regulation of emotion and functional connectivity in the brain," *PLoS ONE* 9, no. 9 (2014), https://doi.org/10.1371/journal.pone.0104550.

3. Daniel Goleman, *Emotional Intelligence — Why It Matters More Than IQ* (New York: Bloomsbury, 1996).

4. Jacob A. Nota and Meredith E. Coles, "Duration and timing of sleep are associated with repetitive negative thinking," *Cognitive Therapy and Research* 39, no. 2 (2014), https://doi.org/10.1007/s10608-014-9651-7.

5. William F. Hart, *Life, Leadership and the Pursuit of Happiness,* (Victoria, Canada: Trafford Publishing, 2010).

6. Bruce Lipton, *The Biology of Belief: Unleashing The Power Of Consciousness, Matter and Miracles* (London, U.K.: Hay House, 2013).

7. Gary John Bishop, *Unfu\*k Yourself: Get Out of Your Head and into Your Life* (self-pub., CreateSpace, 2016).

8. Eric Barker, "The science behind why everything you know about success is (mostly) wrong," *Dr. Bubbs Performance Podcast,* Podcast audio, October 12, 2017, https://drbubbs.com/podcast episodes/2017/10/episode-41-the-science-behind-why-everything-your-know-about-success-is -mostly-wrong-eric-barker.

9. Ian McMahan, "Hacking the free throw: the science behind the most practiced shot in sports," *The Guardian,* November 22, 2017.

10. Marcus E. Raichle et al., "A default mode of brain function," *Proceedings of the National Academy of Sciences* 98, no. 2 (2001), https://doi.org/10.1073/pnas.98.2.676.

11. M. F. Mason et al., "Wandering minds: the default mode network and stimulus-independent thought," *Science* 315, no. 5810 (2007), https://doi.org/10.1126/science.1131295.

12. Michael D. Mrazek et al., "Mindfulness training improves working memory capacity and GRE performance while reducing mind wandering," *Psychological Science* 24, no. 5 (2013), https://doi.org/10.1177/0956797612459659.

13. Catherine Kerr et al., "Effects of mindfulness meditation training on anticipatory alpha modulation in primary somatosensory cortex," *Brain Research Bulletin* 85, no.3-4 (2011), doi:10.1016/j.brainresbull.2011.03.026.

14. Kent G. Bailey, "The sociopath: cheater or warrior hawk?," *Behavioural and Brain Sciences* 18, no. 3 (1995), https://doi.org/10.1017/s0140525x00039613.

15. Belinda Jane Board and Katarina Fritzon, "Disordered personalities at work," *Psychology, Crime and Law* 11, no.1 (2005), https://doi.org/10.1080/10683160310001634304.

16. Kevin Dutton, *The Wisdom of Psychopaths* (London, U.K.: Penguin Random House, 2012).

17. Kristin D. Neff, "The development and validation of a scale to measure self-compassion," *Self and Identity* 12, no. 3 (2013), https://doi.org/10.1080/15298860309027.

18. David A. Sbarra, "Divorce and health: current trends and future directions," *Psychosomatic Medicine* 77, no. 3 (2015), https://doi.org/10.1097/psy.0000000000000168.

19. Filip Raes, "Rumination and worry as mediators of the relationship between self-compassion and depression and anxiety," *Personality and Individual Differences* 48 (2010), https://doi.org/10.1016/j .paid.2010.01.023.

20. Juliana G. Breines and Serena Chen, "Self-compassion increases self-improvement motivation," *Personality and Social Psychology Bulletin* 38, no. 9 (2012), https://doi.org/10.1177/0146167 212445599.

## Chapter 12: Leadership and Great Coaching

1. Justin Peter Brienza and Igor Grossmann, "Social class and wise reasoning about interpersonal conflicts across regions, persons and situations," *Proceedings of the Royal Society B: Biological Sciences* 284, no. 1869 (2017), https://doi.org/10.1098/rspb.2017.1870.

2. Herman A. Witkin, "Social influences in the development of cognitive style," in *Handbook of Socialization Theory and Research*, ed. David A. Goslin (Chicago: Rand McNally, 1969), 687–706; Jeanne Brooks-Gunn, Pamela K. Klebanov, and Greg J. Duncan, "Ethnic differences in children's intelligence test scores: role of economic deprivation, home environment, and maternal characteristics," *Child Development* 67, no. 2 (1996), https://doi.org/10.1111/j.1467-8624.1996 .tb01741.x; Johannes Haushofer and Ernst Fehr, "On the psychology of poverty," *Science* 344, no. 6186 (2014), https://doi.org/10.1126/science.1232491.

3. Paul B. Baltes and Jacqui Smith, "The fascination of wisdom: its nature, ontogeny, and function," *Perspectives in Psychological Science* 3, no. 1 (2008), https://doi.org/10.1111/j.1745-6916.2008.00062.x; Igor Grossmann, "Wisdom in context," *Perspectives on Psychological Science* 12, no. 2 (2017), https:// doi.org/10.1177/1745691616672066; Robert J. Sternberg, "A balance theory of wisdom," *Review of General Psychology* 2, no. 4 (1998), http://psycnet.apa.org/doi/10.1037/1089-2680.2.4.347.

4. Paul B. Baltes and Ursula M. Staudinger, "Wisdom: a metaheuristic (pragmatic) to orchestrate mind and virtue toward excellence," *American Psychologist* 55, no. 1 (2000), https://doi.org /10.1037/0003-066x.55.1.122; Ursula M. Staudinger and Judith Glück, "Psychological wisdom research: commonalities and differences in a growing field," *Annual Review of Psychology* 62, no. 1 (2011), https://doi.org/10.1146/annurev.psych.121208.131659.

5. Thomas Gilovich and Lee Ross, *The Wisest One in the Room: How You Can Benefit from Social Psychology's Most Powerful Insights*, (New York: Free Press, 2016).

6. Gillian V. Pepper and Daniel Nettle, "The behavioural constellation of deprivation: causes and consequences," *Behavioral and Brain Sciences* 40 (2017), https://doi.org/10.1017/s0140525 x1600234x.

7. Michael W. Kraus, Stéphane Côté, and Dacher Keltner, "Social class, contextualism, and empathic accuracy," *Psychological Science* 21, no. 11 (2010), https://doi.org/10.1177/0956797610387613; Margie E. Lachman and Suzanne L. Weaver, "The sense of control as a moderator of social class differences in health and well-being," *Journal of Personality and Social Psychology* 74, no. 3 (1998), https://doi.org/10.1037//0022-3514.74.3.763; Michael W. Kraus, Paul K. Piff, and Dacher Keltner, "Social class, sense of control, and social explanation," *Journal of Personality and Social Psychology* 97, no. 6 (2009), https://doi.org/10.1037/a0016357.

8. Nicole M. Stephens, Hazel Rose Markus, and L. Taylor Phillips, "Social class culture cycles: how three gateway contexts shape selves and fuel inequality," *Annual Review of Psychology* 65, no. 1 (2014), https://doi.org/10.1146/annurev-psych-010213-115143; Jennifer E. Stellar et al., "Class and compassion: socioeconomic factors predict responses to suffering," *Emotion* 12, no. 3 (2012), https://doi.org/10.1037/a0026508.

9. Igor Grossmann et al., "A route to well-being: intelligence versus wise reasoning," *Journal of Experimental Psychology: General* 142, no. 3 (2013), https://doi.org/10.1037/a0029560; Ursula M. Staudinger, David F. Lopez, and Paul B. Baltes, "The psychometric location of wisdom-related performance: intelligence, personality, and more?," *Personality and Social Psychology Bulletin* 23, no. 11 (1997), https://doi.org/10.1177/01461672972311007.

10. Henri Carlo Santos, Michael E. W. Varnum, and Igor Grossmann, "Global increases in individualism," *Psychological Science* 28, no. 9 (2017), https://doi.org/10.31234/osf.io/hynwh.

11. Andrew King (Director of the Sociality, Heterogeneity, Organisation, And Leadership (SHOAL) research group at Swansea University, Wales, U.K.), in discussion with the author, February 2018.

12. Mark Shapiro, "My biggest mistake" (presentation, Leaders in Performance, London, England, November, 2017).

13. Emine Saner, "How the psychology of the England football team could change your life," *The Guardian*, July 10, 2018.

14. Noel E. Brick, Megan J. McElhinney, and Richard S. Metcalfe, "The effects of facial expression and relaxation cues on movement economy, physiological, and perceptual responses during running," *Psychology of Sport and Exercise* 34 (2018), https://doi.org/10.1016/j.psychsport.2017.09.009.

15. Peter J. Bayley, Jennifer C. Frascino, and Larry R. Squire, "Robust habit learning in the absence of awareness and independent of the medial temporal lobe," Nature 436, no. 7050 (2005), https://doi.org/10.1038/nature03857; Clark L. Hull, *Principles of Behavior: An Introduction to Behavior Theory* (New York: Appleton-Century-Crofts,1943); Phillippa Lally et al., "How are habits formed: modelling habit formation in the real world," *European Journal of Social Psychology* 40, no. 6 (2010), https://doi.org/10.1002/ejsp.674.

16. Phillippa Lally, Jane Wardle, and Benjamin Gardner, "Experiences of habit formation: a qualitative study," *Psychology, Health and Medicine* 16, no. 4 (2011), https://doi.org/10.1080/13548506 .2011.555774.

17. Benjamin Gardner, Gert-Jan de Bruijn, and Phillippa Lally, "A systematic review and meta-analysis of applications of the Self-Report Habit Index to nutrition and physical activity behaviours," *Annals of Behavioral Medicine* 42, no. 2 (2011), https://doi.org/10.1007/s12160-011-9282-0.

18. Phillippa Lally, A. Chipperfield, and J. Wardle, "Healthy habits: efficacy of simple advice on weight control based on a habit-formation model," *International Journal of Obesity* 32, no. 4 (2008), https://doi.org/10.1038/sj.ijo.0803771.

19. Rebecca J. Beeken et al., "Study protocol for the 10 Top Tips (10TT) trial: randomised controlled trial of habit-based advice for weight control in general practice," *BMC Public Health* 12, no. 1 (2012), https://doi.org/10.1186/1471-2458-12-667.

20. Alexander J. Rothman, Paschal Sheeran, and Wendy Wood, "Reflective and automatic processes in the initiation and maintenance of dietary change," *Annals of Behavioral Medicine* 38. Supplement 1 (2009), https://doi.org/10.1007/s12160-009-9118-3.

21. Benjamin Gardner, Phillippa Lally, and Jane Wardle, "Making health habitual: the psychology of 'habit-formation' and general practice," *British Journal of General Practice* 62, no. 605 (2012), https://doi.org/10.3399/bjgp12x659466.

22. Matthew Syed, "Charismatic sporting mentors can change lives," *The Times*, May 1, 2018.

23. Rick Bonnell, "Here's what Hornets coach Steve Clifford did when his body screamed 'Enough!,'" *Charlotte Observer*, January 12, 2018, www.charlotteobserver.com/sports/nba/charlotte-hornets /article194479034.html.

# INDEX

Note: Page numbers followed by "f" refer to figures. Page numbers followed by "t" refer to tables.

# ABOUT THE AUTHOR

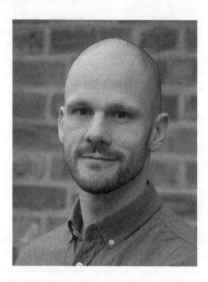

**Dr. Marc Bubbs**, ND, MSc, CISSN, CSCS, is the Performance Nutrition Lead for the Canadian men's national basketball team, a speaker, and a former strength and conditioning coach. He is also the host of the *Dr. Bubbs Performance Podcast*, connecting listeners with world experts in nutrition, training, functional health, and mental performance. Dr. Bubbs regularly presents at health, fitness, and medical conferences across Canada, the United States, the U.K., and Europe and consults with professional sports teams in the NBA, NFL, NHL, and MLB. He practices in Toronto, Canada, and London, England, helping athletes and clients who struggle with obesity, diabetes, and metabolic syndrome improve their health.